TRANSITION TO NURSING PRACTICE

FROM STUDENT TO PROFESSIONAL

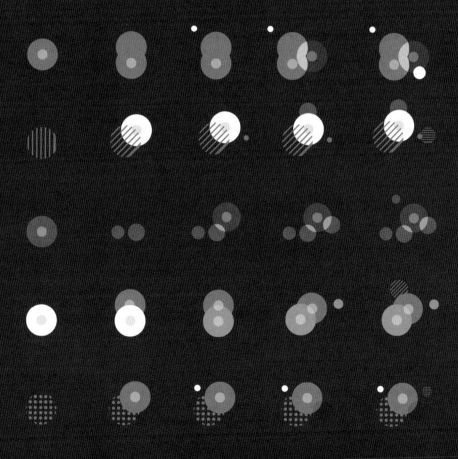

So, I've made it … I'm a registered nurse AND working in an emergency department. To think only 10 months ago I was up till 1am cramming for exams thinking I was killing it. Sure, good grades and performing well as a student are huge ego boosts, but not until I started working did all those late nights begin paying off. This is an endless learning experience with every ounce of fear, anxiety, and self-doubt consciously exploited as new areas for improvement.

Cameron, Graduated 2018, Australia

TRANSITION TO NURSING PRACTICE

FROM STUDENT TO PROFESSIONAL

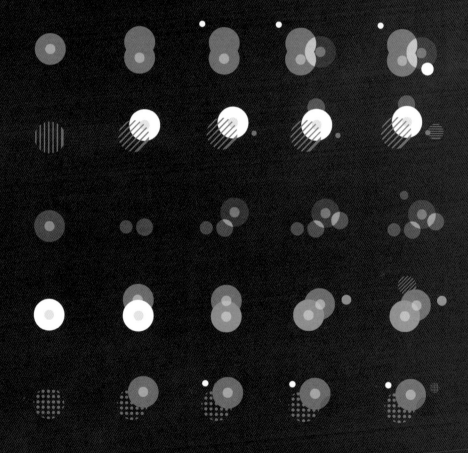

EDITED BY

HELENA HARRISON

MELANIE BIRKS

JANE MILLS

OXFORD

OXFORD
UNIVERSITY PRESS

Oxford University Press is a department of the University of Oxford.
It furthers the University's objective of excellence in research,
scholarship, and education by publishing worldwide. Oxford is a registered
trademark of Oxford University Press in the UK and in certain other countries.
Published in Australia by
Oxford University Press
Level 8, 737 Bourke Street, Docklands, Victoria 3008, Australia.

© Oxford University Press 2021

ISBN 9780190325695

A catalogue record for this
book is available from the
National Library of Australia

Reproduction and communication for educational purposes
The Australian *Copyright Act 1968* (the Act) allows educational institutions that
are covered by remuneration arrangements with Copyright Agency to reproduce
and communicate certain material for educational purposes. For more information,
see copyright.com.au.

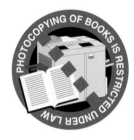

Edited by Adrienne de Kretser, Righting Writing
Typeset by Integra Software Services Pvt. Ltd.
Proofread by Liz Filleul
Indexed by Mary Russell
Printed in China by Sheck Wah Tong Printing Press Ltd

Links to third party websites are provided by Oxford in good faith and for information only.

Oxford disclaims any responsibility for the materials contained in any third party website referenced in this work.

Contents

Part I Being a Registered Nurse – The Nurse in Contemporary Healthcare

Part II Becoming a Registered Nurse – A Development Continuum

Part III Being Practice Ready – The Essential Capabilities

Part IV Joining the Profession – Making the Transition

OXFORD UNIVERSITY PRESS

Figures

Tables

OXFORD UNIVERSITY PRESS

About the Authors

Editors

Dr Helena Harrison is a Lecturer in nursing at James Cook University, with an interest in nursing education at undergraduate and postgraduate levels. She is strongly committed to the preparation of the future nursing workforce through quality nursing education. In particular, Dr Harrison recognises that investment in the development of future nurse educators is critical to the development of the profession and safe, high-quality healthcare. This book was inspired by her PhD research, which focused on practice readiness of registered nurses.

Professor Melanie Birks is an experienced academic with an extensive record in research and publication, having authored numerous peer-reviewed journal articles as well as textbooks and book chapters. She has been educating nursing students for more than 25 years. Professor Birks teaches Nursing, Quality and Strategy at James Cook University. She is passionate about learning and teaching, and believes that quality education can be a life-changing experience. Her research interests are in the areas of accessibility, innovation, relevance and quality in health professional education.

Professor Jane Mills is the Dean and Head of the La Trobe Rural Health School. Considered one of Australia and New Zealand's foremost nurse academics, with extensive experience leading and managing teams in both government and tertiary sectors, her research portfolio focuses on rural and public health, nurse education, the health workforce, and health system strengthening. With a career vision to contribute to a just society by fostering research and graduates who make a positive difference, Professor Mills believes that education and research are powerful vehicles for change.

Contributors

Naomi Byfieldt has worked as a registered nurse since 2004. After completing her Bachelor of Nursing, she completed a Bachelor of Health Science (Hons) in Nursing and a Master of Health Service Management and Planning. Ms Byfieldt has worked in various areas of nursing and has a strong research interest in the areas of palliative care and correctional health. She has been involved in the development and delivery of course content at hospital, regional and university levels since 2011 on the topics of palliative and end of life care and various aspects of research.

Catherine Caballero is an Australian-based health professional and organisational psychologist. In private practice, Ms Caballero delivers career counselling, assessment, development and transitioning services for individuals at various stages of life. She is a Lecturer and Placement Coordinator in Organisational Psychology at Deakin University. As part of this role, she chairs postgraduate teaching units in the Master of Psychology (Organisational) degree. She manages student placements and delivers high-quality placement/work readiness preparation, career development and mentoring activities for provisional psychologists. Her research focus is work readiness. She has developed the Work Readiness Scale for assessment and development, in collaboration with Associate Professor Arlene Walker.

Dr Vicki Cope is a general trained nurse and midwife with a background in teaching, a postgraduate Diploma in Nursing, a Master of Health Science (Nursing) and a PhD focusing on resilience in nursing. Dr Cope has taught nationally and internationally in nursing and midwifery, with research publications concerning leadership, resilience, research methodologies, professionalism, academic writing and safety leadership. Dr Cope is a Fellow of the Royal College of Nursing Australia and of the Australian College of Nursing, and a Board Director of Sigma. She is Academic Chair for postgraduate courses in nursing at Murdoch University.

Dr Lynette Cusack's research focus is on the contemporary role of the nurse in a range of different contexts, exploring models of practice, including impact on the healthcare system, interdisciplinary teams and patients' experience. She provides practice-based research support to nurses and midwives at a major metropolitan hospital in South Australia.

Dr Hugh Davies is a Lecturer in the School of Nursing and Midwifery at Edith Cowan University. His research interests include simulation and clinical competency. He continues to practise as a nurse with over 25 years of experience in critical care.

Tania Dufty is a highly respected nursing executive with a distinguished nursing career that spans almost three decades, across different healthcare jurisdictions including tertiary, rural and remote settings. Her extensive experience in strategic and operational management and her record of leading large-scale organisational change has resulted in transformative outcomes, including her most notable accomplishment – the implementation of the first Australian public nurse-led Walk-in Centre. Ms Dufty has a Master's degree in health administration and was awarded the 2/5 Australian General Hospital Association Prize. She is a Fellow of the Australian College of Nursing and Australasian College of Health Service Managers.

Dr Judy Boychuk Duchscher has been an active researcher and consultant for 20 years in the area of new graduate professional role transition – work for which she has received over 30 national and international grants, awards and scholarships. The findings of her research have generated a theory of transition shock and a model of the stages of transition, resulting in the publication of many peer-reviewed articles, two books, eight book chapters and the delivery of over 250 guest lectures throughout Canada, the US, Australia and Asia on the topic of new nurse integration.

Dr Fiona Foxall is the Associate Dean of Teaching and Learning in the School of Nursing and Midwifery at Edith Cowan University. She is also a registered nurse and a qualified teacher with a Master's degree in medical ethics. Her background is in critical care nursing and her research interests relate to end of life care in the intensive care unit. Dr Foxall has been an educator for 30 years in the UK and Australia. As Associate Dean, she oversees the quality of teaching and learning, accreditation processes and major course reviews to ensure the student experience, retention and success are as good as they can be.

Jayne Hartwig is the Transition Support Educator – Nursing and Midwifery at the Women's and Children's Hospital, North Adelaide. After starting her career in paediatric nursing she became a nurse educator, supporting new nurses and midwives. She is passionate about transition support, helping to ensure that all staff experiencing transition are supported to reach their full potential, from graduates through to senior staff moving into new roles. She also provides education to teams and managers, creating a supportive culture for staff experiencing transition. She has worked with nurses, midwives, allied health and other professionals experiencing transition locally, interstate and overseas.

Major Kylie Hasse is a registered nurse with the Australian Army. She has served both domestically and abroad, completing two operational tours in Afghanistan and Iraq. During her tour of Iraq, Major Hasse's distinguished leadership in war-like operations and her dedication as a nursing officer and health planner were recognised with a Distinguished Service Medal. Her career has involved a variety of roles including command/leadership, management and clinical. Until recently she worked as a career advisor, managing over 400 health professionals including nurses, psychologists and dentists. Her current role is Enoggera Health Centre Manager at Gallipoli Barracks.

Associate Professor Karen Hoare is a nurse practitioner who works clinically in a practice in New Zealand. She has implemented models of care into the general practice, that have resulted in improved health outcomes for children and young people. Her development of the theory of reciprocal role modelling, where new graduate nurses role-model technology skills to experienced practice nurses, who in turn role-model clinical and communication skills back to graduate nurses, led to the award of her doctoral degree. Associate Professor Hoare is the Director of the postgraduate nursing program at Massey University. Originally, she trained as primarily a children's nurse at Great Ormond Street Hospital, London.

Associate Professor Elisabeth Jacob commenced at Australian Catholic University in 2020 as Head of the School of Nursing, Midwifery and Paramedicine (Victoria). She has practised as a registered nurse in both rural and metropolitan health services as well as in several universities. With a strong history in nurse education, Associate Professor Jacob has experience in curriculum development, accreditation and program reviews and has published more than 40 papers in reputable journals. Her research interests include development of the health workforce, skill mix and its effect on patient outcomes, critical thinking and patient outcomes, acute nursing and mixed methods research.

Dr Michael P. Leiter is an organisational psychologist interested in the relationships between people and their work. He has been Professor of Organisational Psychology at Deakin University, where he continues as Honorary Professor, and Canada Research Chair in Occupational Health at Acadia University. Professor Leiter has received ongoing research funding for 30 years from the Social Sciences and Humanities Research Council of Canada, as well as from international foundations, for his internationally renowned work on job burnout and work engagement. His current research and consulting work focus on improving collegiality within workgroups.

Professor Lisa McKenna is Dean and Head of the School of Health at La Trobe University. She has an extensive record in undergraduate and postgraduate nurse education and research with over 200 refereed publications, as well as several books and book chapters, particularly in the areas of nurse education and graduate workforce issues. Professor McKenna has been Editor-in-Chief of *Collegian: The Australian Journal of Nursing Practice, Scholarship and Research* since 2014.

Dr Karen Missen is a Senior Lecturer in the School of Health at Federation University, and has been a nursing academic for over 14 years. Her clinical background is diverse, but she has postgraduate qualifications in intensive care and nursing education, with significant expertise in clinical education at both postgraduate and undergraduate levels. Her PhD study examined the practice readiness of newly graduated registered nurses. It provided insight into key areas in which graduates were deemed not proficient, such as critical thinking and problem-solving, working independently and physical assessment. Dr Missen has been involved in a number of successful research projects and grant applications, resulting in an extensive list of publications and conference presentations.

Dr Melanie Murray is a registered nurse who has worked as a tutor, clinical facilitator, sessional lecturer, clinical nurse and quality manager (ISO 9001 and NSQHS standards). Clinically, her specialty is post anaesthesia care (recovery room) nursing and she has worked in post anaesthetic care units around Australia. Dr Murray completed her PhD in the area of new graduate nurse insights concerning patient safety, and has a passion for all things quality and safety.

Caroline Rosenberg is an organisational psychologist, experienced in leading cross-disciplinary projects. She is currently completing her PhD in leadership. Ms Rosenberg advocates for better integrated career education and experience, so graduates are well equipped to make individual strength-based career decisions. She believes rapid industry-based research is essential to keep tertiary career education and experience relevant to current industry demand and employment climate, and that it is a crucial first step to identify and resolve systematic issues in the workplace.

Dr Morgan Smith is a Senior Lecturer in the Nursing School, University of Adelaide. She has considerable experience in both undergraduate and postgraduate nursing education. Her nurse education research expertise includes nursing students' perspectives on their studies, engagement with learning, and satisfaction with their educational experiences. Dr Smith uses portfolio related concepts to engage students in their learning and thus enhance their nursing related knowledge and expertise. She is also interested in consumer perspectives of healthcare. Her specific areas of nursing interest are public health, primary healthcare and nursing in the community.

Professor Di Twigg is Executive Dean of the School of Nursing and Midwifery at Edith Cowan University. She combines her extensive experience in health service leadership with more recent research and policy development to make a contribution to issues related to nursing workforce, hospital staffing and cost-effective care. She was awarded the Life Time Achievement honour in 2017, and in 2019 was made a Member of the Order of Australia for significant service to nursing through a range of leadership, education and advisory roles.

Associate Professor Arlene Walker is a registered Australian psychologist with a PhD in organisational psychology. She formerly worked as an employee support psychologist in health, providing staff with strategies to manage work-related issues. She is an Associate Head of School at Deakin University, an Associate Professor in organisational psychology and a former co-editor of the *Australasian Journal of Organizational Psychology*. Her research interests include the psychological contract, graduate work readiness, the impact of violence on the workplace, and employee health and well-being. Together with colleague Catherine Caballero, Associate Professor Walker developed the Work Readiness Scale that assesses four dimensions of work readiness.

Adjunct Professor Kylie Ward has served as CEO of the Australian College of Nursing since 2015. Over that time, the ACN has become Australia's beacon for nurse leadership. Adjunct Professor Ward has led an extensive program of works including establishment of the ACN Foundation and the launch of Nurse Strong and Men in Nursing programs. She has been instrumental in numerous key national policy campaigns which support greater access and equity for all. She holds honorary academic appointments with five Australian universities, and has been appointed to the Australian Digital Health Agency Board and the National Health & Medical Research Council Health Translation Advisory Committee. In 2017 she was recognised as Telstra Businesswoman of the Year in the Australian Capital Territory, for Purpose and Social Enterprise.

Acknowledgments

We wish to acknowledge the work of the authors of each of the chapters in this text and thank them for their collaborative contribution. We also wish to acknowledge staff at Oxford University Press. In particular, the efforts of the publisher, Debra James, who encouraged and supported us throughout the development of this text. We also gratefully acknowledge the work of the copyeditor Adrienne de Kretser and the proofreader, Liz Filleul. Finally, we thank our families for their continued support of our work.

Every effort has been made to trace the original source of copyright material contained in this book. The publisher will be pleased to hear from copyright holders to rectify any errors or omissions.

Preface

Nursing students making the transition to the professional role are at once excited to see the culmination of their years of study, and apprehensive about the significant responsibility that accompanies their chosen profession. This textbook reflects years of experience of the editorial team and authors in preparing nursing students to function effectively as registered nurses in a variety of healthcare contexts. The structure of this text is based on the doctoral work of Helena Harrison,[1] which provides a comprehensive evidence-based understanding of workplace readiness in respect of graduate nurses. Much of the content of this text is drawn from that body of work.

This text benefits from the expertise of experienced nursing educators from Australia, New Zealand and Canada. The focus is on assisting nursing students at all stages of their education, but particularly in the final year, in developing their readiness for practice as they enter their chosen profession. Throughout this text, students are presented with theoretical principles that underpin the concept of readiness and the transition experience. Readers are then challenged to apply these principles in practical ways as they work through the chapters. The intent is to reinforce the rewarding and privileged nature of the professional nursing role while preparing nursing graduates for the reality of the practice context.

Part I of this book discusses the professional role of the registered nurse in contemporary healthcare. Familiar concepts are reinforced and presented in the context of preparing for practice. Part II describes the process of transition through an exploration of the theory of transition, the continuum along which transition occurs, and the factors that contribute to practice readiness across this continuum. Part III unpacks the nature of practice readiness through an exploration of the types of readiness that nursing students must develop in preparation for the professional role. These chapters provide practical guidance to assist students in developing readiness in personal, professional, clinical and industry domains. The final section, Part IV, focuses on the ways in which students can maximise readiness for practice during their nursing program, find the right environment in which to flourish as a graduate, and execute a plan that will support a career in nursing.

Pedagogical features are included throughout the text to reinforce key concepts and promote application of learning. Learning outcomes are included in each chapter to assist the reader in understanding the context of the content. Key terminology is captured and defined to aid understanding, both within each chapter and in a comprehensive glossary. Each chapter features an unfolding case study to promote reflection on content. The reader is also encouraged to 'stop, reflect and think' through the use of questions posed in key sections of the discussion. In addition, 'making the transition' activities promote tailored consideration of concepts discussed in each chapter by each student, with reference to their own stage and degree of readiness. These activities provide useful additions for developing a professional nursing portfolio, as discussed in Chapter 3. Each chapter concludes with critical thinking exercises that aim to integrate relevant content in useful ways. Finally, each chapter provides activities for use by instructors in both classroom and online environments.

---

[1] Harrison, H.C. (2018). New graduate registered nurse practice readiness for Australian healthcare contexts: A collective instrumental case study. PhD dissertation, James Cook University.

This textbook is a comprehensive, evidence-based resource that assists nursing students to develop the necessary capabilities to transition effectively to the professional role. This textbook is not a clinical nursing manual that focuses on specific knowledge and skills required for nursing practice. The reader is referred to the wealth of other available material that is designed to assist students to develop fundamental nursing knowledge and skills. We believe this text will make a significant contribution to the development of nursing graduates and assist them in making a smoother, more seamless transition to their professional role. We trust that students will find it a valuable resource as they embark on their career as registered nurses.

Helena Harrison

Melanie Birks

Jane Mills

Guided Tour

Transition to Nursing Practice: From Student to Professional combines the theoretical principles that underpin transition to practice with thought-provoking insights and activities to challenge and promote reflective practice.

All the features included throughout the text aim to reinforce key concepts and demonstrate the application of learning.

Learning Outcomes are included in each chapter to assist in understanding the context of the content.

Learning Outcomes

Following completion of this chapter, you will be able to:

1. Explain the concept of transition.
2. Outline the process and stages of transition for new graduate nurses.
3. Identify strategies to mitigate challenges new graduate nurses can experience with transition.
4. Describe factors that enhance learning and support a positive transition process.

Key terminology is captured and defined to aid understanding, both within each chapter and in a comprehensive **Glossary**.

Interprofessional practice

Two or more health professionals collaborating as a team toward a common purpose with a mutual respect for each other's expertise and a commitment toward achieving this purpose.

Each chapter features an unfolding **Case Study** to promote reflection on content.

Case Study 1.1: Introducing Ben

Ben is a 38-year-old nursing student who has studied his nursing degree part-time. He previously worked as a teacher but was seeking a career change. Ben is in his third year at university and has really enjoyed his studies. He feels very confident about his role and responsibilities and thinks he would do well in a clinical leadership role of some sort later in his career. He is about to go on his final placement and wants to be well prepared – he is keen to make a good impression as he wants to secure a position in the local health service as a graduate nurse.

Portfolio Activity: stop, reflect and think boxes pose questions and encourage reflection about nursing practice, within the context of Portfolio preparation.

 Portfolio Activity 1.1: Stop, reflect and think

Drawing on your experience as a nurse and with nurses, think about the multifaceted role of the nurse. Can you concisely define nursing in a way that embraces all aspects of the role in all contexts?

OXFORD UNIVERSITY PRESS

Portfolio Activity: Making the transition

Review the application process for graduate year positions in your area. What type of evidence would be appropriate to support your application for a graduate program? Audit your existing portfolio to determine whether it is suitable for this purpose. Where are the gaps? How will you fill these to give you the best chance of success in a competitive environment?

Portfolio Activity: Making the transition activities promote tailored consideration of concepts discussed in each chapter and build in complexity as the reader progresses through the text.

Clinical Readiness
Capability to provide a safe basic level of clinical care within scope of practice.

Professional Readiness
Capability to work efficiently and provide care in accordance with registered nurse professional standards and codes of practice.

Personal Readiness
Capability to manage the role and responsibilities of a registered nurse, oneself, and one's environment.

Confidence, emotional competence and performance

Industry Readiness
Capability to navigate the healthcare system, organisations, healthcare parameters, and resources in the provision of care.

Figure 7.1 Professional readiness

Often an image is the best method of conveying information. The text provides useful **tables and figures** to help digest the more complex aspects of transition to professional practice.

Appendix 2: Worksheet – Making the Transition

As you review Figure 1.1 and Table 1.1, consider the following ideas and make some notes in the sections below.

1. Are there similarities and/or differences between the two professional guidelines?

Registered nurse standards for practice – Australia	Competencies for registered nurses – New Zealand

Appendices at the end of the text contain **worksheets** and **templates** selected by the authors, to help you make your transition to practice a successful one.

Appendix 3: The CPD Summary Template

Guidelines for completing the template

Item	What to include
Date	Insert the date the activity was undertaken. If it was over several dates, insert the date range.
Practice standard or competency	Check the standards or competencies for practice relevant to your country and identify the areas of practice you want to develop. Insert the practice standard number you plan to develop in the box. If it is for career advancement, you may choose to use the specialisations national practice standards or certification requirements.
Identified learning need	Insert a statement indicating the area of learning you need to develop.
Activity	State what you did to address your learning need.
Reflective evaluation	State what you learnt, how you plan to change your practice as a result of your learning, and what else you may need to learn.
Evidence	State the form of evidence that supports your claim of learning. Include the title or name of the evidence for easy reference.
Appendix number	Attach the evidence to the CPD summary as an appendix. State the appendix number and title for easy reference.
CPD hours	Number of hours spent on the CPD activity should be provided in this column.

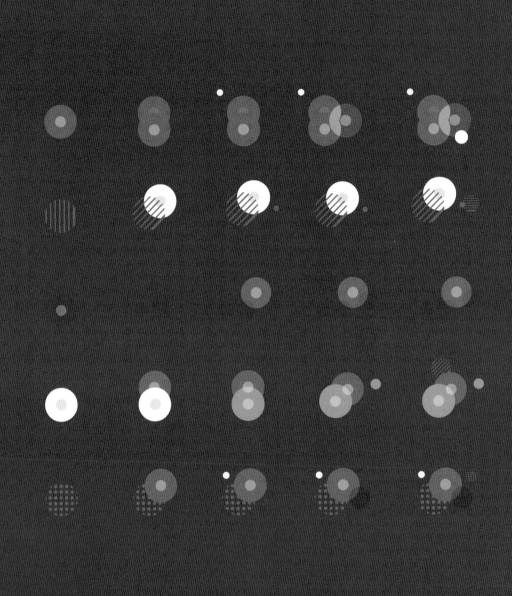

PART I

BEING A REGISTERED NURSE

The Nurse in Contemporary Healthcare

As an undergraduate student, I always knew who I wanted to be and how I wanted to represent myself and be seen as a registered nurse ... that had developed and evolved by the end of third year. That identity is still challenged every day and I need to continually remind myself of how I want my professional identity seen by others.

Natalee, Graduated 2019, Australia

Chapter 1

Nursing – A Professional Role

Fiona Foxall and Di Twigg

Learning Outcomes

Following completion of this chapter, you will be able to:

1. Define and describe the development of nursing as a profession.

2. Analyse the role of the nursing profession in relation to contemporary healthcare in a global and local context.

3. Describe the legislative, professional, industrial and organisational regulation and governance of the nursing profession.

4. Discuss nursing roles and responsibilities and levels of registered nurse practice within the healthcare system.

Key terms

Advocacy

Interprofessional practice

Person-centred care

Profession

Scope of practice

Introduction

As a registered nurse, you are a member of a profession that is at the forefront of healthcare worldwide. Nursing represents the largest segment of the healthcare professions and makes an enormous contribution to the provision of efficient, cost-effective and high-quality healthcare. Nurses are vital to the health and well-being of individuals, families and communities and are reputed to be the most trusted of all healthcare professionals. As a nurse, you have the ability to make a difference to the quality of people's lives. While this is a role that is at times challenging, it is also a privileged, fulfilling position that offers a diverse depth and breadth of rewarding experiences. In this chapter, we reflect on the professionalisation of nursing over time and the major role nurses play in the provision of global, Australian and New Zealand healthcare. Professional regulation, why it is required and how it occurs will be examined along with the various roles nurses occupy, their scope of practice and the standards they are expected to meet. As a profession, we celebrate the contribution made by nurses and the benefits that nursing brings to the health of the global population because, without nurses, universal health coverage cannot be achieved.

Case Study 1.1: Introducing Ben

Ben is a 38-year-old nursing student who has studied his nursing degree part-time. He previously worked as a teacher but was seeking a career change. Ben is in his third year at university and has really enjoyed his studies. He feels very confident about his role and responsibilities and thinks he would do well in a clinical leadership role of some sort later in his career. He is about to go on his final placement and wants to be well prepared – he is keen to make a good impression as he wants to secure a position in the local health service as a graduate nurse.

Defining nursing

Almost every person has contact with a nurse at some point in their lives. According to the World Health Organization (WHO), there are approximately 28 million nurses worldwide, accounting for close to 50% of the global healthcare workforce (WHO, 2020). But what do nurses do? Everyone thinks they know what nurses do – but do they? The traditional image of the nurse is associated with Florence Nightingale, the founder of modern nursing, with a role focused on keeping a sick person safe, comfortable and clean. This image and role of a nurse, however, has changed and expanded significantly over time, contributing to the challenge of clearly defining or describing nursing. Ask anyone to define nursing or to articulate what nurses do and they will struggle to give a concise and realistic answer – try it yourself. The typical answer is 'nurses care for people who are sick' but what does that mean and is that what all nurses do?

 ## Portfolio Activity 1.1: Stop, reflect and think

Drawing on your experience as a nurse and with nurses, think about the multifaceted role of the nurse. Can you concisely define nursing in a way that embraces all aspects of the role in all contexts?

Virginia Henderson has been described as the first lady of nursing and was referred to as arguably the most famous nurse of the 20th century (McBride, 1996). Halloran (1996) likened Henderson's written works as the 20th-century equivalent of those of the founder of modern nursing, Florence Nightingale. Henderson is famous for her definition of nursing:

> The unique function of the nurse is to assist the individual, sick or well, in the performance of those activities contributing to health or its recovery (or to peaceful death) that he [sic] would perform unaided if he had the necessary strength, will or knowledge (Henderson, 1978).

The definition of nursing developed by the WHO in response to the strategy of *Health for All by the Year 2000* (WHO, 1981) highlighted a number of key concepts related to the practice of nursing:

> The mission of nursing in society is to help individuals, families and groups to determine and achieve their physical, mental and social potential, and to do so within the challenging

context of the environment in which they live and work. This requires nurses to develop and perform functions that relate to the promotion and maintenance of health as well as to the prevention of ill-health. Nursing also includes the planning and implementation of care during illness and rehabilitation, and encompasses the physical, mental and social aspects of life as they affect health, illness, disability and dying. Nursing is the provision of care for individuals, families and groups throughout the entire lifespan – from conception to death. Nursing is both an art and a science that requires the understanding and application of the knowledge and skills specific to the discipline. It also draws on knowledge and techniques derived from the humanities and the physical, social, medical and biological sciences.

Later, the International Council of Nurses (ICN, 2020) captured the diversity and essence of nursing in the following definition:

> Nursing encompasses autonomous and collaborative care of individuals of all ages, families, groups and communities, sick or well and in all settings. It includes the promotion of health, the prevention of illness, and the care of ill, disabled and dying people. Advocacy, promotion of a safe environment, research, participation in shaping health policy and in patient and health systems management, and education are also key nursing roles.

These definitions illustrate how nursing has developed over time, as well as the multifaceted role of the nurse, giving us a clearer indication of what nurses do. In summary, nurses:

- provide autonomous and collaborative care;
- focus on health and wellness not only sickness; and,
- include people of all ages and backgrounds, in all settings, as individuals, families and communities in the care they provide.

The development of nursing as a profession

Profession

An occupation, practice or vocation that requires mastery of a complex set of knowledge and skills developed through formal accredited education and/or practical experience, and is governed by its own professional body.

A **profession** is characterised by a high level of responsibility and accountability; is based on specialised, theoretical and/or practical knowledge developed through institutional preparation; has a high level of autonomy; and is, or should be, altruistic. The development of nursing as a profession has been inspiring. It stems from nurses establishing their position as accredited partners in the provision of healthcare, outside the influence of the medical profession, and educated through institutes of higher education.

The pre-Nightingale position of nursing was as a lowly paid, arduous occupation, for those such as criminals, vagrants, and immoral women who were considered unfit for better jobs (Hein, 2001). Post-Nightingale, while the position of nurses in society improved, they functioned in the shadow of the medical profession and were considered dependent on doctors, carrying out tasks under their instruction, associated with medical treatment (Royal College of Nursing [RCN], 2014); they were doctors' handmaidens. Nurses were expected to cooperate with doctors, while doctors made most decisions about patients' treatment and care (Schalemberg & Kramer, 2009a). Historically, nursing literature has alluded to this relationship between doctors and nurses as forming a barrier to nursing's professionalisation.

Over time, nurses and doctors have been involved in a complex relationship, shaped by gender, perspectives, social status and power (Salvage & Smith, 2000). The 'doctor–nurse game' first described by Stein in 1967 demonstrated the traditional relationships between doctors and nurses, featuring nursing subservience and medical dominance (Stein, 1967). In this arrangement, nurses were expected to carry out a doctor's orders without question (Vazirani et al., 2005). In 1989, Hagell asserted that nursing had a distinct knowledge base, not grounded in empirico-analytical science but stemming from the lived experience of nurses as (predominantly) women and as professionals involved in caring relationships with their clients. In 1993, Chellel argued that the traditional authoritarian power of the medical profession can and should be challenged by nurses when making judgments about patient care (Chellel, 1993).

Several studies have highlighted ethical shortcomings in decision-making processes that seem to reflect the 'arrangement' described by Vazirani et al. (2005). These include a failure to consider nurses' opinions (Breau & Rhéaume, 2014; Ferrand et al., 2003) and that nurses' opinions were not respected (Beckstrand & Kirchhoff, 2005; Elpern et al., 2005). As far back as 1983, Murphy and Hunter argued that the nurse's opinion is important, especially when decisions being made are not purely medical but concern values and ethics (Murphy & Hunter, 1983). In 1988, Stenberg highlighted this as a concern that she framed as a feminist issue as, historically, nurses were predominantly female and doctors were predominantly male. Stenberg stated that, unlike physicians, the reasoning skills of nurses were not often appreciated and their values were not often sought. The reasons for this were inextricably linked to nursing's history, its internal divisions and, perhaps most pertinently, its subjugation to medicine (Stenberg, 1988).

Grundstein-Amado (1992) argued that conflict surrounding ethical issues often arose between nurses and doctors as they held divergent beliefs, values and outlooks and that there was a communication gap between each group. Also noted within this study was that nurses were primarily concerned with *care*, involving responsiveness and sensitivity to the patient's wishes. In contrast, doctors' primary concern was *cure*. The knowledge held by doctors was seen as impersonal and universal, based on established ideas of medical practice and patients' rights. Nurses' knowledge, however, was created through interactions with the patient.

Further studies extended Grundstein-Amado's argument (1992) that physicians were primarily concerned with curing their patients, whereas nurses focused on the impact of medical treatment and the provision of holistic care to their patients (Baggs et al., 1992; Sjökvistet et al., 1999). Sirota (2007) and Hughes and Fitzpatrick (2010) asserted that physicians have been traditionally trained to develop technical skills with a focus on curing disease, while nurses have been educated to develop interpersonal skills with patients and colleagues and to provide holistic care for their patients.

Lawrence and Farr (1982) found that nurses often played the role of 'double agent', by acting as patient advocate as well as upholding the doctors' authority. Rodney (1991) found that the role of the nurse may be limited to that of 'information broker', leaving decision-making to doctors. Rodney (1991) found that nurses who were unable to participate in decision-making had feelings of anger, frustration and powerlessness. These findings have been echoed over time by Wilkinson (1989), Storch (2004) and Wiegand and Funk (2012). The inability to participate in decision-making is, according to Rodney (1991), a violation of the nurse's role as advocate. In healthcare, patient **advocacy** is about the promotion and protection of a patient and their rights in relation to their healthcare. An individual who advocates for a patient helps the patient understand healthcare options and processes related to their diagnosis, treatment and outcomes and ensures their human and healthcare rights are upheld.

Advocacy

Publicly speaking up and supporting an individual, cause or course of action.

The need for collaboration

Supporting Grundstein-Amado's (1992) findings, Schalemberg and Kramer (2009a) reported that each professional group in healthcare seemed to have a limited understanding of the other's role and expectations and there was limited communication and collaboration between them. It was suggested that healthcare organisations need to foster interdisciplinary collaboration, based on mutual respect and trust, particularly between physician and nurse (Schalemberg & Kramer, 2009b). Effective interdisciplinary collaboration relies on well-developed **interprofessional practice** (IPP). Effective IPP occurs when two or more health professionals collaborate as a team toward a common purpose, with a mutual respect for each other's expertise and a commitment toward achieving this purpose (IPEC, 2020).

Collaboration, or a lack thereof, between physicians and nurses can influence patient outcomes (Breau & Rhéaume, 2014). Conflicting views between nurses and physicians lead to inconsistencies in effective care (Holms et al., 2014). Importantly, it has been highlighted that ineffective collaboration compromises quality of care and patient safety because of frustration and dissatisfaction among both nurses and doctors (Messmer, 2008; Rosenstein & Naylor, 2012).

All decisions relating to care and treatment require deliberation, with the appropriate weighing of benefits and burdens of treatments being imperative to determine consistency with established treatment goals (Gourgiotis & Aloizos, 2013; Siegel, 2009). Although issues are usually resolved over time, the mechanism by which resolution is facilitated is unclear (Kissoon & d'Agincourt-Canning, 2014). Rodney (1991) suggested that nurses should know the needs of the patient and family and communicate this to the team. The unique relationships developed between nurse and patient and the patient's family, together with nurses' interactions with physicians, confer considerable moral responsibility on the nurse, which provides strong arguments in favour of including nurses in decision-making about patients' care (Baggs, 1993; Kryworuchko et al., 2012; Simpson et al., 1989; Sjökvistet et al., 1999). Nurses spend more time than doctors with the patient and family and should, therefore, be involved in decision-making concerning treatment and care (Baggs, 1993). Interdisciplinary collaboration allows input from the perspectives of all members of the healthcare team, with each profession having special expertise that can lead to enlightened patient management (Baggs & Ryan, 1990; Hughes & Fitzpatrick, 2010; Rose, 2011).

Interprofessional practice

Two or more health professionals collaborating as a team toward a common purpose with a mutual respect for each other's expertise and a commitment toward achieving this purpose.

⬛ Portfolio Activity 1.2: Stop, reflect and think

Think of a situation where you have witnessed nurses and doctors collaborating effectively and a situation where they did not collaborate very well. Now consider the following.

- What were the differences in the outcomes of each situation?
- How could collaboration between the doctors and nurses in these situations have been improved?

During the 1980s and 1990s, the viewpoint that nurses were dependent upon doctors changed quite dramatically. Nurses emerged as professionals, with an increasingly respected voice within the healthcare system and society (Porter, 1991). In 2009, Germov and Freij reported that the doctor–nurse game changed during the 1990s with the professionalisation of nursing, with nurses challenging doctors, offering advice and, as a result, being regarded more respectfully. Also, with the professionalisation of nursing, the view of the nurse as the doctor's handmaiden has changed, with Shields and Watson (2007) arguing that 'medicine without nursing is an untenable concept' (p. 70) and that medicine is dependent upon 'highly educated, intelligent and motivated nurses to enable it to function' (p. 70).

University-educated nurses

The change in viewpoints and the professionalisation of nursing was bolstered with changes in nurse education to meet evolving healthcare needs. In Australia and New Zealand, initial nurse training began in the 1800s under an apprenticeship model of nursing (Godden, 2006). In this model, pre-service nursing programs were generally based in Schools of Nursing located in hospitals; nurses learnt on the job and earned a wage. Commonly, programs were three years in duration, involved theory and practice and were managed by hospital matrons (directors of nursing). Registration relied on passing a state-based examination at the end of the nurse training program, after which new nurses were awarded a certificate. In this model, nursing programs and students' learning experiences were overseen by nursing administrators and the medical profession and driven by the service

OXFORD UNIVERSITY PRESS

needs of hospitals, rather than for educational purposes (Cunich & Whelan, 2010). This remained the mainstay of nurse education until the early 1970s in New Zealand and the 1980s in Australia. As healthcare demand has altered with epidemiological, technological and social development, the need for more qualified nurses to manage advances in medicine and healthcare was identified (Godden, 2006). Concerns about the ability of nurses to meet these needs, a rapidly changing healthcare environment, inequitable recognition of nursing among other health professionals and a need for greater professionalism led to the push for nurses to be educated through universities (Cunich & Whelan, 2010). Hence began the move of nurse education from hospitals to higher education.

In both Australia and New Zealand, this need for more qualified nurses was recognised early in the 1900s; however, it was not until the 1960s that the push for university gained momentum. Inquiries into nurse education and healthcare led to the publication of key reports in both countries: in Australia the Truskett (1970) and Sax (1978) reports and in New Zealand the Carpenter (1972) report identified shortfalls in nurse education. Hospital-based nurse training was criticised for its inability to prepare nurses with the essential knowledge and ability to keep pace with population growth, and societal, medical and technology advancements and evolution. A shortage of qualified nurse educators (NEs) to address training needs, the poor integration of theory and practice and denial of independent decision-making, meant nurses could not provide the level of care consumers would require. Apprenticeship models of nursing were not successful in producing practice-ready nurses and were diminishing the status of RNs. Nurse training needed to be, like other healthcare professions, fully integrated within a tertiary education framework (Duffield, 1986).

In Australia, a key milestone was the transfer of nursing to the higher education sector, which began in 1985. New Zealand started this process earlier, moving training from being hospital-based to university- or polytechnic-based in the 1970s. Over time, regulatory bodies were established, creating standards of practice, education and accreditation processes that simultaneously guided and governed nurse education. These factors influenced viewpoints of nursing and paved the way for establishment of nursing as a profession, one characterised by a high level of responsibility, accountability and autonomy and based on specialised, theoretical and/or practical knowledge developed through institutional preparation.

Case Study 1.2: Nurse as a professional

Ben is in the middle of his extended third-year clinical placement in a surgical ward at a healthcare facility where he has had previous clinical placements. Throughout his degree, he has worked in the unit as a Student in Nursing (SIN), so the staff know him well. This is the area that he would like to work in in the future. Ben enjoys a collegial relationship with Philippa, a resident medical officer. One Friday afternoon, Sarah, a 29-year-old single female, is admitted for a hysterectomy because of a large tumour in her uterus. Following a request from Philippa, Ben is preparing Sarah for surgery. Sarah tells Ben that she doesn't want the procedure because she wants to have children one day. Ben relates this information to his clinical coach and together they approach Philippa to discuss the issue. Philippa does not appear interested, saying that, while there are alternative treatments, the surgeon has decided on this course of action and they should not question it.

- What should Ben do next?

- What are the responsibilities of all those involved in Sarah's care?

- Can you recall a situation where you as a nursing student, or a nurse you have worked with, made a suggestion to a doctor about a patient's care, based on a patient's wishes? What was the response?

- Explain how Ben's education contributed to his ability to understand and act on Sarah's concerns.

The nursing profession's role in healthcare

The importance of nursing to the national and international infrastructures of healthcare is well recognised (WHO, 2015, 2020). The nursing profession is integral to the delivery of healthcare globally and, as a diverse discipline, it encompasses a range of interconnected responsibilities. These responsibilities vary with the context of practice in which nurses work. Commonly, nurses work across broad domains of practice (clinical, education, research, management and policy), locations (metropolitan, regional, rural and remote) and facilities, services or organisation (health service, hospital, school or university). For example, a nurse can work as a manager within a clinical, university or management context in a metropolitan, regional, or rural and remote location. A nurse's responsibilities can include leading, managing services, research for evidence-based practice, delivering clinical interventions and nursing care, and promoting health, education and policy development. Nurses provide a wide range of healthcare in hospital settings, from critical care to accident and emergency and palliative care, and bring person-centred care closer to the communities where it is needed most, including primary healthcare services and aged care facilities. As leaders and managers in healthcare, nurses act as both members and coordinators of interprofessional teams and healthcare services. Nurses drive safety and quality improvements, health service development, systems management, research and education, thereby helping to improve health outcomes and the overall cost-effectiveness of services.

Person-centred nursing

All nursing roles incorporate evidenced-based **person-centred care**. The provision of nursing care is evolving from a traditional approach of 'the nurse knows best' to a patient-centred care approach. Under the traditional approach, nurses undertook treatment and instructed patients, with limited input from patients and families. Person-centred care changes this dynamic. It is a collaborative and respectful partnership built on mutual trust and understanding through good communication. In person-centred care, care is about addressing the individual's healthcare needs, underpinned by the values of respect and an individual right to self-determination.

Each person is treated as an individual, with the aim of respecting people's ownership of their health information, rights and preferences while protecting their dignity and empowering choice. Person-centred care recognises the role of family and community with respect to cultural and religious diversity (McCormack et al., 2013). The Australian and New Zealand governments and professional bodies that regulate the practice of nurses recognise the importance

Person-centred care

An approach to practice whereby the individual is the focus of healthcare and an active partner in their healthcare decisions.

of a person-centred approach in the provision of healthcare and professional practice (Australian Commission for Safety and Quality in Healthcare [ACSQHC], 2019b; Health Quality and Safety Commission New Zealand [HQSC], 2020; Nursing and Midwifery Board of Australia [NMBA], 2016c; Nursing Council of New Zealand [NCNZ], 2012a). The following quote from the ACSQHC (2019b) reflects the commitment of both countries to the provision of quality care that is person-centred.

> A person's care experience is influenced by the way they are treated as a person, and by the way they are treated for their condition. The ultimate goal of our health system is to deliver high-quality care that is safe, of value and to provide an ideal experience for patients, their carers and family (ACSQHC, 2019b).

Healthcare change and the evolution of nursing

Globally and locally, healthcare is constantly changing. These changes contribute to the evolution of the nursing profession and the nurse's role. With advances in health and medical research and new technology, come changes in how healthcare professions organise, provide, deliver and evaluate healthcare. Coupled with an ageing population and growing rates of chronic disease, the demand for flexible, person-centred treatment models has increased. Consumer expectations of the health system and healthcare professionals have changed, resulting in the need for involvement and transparency in decision-making and increased professional accountability. In response to these changes, reforms within the Australian and New Zealand healthcare systems have resulted in a stronger focus on restorative health, disease prevention, coordinated care and chronic disease management across the healthcare sector. The use of electronic and telecommunication in technology-based healthcare has also had a significant impact on the delivery and quality of healthcare in Australia and New Zealand. Telehealth fills an important gap in remote and rural settings where access to healthcare and medical facilities is limited (Gill, 2012; Australian Institute of Health & Welfare [AIHW], 2018; Ministry of Health, 2016).

The nursing profession, as the largest and most prominent division in healthcare, has taken a leading role in adapting to these changes, with nurses attaining the knowledge, attributes and abilities to support service innovation, drive service efficiencies and effect positive change in the way healthcare is delivered. Nurses are working more autonomously in advanced practice and leadership roles, and more recently are delivering health services through technology including increased use of digital tools, eHealth, eLearning and telehealth. Nurses are responding to consumer need for greater involvement and autonomy in decision-making. As the profile of healthcare consumers changes, inclusive practice and person-centred care have become fundamental philosophies underpinning the education and practice of nurses. Health reform related to improving the quality and standards of healthcare has placed nurses at the centre of quality and safety in healthcare (ACSQHC, 2017b). Nurses occupy leadership positions in developing and implementing systems and processes that guide all health professionals in the provision of a safe standard of clinical care (Australian College of Nursing [ACN], 2016). They have worked to reduce medical errors and improve patient safety, promote wellness and expand preventive care, and engage in research with practical applications and impact.

The changing nature of nursing practice in the global context is evident in the literature examining changing nursing roles and practice settings (Birks et al., 2019; Casey et al., 2015; Castner et al., 2013; Duffield et al., 2009; Gardner et al., 2017). The roles are becoming increasingly complex and diverse and, increasingly, independently managing all aspects of care for certain patients and services (Birks et al., 2019; Casey et al., 2015; Castner et al., 2013; Duffield et al., 2009; Gardner et al., 2017).

The nurse's role and scope of practice is multidimensional, enabling nurses to fill gaps in service delivery and improve access for under-served and vulnerable communities. As a result, in Australia and New Zealand, nurses play an integral role in providing comprehensive primary healthcare, particularly to rural and remote communities. For many of these communities, nurses are the first point of contact in primary health and often act as the sole provider of primary healthcare services. Nurses have advanced and expanded their scope of practice to ensure communities in rural and remote areas have access to quality care as close to their homes as possible. Further, nurses play an essential role in helping to empower people to participate in, and manage, their personal healthcare. Consequently, they are in a unique position to identify and intervene in challenges related to the social determinants of disease, through holistic and collaborative approaches.

Such an approach is central to all models of care deployed by, but not limited to, community, school and child health nurses.

An increase in the specialisation of healthcare has also led to changes within nursing. Nurses have developed skills and expertise across a narrower range of areas, leading to an improved quality of care; however, the downside of this increasing specialisation has been increased coordination costs, leading to inefficiency and problems with continuity of care (Duckett & Willcox, 2015). Further, nurses working within specialised areas require education specific to the specialty. The education, standards and competencies relevant to specialty areas of practice can vary between countries, organisations and locations, and the range of education offered is diverse in qualification level and content. Consequently, while spoilt for choice, in some instances, determining what education is most appropriate and relevant can be difficult. Fortunately, the establishment of leading organisations representing specialty areas is growing, and this has led to a more consistent approach. As a result, more nurses are engaging in continuing education and undertaking postgraduate degrees, thus becoming more qualified and independent in their professional roles. This is one of the exciting opportunities that a career in nursing offers. The range of specialty areas is diverse. Box 1.1 provides a list of some of clinical areas in which nurses specialise. While not an exhaustive list, it provides some insight into the breadth of areas in which nurses can work. In many instances, each of these areas diversifies to other areas of specialisation; for example, critical care can include various types of intensive care areas, and similarly paediatrics can include neonatal care and child health.

Box 1.1   Specialty areas of practice

Critical care	Oncology care
Emergency care	Palliative care
Paediatric care	Neurological care
Neonatal care	Perioperative nursing
Community health	Renal care
Family health	Orthopaedics
Gerontic health	Rural and remote health
Mental health	Radiology
Medical	Surgical
Cardiac care	Pain management

OXFORD UNIVERSITY PRESS

Portfolio Activity: Making the transition

How has your perception of nursing and its role in healthcare changed since you first commenced your studies? How has this changing perception influenced the contribution you believe you can make to both the profession and the healthcare context as a registered nurse?

Nurses have a global reputation as the most trusted professionals and are highly regarded for their ethics and honesty (Roy Morgan, 2017). Their role and scope of practice has constantly evolved in response to healthcare reform and client needs. Nurses consistently make an enormous contribution to the development of cost-effective and high-quality healthcare and consequently lead the way in creating universal access to healthcare and, as a result, healthy and productive communities.

Regulation of the nursing profession

By now you will be aware that the nursing profession is governed by a legal, professional, industrial and organisational framework, where the responsibilities of nurses as healthcare professionals are defined and informed by laws, regulations, standards and policies. Nurses as employers, employees, managers and nurse representatives must be aware of and adhere to the laws and regulations under which they practise. It is in the interest of nurses worldwide to understand the content and implications of the legal responsibilities, professional standards and healthcare frameworks which inform their practice. This next section presents an overview of these elements, many of which you will be familiar with. They are important to know and understand as you begin your practice as a registered nurse.

Legal and professional framework

Nursing regulation involves four interrelated elements: accreditation; registration; codes and guidelines; and complaints and notifications (Chiarella & White, 2013). Approved education programs, together with professional standards, guidelines and codes of practice, inform the regulation and education of nurses and set the benchmark expectations for the provision of nursing care to the public.

Nursing is a complex interplay of knowledge and skill acquisition, competence development and increasing capability throughout each nurse's professional life (Benner, 1984, 2004; Benner et al., 2010; NMBA, 2020a, NCNZ, 2020a; ICN, 2020). Eligibility for registration as a nurse is dependent upon the educational qualification. Education programs are designed for nursing students to develop the range of capabilities and competencies relevant to their role and to learn how to perform according to the level of practice outlined by professional standards.

Nurse education in Australia and New Zealand is delivered through the tertiary and vocational education sectors in partnership with healthcare organisations. Individuals must complete an accredited program of study to be eligible for registration as a registered or enrolled nurse. In Australia, approved programs of study for nursing involve the intersection of the *Health Practitioner Regulation National Law Act 2009* (ANMAC, 2012), the Australian Qualifications Framework (AQF), which is the national policy for education qualifications regulated in Australia (AQF, 2013), and the Tertiary Education Quality and Standards Agency, Australia's national regulatory agency for higher education.

As part of legislation governing healthcare, the Australian Health Practitioner Regulation Agency (AHPRA) regulates health practitioners in Australia. AHPRA manages the registration processes for health practitioners and students around Australia and supports National Boards in the development of registration standards, codes and guidelines that inform practice (AHPRA, 2015). AHPRA regulates nurses and midwives through the NMBA, the national board for nursing and midwifery that works with other agencies and state and territory boards in the regulation, registration and accreditation of the nursing profession (NMBA, 2019). In New Zealand, the NCNZ, under the *Health Practitioner Competence Assurance Act 2003*, holds responsibility for the registration of enrolled nurses, registered nurses and nurse practitioners (NCNZ, 2020c). The Council works with nursing education providers and government quality assurance agencies including the Committee on University Academic Programmes (CUAP) and the New Zealand Qualifications Authority (NZQA) in overseeing nurse education, registration and practice competencies that outline the scope of practice for registered nurses.

Regulated nursing roles

In Australia and New Zealand, the nursing workforce consists of three regulated groups of nurses: enrolled nurses (ENs), registered nurses (RNs) and nurse practitioners (NPs). Each nursing role encompasses different levels of responsibility in the provision of care as a result of their education, and each group works at a different level depending on their position and experience.

Enrolled nurses

The minimum requirement for enrolled nurses is the completion of an approved diploma of nursing course delivered through the vocational education and training (VET) sector. Enrolled nurses work under the supervision and direction of registered nurses and contribute to the assessment, planning implementation and evaluation of healthcare delivered to consumers (NMBA, 2016b; NCNZ, 2012a). This can include observing and reporting healthcare changes in consumers, assisting with activities of daily living and administering medication. The overall responsibility for care, however, is maintained by the registered nurse (NMBA, 2016b; NCNZ, 2012a).

Registered nurses

The minimum requirement for registration as a registered nurse in Australia is the completion of a three-year Bachelor of Nursing (BN) degree program (Level 7 on the Australian Qualifications Framework) or equivalent, or a two-year graduate entry Masters degree program in nursing (Level 9 on the Australian Qualifications Framework) (NMBA, 2016a). In New Zealand, an individual must complete a Nursing Council-approved Bachelor of Nursing degree (Level 7 program on the New Zealand Qualifications Authority Framework) or a two-year graduate entry Master's degree (Level 8 on the New Zealand Qualifications Framework) from a polytechnic, institute of technology or university to register as a nurse (NCNZ, 2017). At the completion of an accredited nursing degree program, a student is considered ready to apply for registration to practise nursing in Australia or Aotearoa New Zealand. After initial registration, registered nurses continue to enhance and develop their practice within the workplace. The responsibilities of registered nurses are broad and include planning, implementing and evaluating nursing care. Registered nurses initiate healthcare and are responsible for the ongoing assessment of nursing care needs. They coordinate the care prescribed and/or provided by other health workers and are responsible and accountable for the coordination, delegation and supervision of enrolled nurses and other team members who assist them in the provision of care (NMBA, 2016c; NCNZ, 2012).

When graduating from an approved course of study, graduate nurses are deemed competent to work in any area of nursing at a beginning competency level, in a generalist capacity (NMBA, 2016c; NCNZ, 2012b). When entering the nursing workforce, however, most new nurses may find that they practise at either a novice or beginner level of competence depending on where they commence work (Benner, 1984; El Haddad, 2016; Harrison et al., 2020). Many nurses are generalists but specialisation has become more common in nursing, as the roles and scope of nursing within different areas of practice expand and become more specialist in nature. Over time, with support and ongoing education and experience, a new nurse's breadth and depth of capability increase. The nurse can become more specialised in accordance with the context of practice and personal career aspirations. Specialisation, where it is appropriate, occurs through graduate programs, graduate practice, postgraduate study and experience. In Chapters 5 and 12 we explore these ideas in more depth.

Nurse practitioners

Nurse practitioners are registered nurses who have completed additional prescribed, accredited education at a Masters level and have a minimum three years of experience in their field of practice (NMBA, 2016a; Ministry of Health, 2020). A nurse practitioner's standard of practice builds upon those required by a registered nurse. These registered nurses are authorised to provide advanced nursing care and work with enhanced autonomy and decision-making capacity. Consequently, they function autonomously and collaboratively in an advanced and extended clinical role (NMBA, 2018; Ministry of Health, 2020). This role includes assessment and management of clients and may include but is not limited to the direct referral of patients to other healthcare professionals, prescribing medications and ordering diagnostic investigations (NMBA, 2018). In Australia and Aotearoa New Zealand, advanced practice nursing as a nurse practitioner can be delineated from other areas of advanced practice by the additional legislative functions and regulatory requirements of the nurse practitioner endorsement: a prescribed educational level, a specified advanced nursing practice experience, and continuing professional development (NMBA, 2016a, 2018; NCNZ, 2020a).

Advanced nursing practice (ANP) is demonstrated by the level of practice, not a job position or title (NMBA, 2020b). Advanced practice nurses develop their professional knowledge, critical thinking and clinical reasoning and autonomous practice to a higher level of capability. Nurses practising at an advanced level are described as safe and effective and 'incorporate professional leadership, education and research into their clinically based practice' (NMBA, 2020b, p. 1). Nurses with advanced nursing practice can work within both generalist and specialist contexts, and are responsible and accountable in managing people who have complex healthcare requirements. Many nurses work at an advanced level as they develop along a continuum of practice, but may not be endorsed as a nurse practitioner. Therefore, advanced nursing practice is a level of practice, not a role, and it is acknowledged that it is specific to the individual within their context of practice (enrolled nurse, registered nurse or nurse practitioner) (NMBA, 2020b). This is often the case for nurses working in specific contexts of practice where practice becomes concomitantly more advanced and specialised. The knowledge and practice the nurse develops is related to the specific area of nursing, and in some areas specific standards or competencies may have been developed for the specialty; for example, in perioperative care, the Australian College of Operating Room Nurses (ACORN) develops competencies and contributes to the development of education programs for the specialty (Laws, 2012).

Case Study 1.3: Nursing roles

Ben is keen to take on a clinical leadership role as a nurse practitioner and has expressed his career aspirations to his clinical coach. The coach advised him to speak with the clinical nurse consultant and the nurse practitioner who works on their unit. His coach also asked him about his professional portfolio and suggested he keep good records of his performance as a nursing student and registered nurse, as these would be important in helping him progress to a clinical leadership position.

- What records do you think Ben could include in his portfolio that might help him progress to a nurse practitioner?

- Review the standards and endorsement for a nurse practitioner in your country. What advice would you give Ben to help him as a student and then as a new nurse create a way to advance his career as nurse practitioner?

- What other strategies might be useful to support Ben's progression?

Professional standards, competencies and codes for practice

In Australia, the professional standards for practice for all registered nurses comprise the standards for current practice and inform the development of the scopes of practice and aspirations of registered nurses. Similarly, in Aotearoa New Zealand, the competencies for registered nurses and associated codes and guidelines provide clear and unambiguous guidance on the expectations of professional practice (NCNZ, 2020c). In both countries, registered nurses determine, coordinate and provide safe, quality nursing, including comprehensive assessment, development and implementation of a plan of care, and evaluation of outcomes. As part of their practice, registered nurses are responsible and accountable for supervision and the delegation of nursing activity to enrolled nurses and others (NMBA, 2016c; NCNZ, 2020c). As a new registered nurse, knowing and understanding how the professional standards and competencies apply in your practice will help ensure you practise safely and to the standard expected of the profession and the healthcare system in which you begin your nursing career.

 ## Portfolio Activity 1.3: Stop, reflect and think

Before moving forward, stop and reflect on the professional guidelines that are relevant to your practice as a registered nurse, then consider your response to the following questions.

- Can you provide a description in your own words about each standard or area of competence?
- Think about the professional roles described by the guidelines of your country and reflect on your experiences during clinical placement. Can you provide an example of how your current practice represents each standard or area of competence?

Professional standards and competencies

The Australian registered nurse standards for practice consist of seven standards, as outlined in Figure 1.1. Each standard has specific criteria that describe how that standard is demonstrated. The NMBA explains that the standards are interconnected: standards 1, 2 and 3 are related to each other, as well as to each dimension of practice in standards 4, 5, 6 and 7 as shown in Figure 1.1 (NMBA, 2016c, p. 2).

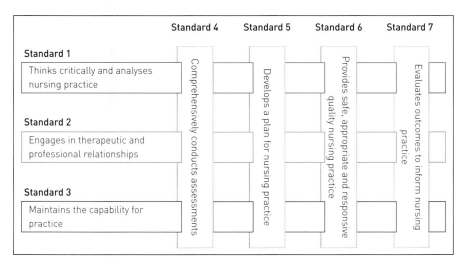

Figure 1.1   Registered nurse standards for practice (NMBA, 2016c)

Conversely, in New Zealand, competencies outline the Scope of Practice for Registered Nurses. The New Zealand Competencies for Registered Nurses fall into four domains of competence. In each domain there are key generic indicators that serve as examples of a registered nurse's evidence of competence (NCNZ, 2012b, p. 6).

Table 1.1 New Zealand competencies for registered nurses (NCNZ, 2012b, pp. 4–5)

Domain 1: Professional responsibility
This domain contains competencies that relate to professional, legal and ethical responsibilities and cultural safety. These include being able to demonstrate knowledge and judgment and being accountable for own actions and decisions, while promoting an environment that maximises health consumer safety, independence, quality of life and health.

Domain 2: Management of nursing care
This domain contains competencies related to assessment and managing health consumer care, which is responsive to the consumers' needs, and which is supported by nursing knowledge and evidence-based research.

Domain 3: Interpersonal relationships
This domain contains competencies related to interpersonal and therapeutic communication with health consumers, other nursing staff and interprofessional communication and documentation.

Domain 4: Interprofessional healthcare and quality improvement
This domain contains competencies to demonstrate that, as a member of the healthcare team, the nurse evaluates the effectiveness of care and promotes a nursing perspective within the interprofessional activities of the team.

Case Study 1.4: Performance standards

Ben is working a morning shift and has received a new admission. He has been asked to conduct a health assessment. Ben believes this is one of his strengths and feels confident about his ability to formulate good care plans for his patients. Ben conducts the assessment and collects physical, observational and verbal data from his patient. He analyses the information and makes some decisions about the patient's situation. He then asks the patient a few more questions and adjusts his care plan. He checks the care plan with the patient and then his clinical coach, who agrees with his assessment decisions. Based on his decisions, he makes a referral to the social worker and a speech pathologist.

• What standards or competencies are illustrated in Ben's performance?

• What key capabilities did Ben use in conducting this health assessment?

Codes of Professional Conduct and Ethics

The Code of Professional Conduct (the Code) for nurses sets out the legal requirements, professional behaviour and conduct expectations for all nurses, in all practice settings in Australia. In New Zealand, this is titled the Code of Conduct. Both documents describe the principles of professional behaviour that guide safe practice, and clearly outline the conduct expected of nurses by their colleagues and the broader community (NMBA, 2018; NCNZ, 2012a). The codes are aligned with national law, detail the specific standards which all nurses are expected to adopt in their practice, and give nursing students an appreciation of and guidance on the conduct and behaviours expected of nurses. These codes support nurses in the delivery of safe practice. Nurses have a responsibility to understand and practise according to their country-specific code.

Table 1.2 Organising frameworks of the registered nurse codes of professional conduct

Australia		Aotearoa New Zealand
Domain: Practise legally	Principle 1: Legal compliance	Principle 1: Respect the dignity and individuality of health consumers
Domain: Practise safely, effectively and collaboratively	Principle 2: Person-centred practice	Principle 2: Respect the cultural needs and values of health consumers
	Principle 3: Cultural practice and respectful relationships	Principle 3: Work in partnership with health consumers to promote and protect their well-being
Domain: Act with professional integrity	Principle 4: Professional behaviour	Principle 4: Maintain health consumer trust by providing safe and competent care
	Principle 5: Teaching, supervising and assessing	Principle 5: Respect health consumers' privacy and confidentiality
	Principle 6: Research in health	Principle 6: Work respectfully with colleagues to best meet health consumers' needs
Domain: Promote health and well-being	Principle 7: Health and well-being	Principle 7: Act with integrity to justify health consumers' trust
		Principle 8: Maintain public trust and confidence in the nursing profession

In Australia, nurses also have a Code of Ethics to follow, as compared to Aotearoa New Zealand where these principles are integrated into the Code of Conduct. From 1 March 2018, the NMBA adopted the ICN Code of Ethics for Nurses (ICN, 2012) for all nurses. The ICN Code of Ethics for Nurses outlines four fundamental responsibilities: to promote health, to prevent illness, to restore health, and to alleviate suffering. The standards of ethical conduct are described in four principal elements, as noted in Figure 1.2 (ICN, 2012).

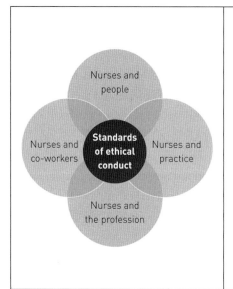

1. **Nurses and people:** In providing care, the nurse promotes an environment in which the human rights, values, customs and spiritual beliefs of the individual, family and community are respected.

2. **Nurses and practice:** The nurse carries personal responsibility and accountability for practice, and for maintaining competence by continually learning.

3. **Nurses and the profession:** The nurse assumes the major role in determining and implementing acceptable standards of clinical nursing practice, management, research and education.

4. **Nurses and co-workers:** The nurse sustains a collaborative and respectful relationship with co-workers in nursing and other fields.

Figure 1.2 ICN Code of Ethics for Nurses (ICN, 2012)

Portfolio Activity: Making the transition

After reviewing the information on the Australian standards and the Aotearoa New Zealand competencies (Figure 1.1, Table 1.1), consider the following ideas and make some notes on the learning plan and worksheet provided in Appendices 1 and 2.

- Are there similarities and/or differences between the two professional guidelines? Note these on the worksheet provided (Appendix 2).
- Consider the practice of registered nurses you have witnessed during your clinical placements. How applicable are the guidelines to the practice of registered nurses? Record your thoughts on the worksheet.
- Think about your education as a nurse in both the university and clinical contexts. Do you have the capabilities to meet the professional standards that are relevant to your practice as a graduate registered nurse? In the space provided on the worksheet, list the standard or area of competence that you need to develop or improve to ensure you meet the professional standards of practice expected on graduation.

- Using the learning plan, list each area and outline two goals with strategies to help you enhance your performance. If necessary, seek help from your university or clinical leaders to help you crystallise your ideas.

Learning Plan

As you read through this book, use the learning plan (Appendix 1) to write down any areas of your performance that you need to develop to ensure that you are ready for your transition to practice. This document will also become a useful tool to add to your professional portfolio. We will talk more about this in Chapter 3.

Scope of practice

The **scope of practice** is the full spectrum of roles, functions, responsibilities, activities and decision-making capacity that individuals within that profession are educated, competent and authorised to perform. The scope of practice of all health professions is influenced by the wider environment, the specific setting, legislation, policy, education, standards and the health needs of the population (NMBA, 2016c). The NMBA and NCNZ standards, codes and frameworks discussed in the previous section, support and direct registered nursing practice and inform its scope of practice. Some functions within the scope of practice of any profession may be shared with other professions, individuals or groups.

Scope of practice

The range of responsibilities and activities that nurses are educated, competent and permitted by law to undertake.

The scope of nursing practice, however, is a concept that defies easy definition (Birks et al., 2016). The NMBA reflects the ambiguity around the concept of scope of practice, stating that, in actuality, scope of practice is influenced by a number of contextual and individual factors (NMBA, 2020a). The ability of the nurse to negotiate these influential factors will determine how well they are able to optimise, or expand, their scope of practice within the confines of this definition. The geographic and clinical contexts in which nurses practise have a major influence on defining the scope of nursing practice (Birks et al., 2016). In Australia, the NMBA established a decision-making framework for nursing and midwifery (NMBA, 2020a) as a way to guide nurses in decisions about scope of practice and their responsibilities associated with delegation and supervision. Similarly, in New Zealand, the NCNZ provides registered nurses with information about their scope of practice and guidelines for decision-making related to expanding the scope of practice (NCNZ, 2010).

Case Study 1.5: Scope of practice

On occasion Ben has been asked to undertake nursing activities that he has not yet been taught. He doesn't mind, because the nurses working with him show him what to do and he is a quick learner. Ben has continued to do the activities despite knowing he should not really be doing them. The nurses really like the fact that he is independent, and praise him for getting the work done. While on his final placement, the clinical coach found Ben with a patient, administering an IV antibiotic bolus. The clinical coach approached Ben and stood by while he finished administering the medication and making the patient comfortable. They then left the patient's bedside and went back to the treatment room. The clinical coach expressed disappointment in Ben's actions and asked Ben to explain what he was doing.

- On an A4 piece of paper, write down any issues about this situation that come to mind.

- Were Ben's actions appropriate and within his scope of practice as a nursing student? What documents could you use to inform your answer to this question?

- Why did the clinical coach express disappointment in Ben's actions, particularly after standing by and watching while Ben completed the procedure. Should the coach have done anything differently?

Portfolio Activity 1.4: Stop, reflect and think

Stop and reflect on your clinical placement experiences. Can you recall an area of practice where you witnessed a registered nurse undertaking an activity beyond their scope of practice? Has there been a situation where you, as a nursing student, have undertaken an activity that is considered beyond what is expected?

OXFORD UNIVERSITY PRESS

Healthcare standards and frameworks

Healthcare organisations and professionals have a duty to consumers to maintain the quality and safety of care. Nurses, as the most ubiquitous profession within healthcare settings and at the point of care, need to be cognisant of healthcare standards and organisational policies and how these inform their practice. This is a key mechanism for ensuring a safe quality of healthcare that meets clients' expectations.

In Australia, regulation of healthcare standards is primarily through the ACSQHC, the peak body that leads and coordinates national improvements in safety and quality in healthcare across the nation (ACSQHC, 2019a). The ACSQHC administers a range of different standards that specify the measures healthcare organisations must implement to ensure safe, high-quality healthcare (ACSQHC, 2017a). The most prominent of these are the National Safety and Quality Health Service (NSQHS) Standards. There are eight NSQHS Standards (Box 1.2) that collectively provide a quality assurance mechanism to ensure expected standards of safety and a nationally consistent message about the level of care clients can expect from health services (ACSQHC, 2017b). Adherence to these standards is essential for all healthcare professionals in all contexts of practice. Importantly, the standards intersect with every aspect of a registered nurse's practice and, together with organisational policies and procedures, regulate and guide nursing practice in Australia.

Box 1.2   National Safety and Quality Health Service Standards (ACSQHC, 2017b)

1. Clinical governance
2. Partnering with consumers
3. Preventing and controlling healthcare-associated infection
4. Medication safety
5. Comprehensive care
6. Communicating for safety
7. Blood management
8. Recognising and responding to acute deterioration

Similarly, in New Zealand, the Health Quality and Safety Commission works with healthcare providers, clinicians and consumers to improve and monitor the quality of health and disability support services. It has a range of frameworks, programs and review committees that collectively contribute to the quality and safety of healthcare across sectors, including processes related to monitoring and evaluation, capacity-building, and consumer engagement and collaboration.

As a new registered nurse, being conversant with your national and local healthcare standards and frameworks is an excellent means of ensuring you are providing a safe quality of nursing care. As a resource, these standards and frameworks can help guide your clinical decision-making, maintain your scope of practice, and alleviate concerns and doubts you might experience related to your responsibilities to provide safe and effective care. This is part of being 'industry ready'. In Chapter 9 we elaborate further on how this knowledge can help you be prepared and ready for practice.

Conclusion

Globally, nursing, as the largest of all healthcare professions, holds a significant position in the provision of healthcare. In Australia and Aotearoa New Zealand, nurses are pivotal in the delivery of cost-effective and high-quality person-centred healthcare. Development of the profession, particularly the regulation related to both the education and practice of nurses, has strengthened the depth, breadth, quality and capacity of healthcare nurses can provide and nursing's position as a leader in healthcare. As a result, nurses have broad responsibilities, and work within a variety of positions and contexts of practice. A range of factors influence and shape the roles and responsibilities of nurses and it is important that, as key contributors to healthcare, the nursing profession continues to be innovative and responsive to healthcare change and challenges to ensure the safe and high-quality provision of healthcare.

Key summary points

- The nursing profession is integral to the delivery of healthcare globally and represents the largest division of the healthcare profession.

- As a diverse discipline, nursing encompasses a range of interconnected responsibilities; however, all nurses assess patients' healthcare needs, plan appropriate therapeutic interventions and care, and implement and evaluate the plan of care.

- The nursing profession is governed by a legal, professional, industrial and organisational frameworks, where the responsibilities of nurses as healthcare professionals are defined and informed by laws, regulations, policies and standards.

- The nursing profession consists of three regulated, interconnected groups of nurses – enrolled nurses (ENs), registered nurses (RNs) and nurse practitioners (NPs) – with different responsibilities and levels of nursing practice.

- Nurses work in a variety of roles in different positions, places, settings and communities. They develop their capabilities over time through accredited education programs and experience in the workplace.

- Knowledge of and adherence to national safety and quality measures and organisational policies and procedures ensure that nurses provide clients with the safe quality of healthcare that is expected and meets their needs.

Critical thinking questions

1. How would you define nursing and the nursing profession?

2. What would you consider as the most significant contribution that the nursing profession has made to the provision of healthcare in Australia and New Zealand?

3. How do you think a person-centred approach to healthcare has improved nursing practice and patient outcomes?

4. As a nursing student, how is your role regulated and what contribution do you think nurse students make to the nursing profession?

5. As a new registered nurse, what particular guidelines and standards do you think would be useful in guiding your beginning practice as a registered nurse?

6. Can you explain the difference between a registered nurse, nurse practitioner and advanced nursing practice?

References

Australian Bureau of Statistics. (2018). *Life tables for Aboriginal and Torres Strait Islander Australians*. https://www.creativespirits.info/aboriginalculture/health/aboriginal-life-expectancy

Australian College of Nursing. (2016). *Nurse leadership: A White Paper by ACN 2015*. Retrieved from https://www.acn.edu.au/wp-content/uploads/2017/10/acn_nurse_leadership_white_paper_reprint_2017_web.pdf

Australian Commission for Safety and Quality in Healthcare. (2017a). *Implementation of the NSQHS standards*. https://www.safetyandquality.gov.au/standards/national-safety-and-quality-health-service-nsqhs-standards/implementation-nsqhs-standards

Australian Commission for Safety and Quality in Healthcare. (2017b). *National safety and quality health service standards second edition.* https://www.safetyandquality.gov.au/sites/default/files/2019-04/National-Safety-and-Quality-Health-Service-Standards-second-edition.pdf

Australian Commission for Safety and Quality in Healthcare. (2019a). *About us.* https://www.safetyandquality.gov.au/about-us

Australian Commission for Safety and Quality in Healthcare. (2019b). *Partnering with consumers: Person-centred care*. https://www.safetyandquality.gov.au/our-work/partnering-consumers/person-centred-care

Australian Government, Department of Health. (2019, August 31). *Health workforce data: Summary statistics: Nursing and midwifery 2018*. https://hwd.health.gov.au/summary.html#part-2

Australian Health Practitioner Regulation Agency. (2015). *Who we are*. http://www.ahpra.gov.au/About-AHPRA/Who-We-Are.aspx

Australian Institute of Health & Welfare. (2016). *Nursing and midwifery workforce 2015.* https://www.aihw.gov.au/reports/workforce/nursing-and-midwifery-workforce-2015

Australian Institute of Health & Welfare. (2018). *Australia's health 2018*. https://www.aihw.gov.au/reports/australias-health/australias-health-2018

Australian Nursing and Midwifery Accreditation Council. (2012). *Registered nurse accreditation standards*. https://www.anmac.org.au/

Australian Qualifications Framework Council. (2013). *Australian qualifications framework* (2nd ed., January). https://www.aqf.edu.au/sites/aqf/files/aqf-2nd-edition-january-2013.pdf

Baggs, J. G. (1993). Two instruments to measure interdisciplinary bioethical decision making. *Heart and Lung, 22*(6), 542–547.

Baggs, J. G., & Ryan, S. A. (1990). ICU nurse–physician collaboration and nursing satisfaction. *Nursing Economics, 8*(6), 386–392.

Baggs, J. G., Ryan, S. A., Phelps, C. E., Richeson, J. F., & Johnson, J. E. (1992). The association between interdisciplinary collaboration and patient outcomes in a medical intensive care unit. *Heart and Lung, 21*(1), 18–24.

Beckstrand, R. L., & Kirchhoff, K. T. (2005). Providing end-of-life care to patients: Critical care nurses' perceived obstacles and supportive behaviors. *American Journal of Critical Care, 14*(5), 395–403.

Benner, P. (1984). *From novice to expert: Excellence and power in clinical nursing practice*. Addison-Wesley.

Benner, P. (2004). Using the Dreyfus model of skill acquisition to describe and interpret skill acquisition and clinical judgment in nursing practice and education. *Bulletin of Science, Technology & Society, 24*(3), 188–199. https://doi.org/10.1177/0270467604265061

Benner, P. E., Sutphen, M., Leonard, V., & Day, L. (2010). *Educating nurses: A call for radical transformation*. Jossey-Bass.

Birks, M., Davis, J., Smithson, J., & Cant, R. (2016). Registered nurse scope of practice in Australia: An integrative review of the literature. *Contemporary Nurse, 52*(5), 522–543. https://doi.org/10.1080/10376178.2016.1238773

Birks, M., Davis, J., Smithson, J., & Lindsay, D. (2019). Enablers and barriers to registered nurses expanding their scope of practice in Australia: A cross-sectional study. *Policy, Politics & Nursing Practice, 20*(3), 145–152. https://doi.org/10.1177/1527154419864176

Breau, M., & Rhéaume, A. (2014). The relationship between empowerment and work environment on job satisfaction, intent to leave, and quality of care among ICU nurses. *Dynamics, 25*(3), 16–24.

Brown, R. A., & Crookes, P. A. (2016). What are the 'necessary' skills for a newly graduating RN? Results of an Australian survey. *BMC Nursing, 15*(1), 23. https://doi.org/10.1186/s12912-016-0144-8

Casey, M., Fealy, G., Kennedy, C., Hegarty, J., Prizeman, G., McNamara, M., O'Reilly, P., Brady, A., & Rohde, D. (2015). Nurses', midwives' and key stakeholders' experiences and perceptions of a scope of nursing and midwifery practice framework. *Journal of Advanced Nursing, 71*(6), 1227–1237. https://doi.org/10.1111/jan.12603

Castner, J., Grinslade, S., Guay, J., Hettinger, A. Z., Seo, J. Y., & Boris, L. (2013). Registered nurse scope of practice and ED complaint-specific protocols. *Journal of Emergency Nursing, 39*(5), 467–473. https://doi.org/10.1016/j.jen.2013.02.009

Chellel, A. (1993). Outcomes, ethics and accountability. *Nursing Standard, 7*(22), 53–55. https://doi.org/10.7748/ns.7.22.53.s48

Chiarella, M., & White, J. (2013). Which tail wags which dog? Exploring the interface between professional regulation and professional education. *Nurse Education Today, 33*(11), 1274–1278. https://doi.org/10.1016/j.nedt.2013.02.002

Cunich, M., & Whelan, S. (2010). Nurse education and the retention of registered nurses in New South Wales. *Economic Record, 86*(274), 396–413. https://doi.org/10.1111/j.1475-4932.2010.00632.x

Duckett, S., & Willcox, S. (2015). The health workforce. In S. Duckett & S. Willcox (Eds.), *The Australian health care system* (5th ed., pp. 91–122). Oxford University Press.

Duffield, C. M. (1986). Nursing in Australia comes of age. *International Journal of Nursing Studies, 23*(4), 281–284. https://doi.org/10.1016/0020-7489(86)90051-9

Duffield, C., Gardner, G., Chang, A. M., & Catling-Paull, C. (2009). Advanced nursing practice: A global perspective. *Collegian, 16*(2), 55–62. https://doi.org/10.1016/j.colegn.2009.02.001

El Haddad, M. (2016). *Grounded theory examination of the perspective of practice and education sectors regarding graduate registered nurse practice readiness in the Australian context*. PhD thesis, University of Wollongong, NSW, Australia.

Elpern, E. H., Covert, B., & Kleinpell, R. (2005). Moral distress of staff nurses in a medical intensive care unit. *American Journal of Critical Care, 14*(6), 523–530.

Eraut, M. (1998). Concepts of competence. *Journal of Interprofessional Care, 12*(2), 127–139. https://doi.org/10.3109/13561829809014100

Ferrand, E., Lemaire, F., Regnier, B., Kutefan, K., Badet, M., Asfar, P., Jaber, S., Chagnon, J-L., Renault, A., Robert, R., Pochard, F., Herve, C., Brun-Buisson, C., Duvaldestin P., & French RESSENTI Group. (2003). Discrepancies between perceptions by physicians and nursing staff of intensive care unit end-of-life decisions. *American Journal of Respiratory and Critical Care Medicine, 167*(10), 1310–1315. https://doi.org/10.1164/rccm.200207-752OC

Gardner, G., Duffield, C., Doubrovsky, A., Bui, U. T., & Adams, M. (2017). The structure of nursing: A national examination of titles and practice profiles. *International Nursing Review, 64*(2), 233–241. https://doi.org/10.1111/inr.12364

Germov, J., & Freij, M. (2009). The doctor/nurse game. In J. Germov (Ed.), *Second opinion: An introduction to health sociology* (4th ed., pp. 347–364). Oxford University Press.

GfK Verein. (2016, March 03). *Trust in professions 2016: A GfK Verein study.* https://www.nim.org/sites/default/files/medien/359/dokumente/pm_gfk_verein_trust_in_professions_2016_eng_fin.pdf

Gill. (2012). *A National Telehealth Strategy for Australia. Australian National Consultative Committee on Electronic Health*. https://www.who.int/goe/policies/countries/aus__support_tele.pdf

Godden, J. (2006). *Lucy Osburn, a lady displaced: Florence Nightingale's envoy to Australia.* Sydney University Press.

Gourgiotis, S., & Aloizos, S. (2013). Making the decision to withdraw or withhold life support: Thoughts and questions. *Hellenic Journal of Surgery, 85*(1), 296–300. https://doi.org/10.1007/s13126-013-0055-z

Grundstein-Amado, R. (1992). Differences in ethical decision-making among nurses and doctors. *Journal of Advanced Nursing, 17*(2), 129–137. https://doi.org/10.1111/j.1365-2648.1992.tb01867.x

Hagell, E. I. (1989). Nursing knowledge, women's knowledge: A sociological perspective. *Journal of Advanced Nursing, 14*(3), 226–233. https://doi.org/10.1111/j.1365-2648.1989.tb01529.x

Halloran, E. J. (1996). Virginia Henderson and her timeless writings. *Journal of Advanced Nursing*, 23(1), 17–27. https://doi.org/10.1111/j.1365-2648.1996.tb03130.x

Harrison, H., Birks, M., Franklin, R., & Mills, J. (2020). An assessment continuum: How healthcare professionals define and determine practice readiness of newly graduated registered nurses. *Collegian, 27*(1), 198–206. https://doi.org/10.1016/j.colegn.2019.07.003

Health Quality and Safety Commission New Zealand. (2020). *Patient experience.* https://www.hqsc.govt.nz/our-programmes/health-quality-evaluation/projects/patient-experience/

Hein, E. (2001). *Nursing issues in the 21st century: Perspectives from the literature.* Lippincott.

Henderson, V. (1978). The concept of nursing. *Journal of Advanced Nursing, 3*(2), 113–130. https://doi.org/10.1111/j.1365-2648.1978.tb00837.x

Holms, N., Milligan, S., & Kydd, A. (2014). A study of the lived experiences of registered nurses who have provided end-of-life care within an intensive care unit. *International Journal of Palliative Nursing, 20*(11), 549–556. https://doi.org/:10.12968/ijpn.2014.20.11.549

Hughes, B., & Fitzpatrick, J. (2010). Nurse–physician collaboration in an acute care community hospital. *Journal of Interprofessional Care, 24*(6), 625–632. https://doi.org/:10.3109/13561820903550804

International Confederation of Midwives. (2017). *Core document: International definition of the midwife*. https://www.internationalmidwives.org/assets/files/definitions-files/2018/06/eng-definition_of_the_midwife-2017.pdf

International Council of Nurses. (2012). *The ICN code of ethics for nurses*. https://www.icn.ch/sites/default/files/inline-files/2012_ICN_Codeofethicsfornurses_%20eng.pdf

International Council of Nurses. (2020). *Nursing policy: Nursing definitions*. https://www.icn.ch/nursing-policy/nursing-definitions

Interprofessional Education Collaborative. (2020). *Core competencies for interprofessional collaborative practice: 2016 update*. https://www.ipecollaborative.org/core-competencies.html

Kearney, M. H., & Kenward, K. (2010). Nurses' competence development during the first 5 years of practice. *Journal of Nursing Regulation, 1*(1), 9–15. https://doi.org/:10.1016/S2155-8256(15)30360-4

Kissoon, N., & d'Agincourt-Canning, L. (2014). Death in the ICU: When comfort is therapeutic. *Critical Care Medicine, 42*(9), 2147–2148. doi:10.1097/CCM.0000000000000538.

Kryworuchko, J., Hill, E., Murray, M. A., Stacey, D., & Fergusson, D. A. (2012). Interventions for shared decision-making about life support in the intensive care unit: A systematic review. *World Views on Evidence-Based Nursing*, *10*(1), 3–16. https://doi.org/:10.1111/j.1741-6787.2012.00247.x

Lawrence, J., & Farr, E. (1982). The nurse should consider critical care ethical issues. *Journal of Advanced Nursing*, *7*(3), 223–229. https://doi.org/:10.1111/j.1365-2648.1982.tb00234.x

Laws, T. (2012). Perioperative nursing. In A. Berman, S. Snyder, B. Kozier & G. Erb (Eds.), (2012). *Kozier and Erb's fundamentals of nursing* (2nd Australian ed., Vol. 2, pp. 1045–1086). Pearson.

Macri, J. (2016). Australia's health system: Some issues and challenges. *Journal of Health and Medical Economics*, *2*(2), 1–3. https://doi.org/10.21767/2471-9927.100015

McBride, A. B. (1996). *Remembering the first lady of nursing. Reflections, 1. Sigma Theta Tau.* https://www.sigmarepository.org/vhlonrnl/

McCormack, B., Manley, K., & Titchen, A. (Eds.) (2013). *Practice development in nursing and healthcare* (2nd ed.). John Wiley & Sons.

Messmer, P. (2008). Enhancing nurse–physician collaboration using pediatric simulation. *Journal of Continuing Education in Nursing*, *39*(7), 319–327. https://doi.org/10.3928/00220124-20080701-07

Ministry of Health. (2016). *New Zealand health strategy: Future direction.* https://www.health.govt.nz/new-zealand-health-system/new-zealand-health-strategy-future-direction/five-strategic-themes/smart-system

Ministry of Health. (2020). *Nurse practitioners in New Zealand.* https://www.health.govt.nz/our-work/nursing/nurses-new-zealand/nurse-practitioners-new-zealand

Murphy, C., & Hunter, H. (1983). *Ethical problems in the nurse–patient relationship.* Allwin & Bacon Publishing.

Nursing and Midwifery Board of Australia. (2016a). *Endorsement as nurse practitioner.* https://www.nursingmidwiferyboard.gov.au/Registration-Standards/Endorsement-as-a-nurse-practitioner.aspx

Nursing and Midwifery Board of Australia. (2016b). *Registration and endorsement.* http://www.nursingmidwiferyboard.gov.au/Registration-and-Endorsement.aspx

Nursing and Midwifery Board of Australia. (2016c). *Registered nurse standards for practice.* https://www.nursingmidwiferyboard.gov.au/Codes-Guidelines-Statements/Professional-standards/registered-nurse-standards-for-practice.aspx

Nursing and Midwifery Board of Australia. (2018). *Nurse practitioner standards for practice.* https://www.nursingmidwiferyboard.gov.au/Codes-Guidelines-Statements/Professional-standards/nurse-practitioner-standards-of-practice.aspx

Nursing and Midwifery Board of Australia. (2019). *About the NMBA.* https://www.nursingmidwiferyboard.gov.au/About.aspx

Nursing and Midwifery Board of Australia. (2020a). *Decision-making framework for nursing and midwifery.* https://www.nursingmidwiferyboard.gov.au/Codes-Guidelines-Statements/Frameworks.aspx

Nursing and Midwifery Board of Australia. (2020b). *Fact sheet: Advanced nursing practice and specialty areas within nursing.* https://www.nursingmidwiferyboard.gov.au/Codes-Guidelines-Statements/FAQ/fact-sheet-advanced-nursing-practice-and-specialty-areas.aspx

Nursing Council of New Zealand. (2007). *Competencies for registered nurses.* https://www.nursingcouncil.org.nz/Public/Nursing/Standards_and_guidelines/NCNZ/nursing-section/Standards_and_guidelines_for_nurses.aspx?hkey=9fc06ae7-a853-4d10-b5fe-992cd44ba3de

Nursing Council of New Zealand. (2010). *Decision-making process for expanding scope of registered nursing practice.* https://www.nursingcouncil.org.nz/Public/Nursing/Scopes_of_practice/Registered_Nurse/NCNZ/nursing-section/Registered_nurse.aspx?hkey=57ae602c-4d67-4234-a21e-2568d0350214

Nursing Council of New Zealand. (2012a). *Code of conduct.* https://www.nursingcouncil.org.nz/Public/Nursing/Standards_and_guidelines/NCNZ/nursing-section/Standards_and_guidelines_for_nurses.aspx

Nursing Council of New Zealand. (2012b). *Competencies for enrolled nurses.* https://www.nursingcouncil.org.nz/Public/Nursing/Standards_and_guidelines/NCNZ/nursing-section/Standards_and_guidelines_for_nurses.aspx?hkey=9fc06ae7-a853-4d10-b5fe-992cd44ba3de

Nursing Council of New Zealand. (2017). *How to become a nurse.* https://www.nursingcouncil.org.nz/Public/Education/How_to_become_a_nurse/NCNZ/Education-section/How_to_become_a_nurse.aspx?hkey=3e91d756-619a-45b8-a544-2779b93372ef

Nursing Council of New Zealand. (2019). *The New Zealand nursing workforce: A profile of nurse practitioners, registered nurses and enrolled nurses 2018–2019.* Nursing Council of New Zealand.

Nursing Council of New Zealand. (2020a). *Kaiwainga tapuhi nurse practitioner.* https://www.nursingcouncil.org.nz/Public/Nursing/Scopes_of_practice/Nurse_practitioner/NCNZ/nursing-section/Nurse_practitioner.aspx?hkey=1493d86e-e4a5-45a5-8104-64607cf103c6

Nursing Council of New Zealand. (2020b). *Education: Educating and preparing competent nurses.* https://www.nursingcouncil.org.nz/Public/Education/NCNZ/Education.aspx?hkey=ad8e6aed-3834-4aef-bbd2-eaa223a5c113

Nursing Council of New Zealand. (2020c). *Standards and guidelines for nurses.* https://www.nursingcouncil.org.nz/Public/Nursing/Standards_and_guidelines/NCNZ/nursing-section/Standards_and_guidelines_for_nurses.aspx

Porter, S. (1991). A participant observation study of power relations between nurses and doctors in a general hospital. *Journal of Advanced Nursing, 16*(6), 728–735. https://doi.org/10.1111/j.1365-2648.1991.tb01731.x

Reinhart, R. J. (2020). *Nurses continue to rate highest in honesty, ethics.* https://news.gallup.com/poll/274673/nurses-continue-rate-highest-honesty-ethics.aspx

Research New Zealand. (2017). Trust and confidence in Members of Parliament compared with local councillors, lawyers, journalists and others such as those working in the Ambulance Service [media release]. https://www.researchnz.com/

Rodney, P. (1991). Dealing with ethical problems: An ethical decision-making model for critical care nursing. *Canadian Critical Care Nursing, 8,* 8–10.

Rose, L. (2011). Interprofessional collaboration in the ICU: How to define? *Nursing in Critical Care, 16*(1), 5–10. https://doi.org/:10.1111/j.1478-5153.2010.00398.x

Rosenstein, A. H., & Naylor, B. J. (2012). Incidence and impact of physician and nurse disruptive behaviors in the emergency department. *Journal of Emergency Medicine, 43*(1), 139–143. https://doi.org/:10.1016/j.jemermed.2011.01.019

Roy Morgan. (2017). Roy Morgan image of professions survey 2017: Health professionals continue domination with nurses most highly regarded again; followed by doctors and pharmacists [press release]. http://www.roymorgan.com/findings/7244-roy-morgan-image-of-professions-may-2017-201706051543

Royal College of Nursing. (2014). *Defining nursing.* Royal College of Nursing. http://prdupl02.ynet.co.il/ForumFiles_2/24172956.pdf

Salvage, J., & Smith, R. (2000). Doctors and nurses: Doing it differently. The time is ripe for a major reconstruction. *British Medical Journal, 320*(7241), 1019–1020. https://doi.org/:10.1136/bmj.320. 7241.1019

OXFORD UNIVERSITY PRESS

Schalemberg, C., & Kramer, M. (2009a). Types of intensive care units with the healthiest, most productive work environments. *American Journal of Critical Care*, *16*(5), 458–468.

Schalemberg, C., & Kramer, M. (2009b). Nurse–physician relationships in hospitals: 20,000 nurses tell their story. *Critical Care Nurse*, *29*(1), 74–83. https://doi.org/:10.4037/ccn2009436

Shields, L., & Watson, R. (2007). The demise of nursing in the United Kingdom: A warning for medicine. *Journal of the Royal Society of Medicine*, *100*(2), 70–74. https://doi.org/:10.1258/jrsm.100.2.70

Siegel, M. D. (2009). End-of-life decision making in the ICU. *Clinical Chest Medicine*, *30*(1), 181–194. https://doi.org/:10.1016/j.ccm.2008.11.002

Simpson, T. F., Armstrong, S., & Mitchell, P. (1989). American Association of Critical Care Nurses demonstration project: Patients' recollections of critical care. *Heart and Lung*, *18*(4), 325–332.

Sirota, T. (2007). Nurse–physician relationships: Improving or not? *Nursing*, *37*(1), 52–55. https://doi.org/10.1097/00152193-200701000-00040

Sjökvistet, P., Nilstun, T., Svantesson, M., & Berggren, L. (1999). Withdrawal of life support: Who should decide? Differences in attitudes among the general public, nurses and physicians. *Intensive Care Medicine*, *151*, 288–292.

Stein, L. I. (1967). The doctor–nurse game. *Archives of General Psychiatry*, *16*(6), 699–703. https://doi.org/:10.1001/archpsyc.1967.01730240055009

Stenberg, A. (1988). The responsible powerless: Nurses and decisions about resuscitation. *Journal of Cardiovascular Nursing 3*(1), 47–56. https://doi.org/10.1097/00005082-198811000-00009

Storch, J. L. (2004). End-of-life decision-making. In J. L. Storch, P. Rodney & R. Starzomski (Eds.), *Toward a moral horizon: Nursing ethics for leadership and practice* (pp. 262–284). Prentice Hall.

Thomas, S.L., Wakerman, J., & Humphreys, J. S. (2015). Ensuring equity of access to primary health care in rural and remote Australia: What core services should be locally available? *International Journal for Equity in Health*, *14*, 111. https://doi.org/:10.1186/s12939-015-0228-1

Vazirani, S., Hays, R. D., Shapiro, M. F., & Cowan, M. (2005). Effect of a multidisciplinary intervention on communication and collaboration among physicians and nurses. *American Journal of Critical Care*, *14*(1), 71–77.

Wiegand, D. L., & Funk, M. (2012). Consequences of clinical situations that cause critical care nurses to experience moral distress. *Nursing Ethics*, *19*(4), 479–487. https://doi.org/:10.1177/0969733011429342

Wilkinson, J. M. (1989). Moral distress: A labor and delivery nurse's experience. *Journal of Obstetric, Gynaecological and Neonatal Nursing*, *18*(6), 513–519. https://doi.org/:10.1111/j.1552-6909.1989.tb00503.x

World Health Organization. (1981). *Health for all by the year 2000.* https://iris.wpro.who.int/bitstream/handle/10665.1/6967/WPR_RC032_GlobalStrategy_1981_en.pdf

World Health Organization. (2015). *Health workforce 2030: Towards a global strategy on human resources for health.* http://www.who.int/hrh/documents/15-295Strategy_Report-04_24_2015.pdf?ua=1

World Health Organization. (2020). *State of the world's nursing 2020: Investing in education, jobs and leadership*. https://www.who.int/publications/i/item/nursing-report-2020

Chapter 2

Contexts of Nursing Practice

Helena Harrison and Karen Hoare

Learning Outcomes

Following completion of this chapter, you will be able to:

1. Critically reflect upon the political, economic, social and professional factors that influence contemporary healthcare systems.

2. Describe healthcare systems and consumers in Australia and New Zealand.

3. Outline the healthcare professionals working within healthcare systems.

4. Analyse the challenges for healthcare systems in Australia and New Zealand and implications for graduates transitioning to the professional role.

Key terms

Digital health   Healthcare system

Introduction

The healthcare system is the context of practice in which nurses learn, work and develop as professionals. The provision of safe healthcare relies on understanding the system, the factors that contribute to its complexity and the ways in which we can embrace the opportunities such complexities have for professional growth and career development. As a nursing student and a new graduate, understanding how contemporary healthcare is delivered and the associated challenges will help support and prepare you to navigate and manage your responsibilities successfully. This success will manifest as industry readiness for practice, a concept we explore in detail in Chapter 9. This chapter begins with an overview of contemporary healthcare systems and the key factors that influence and shape these. We will then examine the healthcare systems of Australia and New Zealand and explore the key challenges and opportunities that you will encounter as you transition to your new role as a registered nurse.

Case Study 2.1: Introducing Evan

Evan is a mature student aged 28 who has travelled the world as a tour guide for a travel company. He really enjoys working with people, so he decided to become a nurse. He graduated top of his class. His graduate year will consist of two rotations including the Emergency Department, which is where he hopes to work in the future.

Healthcare systems

Healthcare system

An organised, interconnected arrangement of individuals, institutions, organisations and resources that provide healthcare services to meet the health needs of a population.

Kuziemsky (2016) describes **healthcare systems** as complex adaptive systems characterised by 'emergent behaviours, non-linear processes, co-evolution, requisite variety, and simple rules' (p. 5). As a healthcare system grows, internal and external processes related to consumers, care delivery, management and economic, educational and policy directives constantly interact and adapt over time (Kuziemsky, 2016). The degree of interrelatedness between the elements and the emergent and often unpredictable environment makes health management and reform challenging, and healthcare systems complex to negotiate.

As the dominant context of practice, healthcare systems have an important role in the practice and education of registered nurses. In conjunction with universities, healthcare settings are the context in which new nurses are prepared and commonly commence their first year of practice. Many factors impact on the healthcare system and shape how healthcare is delivered. These factors fall into four broad categories illustrated by Figure 2.1 – political, economic, organisational and regulatory (Harrison et al., 2020).

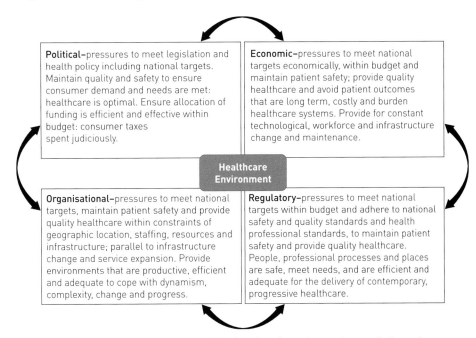

Political–pressures to meet legislation and health policy including national targets. Maintain quality and safety to ensure consumer demand and needs are met: healthcare is optimal. Ensure allocation of funding is efficient and effective within budget: consumer taxes spent judiciously.

Economic–pressures to meet national targets economically, within budget and maintain patient safety; provide quality healthcare and avoid patient outcomes that are long term, costly and burden healthcare systems. Provide for constant technological, workforce and infrastructure change and maintenance.

Healthcare Environment

Organisational–pressures to meet national targets, maintain patient safety and provide quality healthcare within constraints of geographic location, staffing, resources and infrastructure; parallel to infrastructure change and service expansion. Provide environments that are productive, efficient and adequate to cope with dynamism, complexity, change and progress.

Regulatory–pressures to meet national targets within budget and adhere to national safety and quality standards and health professional standards, to maintain patient safety and provide quality healthcare. People, professional processes and places are safe, meet needs, and are efficient and adequate for the delivery of contemporary, progressive healthcare.

Figure 2.1 Political, economic, organisational and regulatory factors influencing healthcare (Harrison et al., 2020, p. 117)

Likely you have experienced the effect of many of these factors during your clinical placement experiences or healthcare work. In the next two sections, we will place these factors into context, by examining the healthcare systems of Australia and New Zealand. This contextualisation will help to explain why, as new nurses, you need to be ready with a multidimensional set of capabilities that enables you to cope with change and manage your workload within dynamic complex environments. The overview of each health system and the challenges they face is not exhaustive. We would encourage you to engage in the activities throughout the chapter to explore the healthcare system that you will be working in, prior to beginning your first year of practice. This will ensure you are well informed about the dynamic elements within the context in which will begin your career as a registered nurse.

Case Study 2.2: Impact of rapid change

The declaration of a pandemic has had a major impact on Evan's workplace. In the Australian ED where he is currently working, they have had to quickly implement changes to clinical practice to reduce the risk of COVID-19 spreading. These changes have been really stressful for staff. At lunchtime, a colleague expresses how confusing they find the government's decision-making process about the lockdown restrictions. How could Evan explain the factors that the government has had to consider in this public health emergency?

Australian healthcare system

The Australian healthcare system is a complex system of governments, organisations, services and consumers (Australian Institute of Health & Welfare [AIHW], 2020a). Federal, state and territory governments, along with their respective local governments, hold joint responsibility for the administration, coordination, funding and regulation of healthcare. In partnership with non-government sectors, these different levels of government develop and implement policy, plan and deliver healthcare services. National health policy, administered via the federal Health Minister, provides the defining framework for decisions related to healthcare delivery (AIHW, 2020a). Governments fund the majority of healthcare (69%) with non-government sources, including individuals, making up the difference (31%). The Australian government is the main source of funds (over 42%), primarily supporting medical and hospital services, subsidised medicines, research, and collecting and disseminating health and welfare information. State and territory governments fund the majority of community health services (AIHW, 2020a). Medicare, Australia's universal healthcare scheme, is funded through taxation and covers costs associated with medical services, public hospitals and medicines through the Pharmaceutical Benefits Scheme (PBS). The PBS subsidises medicines to help lower costs, thus increasing accessibility to medicines and other pharmaceuticals. Similarly, the government Medicare Benefits Schedule (MBS) subsidises health services for the same reasons (AIHW, 2020a). Figure 2.2 illustrates funding sources and expenditure in Australia.

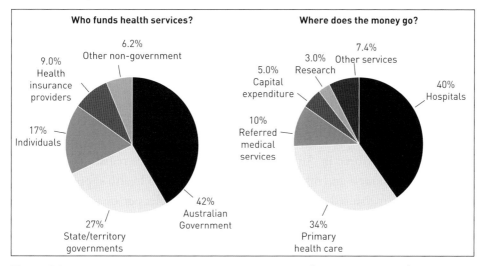

Figure 2.2   Funding sources and expenditure in Australia (AIHW, 2020a, p. 36)

Healthcare services in Australia vary in response to environmental, geographic and population differences between states and territories. The healthcare system is designed to accommodate these variations, resulting in a range of healthcare models and service providers. Healthcare services form a network of institutions, organisations and health professionals that collectively provide healthcare. Institutions include healthcare facilities such as hospitals and aged care facilities, general practice and community clinics, and healthcare agencies. Organisations include specialised healthcare organisations, government-related organisations, and charity and welfare support groups. Community, secondary and tertiary care facilities provide primary and acute care (AIHW, 2020a). These vary in the depth and breadth of services and location. A substantial share of healthcare services is delivered in primary health settings. Primary care services are provided by healthcare practitioners in consumers' homes or in public and private community clinics or centres (AIHW, 2020a).

Geographic dissonance affects the availability, nature and demand for healthcare services. Most tertiary referral facilities in Australia are located in metropolitan centres where a broad scope of services is offered. Regional areas are commonly characterised by secondary care services (AIHW, 2020a). While substantial services may be available in regional centres, access to specialist care often requires travel to tertiary facilities. Many locations in Australia are considered rural and remote. In remote and very remote locations, primary care clinics, often managed by registered nurses or nurse practitioners (NPs), are the most common, and often the only, form of healthcare service (AIHW, 2020a).

Australian health workforce

The health workforce in Australia is diverse. It includes registered regulated health professionals and other health professionals and health support workers who are not registered and/or regulated; for example, personal or healthcare workers and medical technicians (AIHW, 2020a). With the addition of paramedics in 2018, there are now 15 registered healthcare professions, including nursing, that represent the majority of the registered, regulated healthcare workforce (AHPRA, 2020). As the statistics in Figure 2.3 demonstrate, the number of registered healthcare professionals continues to grow each year, indicative of an evolving healthcare system and demand. This is particularly so for allied health professionals employed in the workforce, with steady annual increases of 2.6%–6.7%, the lowest being chiropractors (2.6%) and the highest occupational therapists (6.7%) (Australian Government Department of Health, 2019). In March 2020, the number of registered nurses employed in Australia increased from 274563 in 2016 to 314412 (Nursing and Midwifery Board of Australia [NMBA]). Registered nurses are likely to be women (275282) with the majority aged 35–39 years of age. As discussed in Chapter 1, nurses and midwives make up the majority of the healthcare workforce at 57% of all registered health professionals in Australia.

OXFORD UNIVERSITY PRESS

Profession	Measure	2013	2018	% change
Allied health	Number of practitioners	108 680	133 388	22.7
	FTE total	98 545	119 914	21.7
	FTE per 100 000 population	426	480	12.7
Dental practitioners	Number of practitioners	17 847	20 589	15.4
	FTE total	16 604	19 045	14.7
	FTE per 100 000 population	72	76	5.9
Medical practitioners	Number of practitioners	82 408	98 395	19.4
	FTE total	88 382	103 725	17.4
	FTE per 100 000 population	382	415	8.7
Nurses and midwives	Number of practitioners	295 060	333 970	13.2
	FTE total	267 164	293 711	9.9
	FTE per 100 000 population	1155	1176	1.8
All professions	Number of practitioners	503 995	586 342	16.3
	FTE total	470 695	536 395	14.0
	FTE per 100 000 population	2035	2147	5.5

Figure 2.3 Key workforce statistics for selected health professions (AIHW, 2020a)

Portfolio Activity 2.1: Stop, reflect and think

Reflect on your experiences in the healthcare environment and the range of individuals you have consulted with when providing healthcare. Were these regulated or non-regulated individuals? How was their role different from your own? What do you think are the advantages or disadvantages of being part of a regulated profession?

New Zealand healthcare system

New Zealand's healthcare system is a curious mix of free publicly funded services, subsidised care and private provision. Similar to Australia, a complex, extensive system of organisations and people provide health and disability services for New Zealanders (see Figure 2.4). Healthcare services are managed by District Health Boards (DHBs), under the auspices of the Minister of Health, who leads health policy development through the Ministry of Health. The Ministry of Health is charged with stewardship of the sector and endeavours to provide a fair, trustworthy public health system. Core business of the Ministry is to advise government, purchase health and disability services and provide information and payments for them. Additionally, the Ministry plans, monitors and evaluates the services provided by 20 DHBs, Crown entities, and other governmental and non-governmental organisations.

DHBs are largely responsible for the administration and distribution of health services. They commission health and disability services for their defined geographical location, seeking efficient and effective delivery of health services to meet population needs and promoting effective support and care for individuals needing health and disability services. Every year the government allocates public funds to DHBs with which to purchase and manage health services for New Zealanders. Known as Vote Health, these funds make up approximately one-fifth of government expenditure and in 2019/20 totalled $19 871 million (Ministry of Health, 2019f). In 2019/20 approximately 70.4% of the Vote ($13 980 million) was allocated to the 20 DHBs. The other major source of funding is allocated to Accident Compensation Corporation (ACC) levies and premiums (Ministry of Health, 2019c). The ACC was established in 1974 to provide personal injury cover for all citizens and visitors who have an accident while in New Zealand. Governed by the Ministry of Health, the ACC determines which injuries are covered, provides entitlements for eligible people, helps to prevent injury and supports the recovery of those injured. The ACC is also responsible for collecting levies and premiums and assists professionals to become ACC providers (New Zealand Government, 2018).

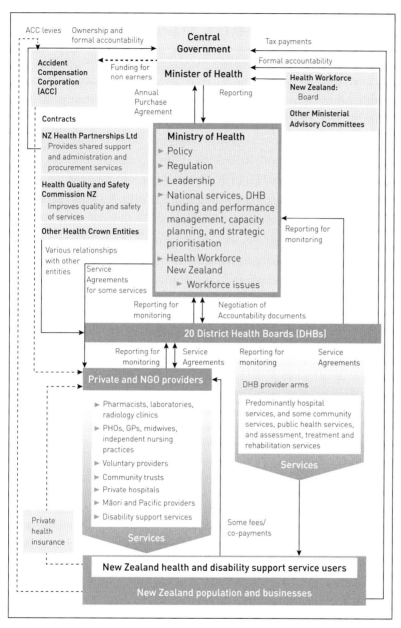

Figure 2.4   New Zealand health and disability sector (Ministry of Health, 2017)

New Zealand health workforce

The Health Quality and Safety Commission, responsible to the Minister of Health, works in conjunction with health regulatory authorities responsible for specific health professions, to regulate the standard of healthcare in New Zealand. The health and disability workforce in New Zealand largely consists of three major regulated professional groups: medical, nursing and midwifery and allied health professions, and kaiāwhina, New Zealand's non-regulated workforce (Ministry of Health, 2017). In 2019, the highest number of registered health professionals were registered nurses, totalling 51 700, a 3.3% increase from 2017 (Nursing Council of New Zealand [NCNZ], 2019a). Like Australia, the majority are female (91%) and ageing, with 51% being 50 years of age or older (median age 46 years). The majority of registered nurses work in acute settings (39%) with 15% working in primary and community care. As at March 2020, 455 NPs were registered in New Zealand (NCNZ, 2019b). In 2018, registration data indicated the size of the medical workforce was 16 292 (approximately 333.5 per 100 000 population), signalling an annual increase of 4.2% (Medical Council of New Zealand, 2019). After initial registration most graduates stay approximately five years and the majority of those who leave, go to Australia. Allied Health Aotearoa New Zealand (AHANZ) is an umbrella group for 27 allied health, science and technical professional associations, representing more than over 30 000 individual allied health professionals (AHANZ, n.d.).

Health system challenges

Inevitably, challenges accompany complex systems characterised by layers of individuals, groups and organisations with multiple arrangements and processes. As we noted at the beginning of the chapter (see Figure 2.1), there are factors that continually add pressure to and result in change across all healthcare systems. In this section we will explore some of the more prevalent challenges all healthcare systems experience, and illustrate their impact with examples from Australia and New Zealand. Some of these challenges you will have already experienced, others may be new to you. Understanding them will help you prepare for the context in which you will commence practice as a registered nurse. You need to develop the capability to work effectively within different systems and, importantly, source them as opportunities for your professional growth and development.

Portfolio Activity 2.2: Stop, reflect and think

As you read through the following section, take some time to reflect on each of the challenges and consider the opportunities inherent in each challenge. Consider how the situations presented might support you in your transition and development as a new registered nurse.

Change and reform in healthcare

Despite being robust, current and future demand means that healthcare systems require continual adjustment to meet the needs of the communities they serve. Healthcare demand is growing, and fast-moving changes in healthcare technology and treatments, consumer expectations and an ageing population with longer life expectancy and more complex, chronic health problems are influencing this demand. At times, health service demand often exceeds workforce capacity and funding arrangements.

Healthy populations and gains in life expectancy are contingent on economic, social and political stability and the absence of catastrophic events. Natural and manmade disasters and an impending health workforce shortage have strained health budgets. In addition, emerging health risks include antimicrobial resistance, and pandemic and epidemic diseases (McCloskey et al., 2014; World Health Organization [WHO], 2020a). In 2019, the WHO listed 10 threats to global health (Figure 2.5), many of which are prominent and have significantly challenged health systems worldwide: the most recent is the impact of COVID-19 (WHO, 2019). The COVID-19 pandemic of 2020 pushed economic and healthcare systems in many countries to the point of collapse, as they struggled to cope. This unprecedented event has highlighted the vulnerabilities not just in our systems but in our preparation, resources and capacity to cope and respond to unpredictable healthcare challenge and change.

Adapting healthcare to meet the needs of sociodemographic change is reliant on integrating current and future trends into government policies and planning. As a result, healthcare is often a focus of significant reform. Reform in itself can be a challenge, with constant change required to manage and mould healthcare systems to align with political, economic and societal evolution. These changes also alter the practice of healthcare professionals and their workplace environment.

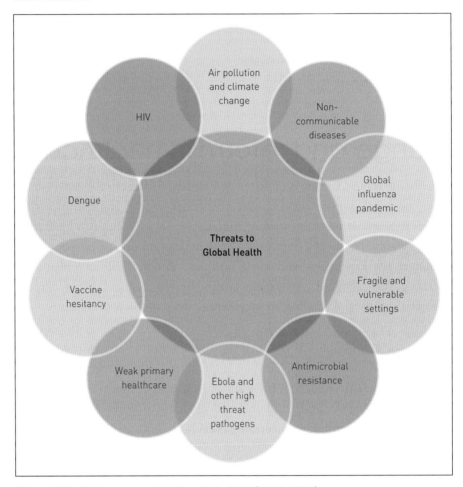

Figure 2.5   10 threats to global health in 2019 (WHO, 2019)

Technological advancement and digital health

To cope with the myriad challenges to the healthcare system, preventative healthcare and mobile health services that utilise technology and link geographic locations will continue to be strategic priorities. Over the last century, technological advancements have had a profound effect on healthcare delivery and changed the way healthcare professionals engage in practice. As a result, **digital health** is now a ubiquitous feature of healthcare systems. Digital health is the use of digital technologies such as wearable and smart devices, eHealth, telehealth and telemedicine, information communication technology (ICT), the internet and robotics in health prevention, promotion, treatment and management (WHO, 2020a).

Digital health

The collective use of digital technologies to deliver, manage, and improve healthcare and promote wellness.

Technology has created considerable change in how society sources and uses information. Thus, individuals and families are more informed and assertive about their own healthcare. How we collect, document and disseminate information and communicate is faster and more multifaceted. The impact of technology has been exemplified in the response to the 2020 COVID-19 pandemic, where swift dissemination of information supported the management of those exposed to the virus, and bolstered research efforts to understand, contain, treat and prevent its spread. Technology related to contact tracing, rapid testing, ventilation and personal protective equipment (PPE) all contribute to managing the disease and preserving human life.

Contemporary nursing practice requires nurses to be adept with technology, and able to utilise it effectively and efficiently in the course of their work. In Australia, the registered nurse accreditation standards require the inclusion of 'health informatics and digital health technologies' in nursing curricula (Australian Nursing and Midwifery Accreditation Council [ANMAC], 2019). As a result, nurses need to be adept at using technology regardless of context and to demonstrate an ability to provide evidenced-based care flexibly and without compromise. For nurses, as principal healthcare providers, technological competence is critical to safe efficient healthcare. It is not just about being able to manage patient equipment and documents electronically, or access databases and seek information. Technologically competent nurses understand how technology can be optimised to support nursing care and make the best use of emerging health technologies and health data. They are adept at integrating technology with person-centred care in contemporary nursing practice.

Population diversity

International migration is a key contributor to population growth and change (United Nations, Department of Economic and Social Affairs [UNDESA], 2019). As a result, national populations worldwide have become more culturally, linguistically and ethnically diverse. Diversity can be defined in many ways. Commonly it is determined by country of birth, ethnicity and language spoken. Age, gender identity, sexual orientation, religiosity, political allegiances and level of ability also characterise diversity. Changes to population diversity require changes to healthcare to ensure systems are responsive and anchored in cultural, traditional and contemporary perspectives of health and wellness. Increased diversity means that nurses need to provide care for a range of ethnic groups with different healthcare needs across broad geographic locations.

Health concerns for some population groups will be distinct, and for others discreet, and at times very different. Language and literacy create barriers that cause health disparities and limit access to healthcare, thus exacerbating health issues. These factors drive change in demand and the types of health services provided. Healthcare for diverse populations requires inclusive practice – interpersonal capability and culturally safe practice to account for unique healthcare needs. In Australia, approximately 26% (6.1 million) of the population is born overseas, with residents migrating from over 200 countries (AIHW, 2019). Migrants in Australia generally cluster in capital cities; however, with increased costs of city living, regional areas are now seeing a growth in migrant populations (AIHW, 2019).

 ## Portfolio Activity 2.3: Stop, reflect and think

Think about your own preconceptions of different groups in society. How have these preconceptions been shaped, and how do they influence your practice?

Indigenous peoples

Australia has a history of major disparities in the health and well-being of Indigenous and non-Indigenous people. Those who identify as Aboriginal and Torres Strait Islander represent 3.3% (787 000) of the population, with a high percentage residing in rural and remote locations (AIHW, 2020b). In 2020, Indigenous Australians experienced a burden of disease that was 2.3 times that of non-Indigenous Australians (AIHW, 2020b). In 2020 there were two significant events that will impact on how nurses work with and care for Australia's Indigenous peoples. The first significant event was the launch of a National Agreement on Closing the Gap in July 2020 (Australian Government, 2020). This agreement was developed through a broad consultation process with Australia's Indigenous peoples. The Coalition of Aboriginal and Torres Strait Islander Peak Organisations, representing Australia's Indigenous people, and Australian governments at all levels committed to improving the lives of Indigenous Australians, including their health and well-being. The agreement replaces the original Closing the Gap agreement started in 2008 by the Council of Australian Governments. The original agreement, known as the National Indigenous Reform Agreement, was monitored and reported on by successive Australian Prime Ministers since its inception. While there was some progress in improving the health and well-being of Australian Aboriginal and Torres Strait Islander peoples under the original agreement, it was slow and failed to achieve many of the original goals. Target 1 in the National Agreement on Closing the Gap is to 'close the gap in life expectancy within a generation by 2031'. While many of the other targets also relate to health and well-being, choosing to close the gap in life expectancy at number 1 indicates the urgency with which we need to address Indigenous health issues in Australia. In saying this, the spiritual and physical interconnection between the social determinants of health and each of the 16 targets is clear. The link between Indigenous well-being and language, culture and the land is indisputable. As nurses, practising in a culturally safe way that supports Indigenous health and well-being in every aspect is central to our practice.

The second significant event was the Black Lives Matter social movement that began in May 2020 in the USA and subsequently swept the globe. In response to the level of racial discrimination that was highlighted by this movement, Geia et al. (2020) proposed four principles that underpinned a call to action from nursing leaders in Australia:

1. Indigenous health is everybody's business;
2. Indigenous nurses should be actively and authentically included in dismantling structures in health and education institutions that perpetrate racism;

3. Nursing curricula should promote the social and cultural determinants of Australia's First Peoples; and

4. We all should celebrate 'belonging' to the caring culture of our discipline.

Aotearoa New Zealand also has a diverse population with an over-arching bicultural framework. Polynesian Māori have lived in New Zealand since about 1000 ACE; the country was first colonised by European migrants in the early 19th century. In 1840, Ti Tiriti Waitangi (The Treaty of Waitangi) was forged with the indigenous Māori population. It is considered to be the founding document of New Zealand. The Treaty's contemporary interpretation ensures participation, protection and partnership with Māori and its influence is evident throughout the healthcare system. Nevertheless, stark inequalities still persist between the health status of Māori and non-Māori.

The most recent report on Māori health trends (Ministry of Health, 2019g) showed that heart disease is the major cause of death for Māori men and women, at rates up to twice as high as those of non-Māori. The largest difference between Māori and non-Māori people was for rates of rheumatic heart disease, which was four times higher for Māori men and women. Commensurate rates of hospitalisation for heart failure were also observed between Māori and non-Māori. Of note in this report was the experience of racism reported by Māori. Māori adults were twice as likely as non-Māori to have experienced a physical attack that was ethnically motivated. Māori women were seven times more likely than non-Māori women to have experienced unfair treatment when renting or buying a house, because of ethnicity. Māori men were twice as likely as non-Māori men to have experienced anxiety or a depressive disorder. This figure was similar but a little lower for Māori women.

The disparities in Māori health and well-being persist regardless of a much more overt policy agenda for Māori in Aotearoa compared to any for Australian Aboriginal and Torres Strait Islander peoples. This disparity in turn is assisted by the smaller scale of government in Aotearoa, compared to Australia's federated system of government. In both countries, the struggle to achieve parity of health and well-being outcomes for Indigenous peoples continues. Nurses are a key part of enacting the policy and practice initiatives, but only when they are competent to practise in a culturally safe way can this come to life in the healthcare system.

Case Study 2.3: Working with diversity

Will Evan's knowledge and skill set as a graduate nurse differ from those of someone with less life experience? If so, how do you think it might influence his interactions with others? What capabilities do you think enable nurses to work with people from diverse backgrounds?

Population growth

The United Nations world population prospects indicate that while the growth rate in many countries has slowed, the global population continues to grow and age (UNDESA, 2019). In 2019, worldwide life expectancy was 72.6 years, eight years higher than in 1990. By 2050, this is expected to increase to 77.1 years (UNDESA, 2019). The current life expectancy in New Zealand is 82.36 years, with an annual growth rate of 0.18% since 2015. In Australia, life expectancy is slightly higher at 83.5 years, with an annual growth rate since 2015 of 0.18–0.2 (UNDESA, 2019, p. 30). In both countries, females have higher life expectancy. By 2050, overall life expectancy for Australia and New Zealand is predicted to reach 87.1 years, one of the highest rates globally. In fact, globally, Australia and New Zealand have shown the largest gains in survival past age 65 for men and women; this is a reflection of the stability, healthcare infrastructure and economic fortitude of both countries (UNDESA, 2019). Globally, the number of persons aged 65 or over is projected to double between 2019 and 2050 and by 2050 persons over 65 years will outnumber those under 24 years. Projections suggest that, by 2030, 19.5% of the combined population of Australia and New Zealand will be 65 years or over and this will grow to 22.9% by 2050. In 2019, Australia's population reached 25.2 million with 15.9% of the population over the age of 65, and in New Zealand, with a population of 4.8 million, 16% of people were aged over 65 (UNDESA, 2019). Improved lifestyle choices and advances in treatments for health and disease contribute to healthier populations that live longer.

Population growth and ageing means health services will need to expand to manage increased demand, the prevalence of illness and population growth and spread. Accompanying population growth and longevity, more chronic illness and disability are predicted. In Australia, chronic conditions are a key contributor to the disease burden. Current figures estimate that almost half (47%) of Australians have a chronic illness, with approximately 20% estimated to have two or more, and the majority of these people are over 65 years (AIHW, 2020a). In 2017, New Zealand reported similar outcomes with the prevalence of people living with chronic illnesses increasing; some with more than one chronic condition (Ministry of Health, 2020a). In both countries, common chronic conditions include cardiovascular disease, cancer, mental health conditions and back pain (AIHW, 2020a; Ministry of Health, 2020a).

Population health

Commensurate with population growth worldwide, the prevalence of communicable and non-communicable diseases is increasing. Non-communicable disease includes obesity, diabetes and certain types of cancers. Obesity and diabetes are risk factors for a number of chronic conditions and are key contributors to the total burden of disease for both Australia and New Zealand. Rising rates of obesity and diabetes in both Australia and New Zealand are particularly problematic. Almost 67% of Australians over 18 years of age are classified as obese (AIHW, 2020a). Similarly, in New Zealand, 30.9% of people over 15 years are identified as obese; New Zealand has the third highest adult obesity rate in the Organisation for Economic Co-operation and Development (OECD) (Ministry of Health, 2019d, 2019e). Obesity can differ with ethnicity; for example, in New Zealand, figures are higher for Pacific (66.5%) and Māori (48.2%) as compared to European New Zealanders 29.1% (Ministry of Health, 2019d). The increasing prevalence of obesity in children is concerning. In Australia, more than 25% of children aged two to 17 and in New Zealand 11.3% of children (under 15 years) are overweight or obese. Similarly, diabetes in children is increasing with both Australia and New Zealand reporting a rise in both type 1 and 2 (AIHW, 2020a; Ministry of Health, 2019d).

Portfolio Activity 2.4: Stop, reflect and think

Think about the implications a growing rate of obesity and diabetes might have for healthcare services in the future. Consider the resources (financial, economic, informational and tangible) that will be needed to provide safe optimal healthcare. What impact do you think these population changes might have on healthcare delivery and, more specifically, nursing practice?

In Aotearoa New Zealand, over 200 000 people are diagnosed with diabetes each year. Again, compared to other New Zealanders, diabetes in Māori and Pacific populations is three times higher (Ministry of Health, 2014). In Australia in 2017, diabetes contributed to 10% of all deaths with one in 20 (1.2 million) adults self-reporting diabetes. Rates of diabetes increase with remoteness and socio-economic disadvantage, with Indigenous Australians four times more likely to have type 2 diabetes when compared to non-Indigenous Australians. Similarly, health issues related to mental health, substance abuse disorders, domestic violence and injuries (both intentional and unintentional) continue to grow; in Australia, mental and substance use disorders comprise the third highest burden of disease group (AIHW, 2020a).

Communicable diseases also have significant impacts on healthcare systems and resources. Diseases including hepatitis, tuberculosis, influenza and SARs-related viruses, vaccine-preventable diseases such as measles and mumps and mosquito-borne diseases such as Zika, dengue fever and malaria require strategic and coordinated responses from healthcare systems that draw upon significant health resources. Emerging threats and increasing drug resistance contribute to the challenge of disease management. For health systems, the COVID-19 response was both significant and unprecedented in terms of financial, physical and practice impact. Along with other measures, the Australian government released a $24 billion health package to protect Australians during the crisis. The plan included the provision of resources for healthcare in hospital and at home, primary and mental healthcare, digital health and research (AIHW, 2020a).

Health workforce

Central to the effectiveness of any healthcare system is the range of professionals that come together to deliver healthcare. At any time, registered nurses can engage with multiple services and individuals within the healthcare system to provide care that meets patients' needs. Figure 2.6 illustrates the wide range of health professionals that may come together in the provision of healthcare (AIHW, 2020a; Ministry of Health, 2019a).

 Portfolio Activity: Making the transition

Think about your own understanding of the different health professionals you have worked with during your clinical placements. How have these individuals shaped your knowledge and understanding of their profession and how you collaborate in practice? Do you need to know more about the groups you work with now and in the future? Think about how you might enhance your knowledge to improve your interprofessional practice.

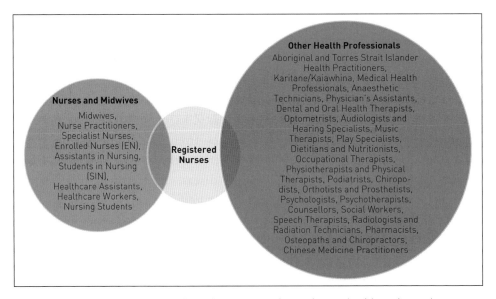

Figure 2.6   Health professionals and support workers who work with registered nurses

OXFORD UNIVERSITY PRESS

Corresponding with global trends, while the Australian and New Zealand healthcare workforces are evolving, evidence suggests they remain undersized, underqualified or inequitably distributed to meet current and future demand (AIHW 2016, 2020a; Health Workforce Australia [HWA], 2012; NCNZ, 2019a; Productivity Commission, 2015). An ageing health workforce and high attrition rates are key factors leading to workforce shortages, with nursing and medical professionals the most prominent shortage. As noted earlier, both Australia and New Zealand have an ageing registered nurse workforce with close to half aged 45 years and over. In Australia, workforce projections detailed in 2014 suggested a shortage of 109 490 nurses and 2701 doctors would occur by 2025 unless measures were taken to improve workforce capability and capacity (HWA, 2014). Of particular concern for both Australia and New Zealand is the need for greater distribution of the health workforce in regional, rural and remote areas. In Australia the majority of people (71%) live in coastal cities and younger people tend to congregate in larger cities where health infrastructure is more robust (AIHW, 2020a). Those living with disabilities (approximately 18%) and chronic conditions, however, more commonly live in regional areas where the availability of and access to healthcare services is limited, particularly specialist services. Table 2.1 illustrates the maldistribution of key health workers across major cities, the regions and remote areas. As you can see, in remote and very remote areas, nurses, midwives and Aboriginal and Torres Strait Islander health practitioners provide the majority of care. The table also shows that the number of allied health professionals such as psychologists and occupational therapists drops significantly in outer regional, remote and very remote areas.

Table 2.1 National health workforce data – remoteness area by number of practitioners 2016 (Australian Government, 2019)

Profession	Major cities	Inner Regional	Outer Regional	Remote	Very Remote	Total
ATSI health practitioners	356	325	896	618	729	2 924
Dental practitioners	101 243	17 861	7 375	829	371	127 679
Medical practitioners	487 197	83 403	34 282	5 495	2 651	613 028
Nurses and midwives	1 548 673	387 422	168 735	26 902	17 020	2 148 752
Occupational therapists	85 100	16 603	7 224	799	419	110 145
Pharmacists	136 511	25 162	10 998	1 389	634	174 694
Physiotherapists	136 160	22 135	8 321	1 099	566	168 281
Psychologists	162 937	23 502	7 942	965	477	195 823
Total	2 658 177	576 413	245 773	38 096	22 867	3 541 326

Internationalisation of the health workforce

Healthcare teams are multicultural and diverse in age, profession and practice. As a result of globalisation, the migration of skilled workforces has increased (UNDESA, 2019). Nurse migration is common for many countries and is often the result of intentional recruitment strategies to address nursing shortages. In healthcare, as populations grow and healthcare demand increases, healthcare systems look to overseas health professionals to bolster health workforce numbers (WHO, 2020b). Nurses are vital to the international infrastructure of healthcare, and worldwide there is a recognised shortage where demand exceeds supply. As a response to nursing shortages, many countries bring in overseas nurses to meet the demand.

Both Australia and New Zealand implement such strategies and have experienced an increase of international registered nurses joining the workforce (Chun Tie et al., 2018; Skaria et al., 2019). Overseas qualified nurses now make a significant contribution to the nursing workforce numbers. For example, in New Zealand, overseas qualified nurses comprise 27% of the total nursing workforce with the majority having qualified in the Philippines (34%) or the United Kingdom (25%) (NCNZ, 2019b). Similarly, in Australia, close to 30% of registered nurses have qualified outside of Australia with the total nursing workforce characterised by over 150 nationalities including nurses from New Zealand (Chun Tie et al., 2019). As a new registered nurse, you are likely to work with nurses from India, Canada, Australia and the Philippines as part of the nursing team providing care.

There are, however, challenges associated with nurse migration and the growth of a multicultural nursing workforce (Chun Tie et al., 2018). In 2011, Nichols, Davis and Richardson reviewed nurse migration in the United States, and reported that, worldwide, the education and regulation of nurses was 'highly diverse and varies considerably in scope and complexity' (p. 566). The authors stressed that this diversity poses significant challenges to the maintenance of practice and regulatory standards, and increases the likelihood of communication errors and misunderstandings in healthcare (Nichols et al., 2011, p. 633). These challenges continue to exist. Issues currently identified with an international workforce relate to variation in the training and education of nurses, health systems and processes, and legal, cultural and language differences. Communication and the provision of culturally appropriate care has been identified as problematic (International Council of Nurses [ICN], 2015; Chun Tie et al., 2018). Furthermore, international nurses face challenges integrating into the workforce (Braithwaite et al. 2017; Chun Tie et al., 2019; Skaria et al., 2019). In Australia and New Zealand, measures are in place to ensure internationally qualified nurses are competent and supported to assimilate into the workplace; however, evidence suggests that further development is needed if nurses are to practise safely and confidently (Chun Tie et al., 2019; Skaria et al., 2019).

Working within such diverse teams can present an opportunity for healthcare teams to develop knowledge that can enhance person-centred care, empathy and interpersonal skills. As new nurses, recognising your own cultural standpoint and biases and respecting the beliefs and values of others can lead to collegial and productive relationships. These factors contribute to more cohesive teamwork that produces a safer quality of healthcare.

Case Study 2.4: Working in diverse teams

Evan has been working in a healthcare team with nurses and doctors from around the world. There are two doctors he regularly works with whose accents he finds difficult to understand. This concerns him because when he receives handover, he is not sure he has the correct information. He doesn't want to say anything because he does not want to come across as being rude or perhaps racist.

- Should Evan say something to his two doctor colleagues about this? Why or why not?

- What might be the consequences if Evan does or does not speak up?

- If Evan feels uncomfortable, what else could he do in this situation?

Health reform, development and change within the context of practice and content of nursing work, leads to changes within professional responsibilities. Ten years ago, Jackson and Haigh noted that the expansion of the nurse's role will continue as nurses work across more 'diverse and innovative contexts' (Jackson & Haigh, 2010, p. 4). In 2020, nurse-led clinics and services, particularly in rural and remote areas, and advanced and specialised nursing roles such as nurse practitioners are ever-present and essential to health service delivery. While it can be challenging to keep up and maintain professional competence, reform has provided the opportunity for nurses to develop and extend their role and to take the lead in the delivery of healthcare. This context heightens the need for you as a new nurse to take the lead, be self-directed in your learning and development and proactive in seeking out opportunities and individuals to support your professional growth.

Case Study 2.5: Managing workplace challenges

Evan has been working now for two months but he is really struggling with his workload. The staff are always busy and one particular nurse complained the other day when she found out he was on her team. He then overheard her in the tearoom complaining about the workloads, saying that 'all these graduates need to be better prepared when they come out of uni – we just don't have time to teach them everything'. After hearing this, Evan does not want to admit he is struggling or ask for help. He doesn't want to be a burden or look stupid. Evan thought he was well prepared and chose the right job but now he is not sure.

- Why do you think the senior nurse made that comment?

- What factors could be contributing to the business of the department?

- What could Evan do to help himself with his workload management and improve his job satisfaction?

- Describe some of the outcomes for Evan if he does not seek help and continues to struggle.

Portfolio Activity: Making the transition

After reading this chapter, identify the challenges within the healthcare system that you think will have the greatest impact on your professional development in your first 12 months of practice as a registered nurse. Set three goals, with associated strategies, to better prepare yourself to manage those challenges. The goals and strategies can be things you can do during your classes before you begin your new role, during your clinical placements or something you will do when you commence practice as a registered nurse.

You can record your goals on the learning plan (Appendix 1) you began developing after reading Chapter 1.

Conclusion

The prospect of working as a healthcare professional in the dynamic and complex healthcare environment can be both exciting and daunting. Political, economic, social and professional factors have contributed to health system change and challenges, and will continue to do so. The evolution of healthcare and society has altered delivery and demand. Healthcare consumers require more complex, specialised, interprofessional care. Economic constraints and the need to moderate costs constantly challenge healthcare managers to balance requirements with available resources. Nurses, as the largest group of healthcare professionals and key stakeholders in healthcare, manage evolving roles and responsibilities in parallel with a need to be resourceful and adaptive in the face of continual change. Positive outcomes in the healthcare environment rely on sufficiently educated and competent healthcare teams. Ensuring new graduate nurses are prepared and ready for the dynamism that characterises the context in which they work, is crucial. As you work through the chapters that follow, you will develop an increasing awareness of the specialist skill set you bring to this environment, and the ways in which you are poised to make a difference in your professional role.

Key summary points

- Political, economic, organisational and regulatory factors shape healthcare systems and influence and inform the education and practice of registered nurses.

- External and internal factors related to the provision of healthcare constantly exert pressure, stimulate change and modify contexts of practice, making them complex systems to navigate.

- Registered nurses need to work effectively with varied health professionals from diverse backgrounds, to provide optimal safe healthcare.

- Understanding the complexity of contemporary healthcare and healthcare systems is critical to being able to work effectively, efficiently and competently as a registered nurse.

- New nurses need to be prepared with the capabilities to adapt to change, seek opportunities for development and manage their responsibilities to provide safe nursing care.

Critical thinking questions

1. Explain how the healthcare system can both influence and inform the education and transition to practice of new nurses.

2. What would you consider as the most challenging aspects of the contemporary healthcare system for new nurses?

3. As a nursing student, how is your role influenced by the healthcare system and how will this change when you become a registered nurse?

4. Can you explain the potential membership of an interprofessional healthcare team and how this contributes to the effectiveness of a healthcare system?

5. As a new nurse, what opportunities do you think a complex challenging workplace environment might offer you to develop your ability to work effectively in the health care system?

OXFORD UNIVERSITY PRESS

References

Allied Health Aotearoa New Zealand. (n.d.). *About us: What we do*. https://www.alliedhealth. org.nz/about-us.html

Australian Government Department of Health. (2019). *Health workforce data*. Australian Institute of Health and Welfare. https://hwd.health.gov.au/publications.html#alliedh17

Australian Government. (2019). *Health workforce data*. Retrieved August 24, 2020 from https:// hwd.health.gov.au/datatool.html

Australian Government. (2020). *National agreement on closing the gap: At a glance*. https:// www.closingthegap.gov.au/national-agreement-closing-gap-glance

Australian Health Practitioner Regulation Agency. (2020). *About*. https://www.ahpra.gov.au/ About-AHPRA.aspx

Australian Institute of Health and Welfare. (2016). *Nursing and midwifery workforce 2015*. https://www.aihw.gov.au/reports/workforce/nursing-and-midwifery-workforce-2015/ contents/who-are-nurses-and-midwives.

Australian Institute of Health and Welfare. (2019). *Australia's welfare 2019 data insights*. Australia's welfare series no. 14. Cat. no. AUS 226. https://www.aihw.gov.au/getmedia/ fe037cf1-0cd0-4663-a8c0-67cd09b1f30c/aihw-aus-222.pdf.aspx?inline=true

Australian Institute of Health and Welfare. (2020a). *Australia's health 2020*. https://www.aihw. gov.au/reports-data/australias-health

Australian Institute of Health and Welfare. (2020b). *Australia's health 2020: Indigenous health and well-being*. https://www.aihw.gov.au/reports/australias-health/indigenous-health-and-well-being

Australian Nursing and Midwifery Accreditation Council. (2019). *Registered nurse accreditation standards 2019*. https://www.anmac.org.au/search/publication

Braithwaite, J., Herkes, J., Ludlow, K., Lamprell, G., & Testa, L. (2017). Association between organisational and workplace cultures, and patient outcomes: Systematic review. *BMJ Open*, *6*(12), Article e017708. http://dx.doi.org/10.1136/bmjopen-2017-017708

Chun Tie, Y., Birks, M., & Mills, J. (2018). The experiences of internationally qualified registered nurses working in the Australian healthcare system: An integrative literature review. *Journal of Transcultural Nursing: Official Journal of the Transcultural Nursing Society*, *29*(3), 274–284. https://doi.org/10.1177/1043659617723075

Chun Tie, Y., Birks, M., & Francis, K. (2019). Playing the game: A grounded theory of the integration of international nurses. *Collegian*, *26*(4), 470–476. https://doi.org/10.1016/j. colegn.2018.12.006

Cox, M., Cuff, P., Brandt, B., Reeves, S., & Zierler, B. (2016). Measuring the impact of interprofessional education on collaborative practice and patient outcomes, *Journal of Interprofessional Care*, *30*(1), 1–3. https://doi.org/10.3109/13561820.2015.1111052

D'Ambra, A. M., & Andrews, D. R. (2014). Incivility, retention and new graduate nurses: An integrated review of the literature. *Journal of Nursing Management*, *22*(6), 735–742. https:// doi.org/10.1111/jonm.12060

Dawson, A. J., Stasa, H., Roche, M. A., Homer, C. S. E., & Duffield, C. (2014). Nursing churn and turnover in Australian hospitals: Nurses' perceptions and suggestions for supportive strategies. *BMC Nursing*, *13*(11), 1–10. https://doi.org/10.1186/1472-6955-13-11

Freeling, M., & Parker, S. (2015). Exploring experienced nurses' attitudes, views and expectations of new graduate nurses: A critical review. *Nurse Education Today*, *35*(2), e42–e49. https://doi.org/10.1016/j.nedt.2014.11.011

Geia, L., Baird, K., Bail, K., Barclay, L., Bennett, J., Best, O., Birks, M., Blackley, L., Blackman, R., Bonner, A., Bryant A. R., Buzzacott, C., Campbell, S., Catling, C., Chamberlain, C., Cox, L., Cross, W., Cruickshank, M., Cummins, A., Dahlen, H., … Wynn, R. (2020). A unified call to action from Australian nursing and midwifery leaders: Ensuring that black lives matter. *Contemporary Nurse*, 1–12. https://doi.org/10.1080/10376178.2020.1809107

Harrison, H., Birks, M., Franklin, R. C., & Mills, J. (2020). Fostering graduate nurse practice readiness in context. *Collegian*, *27*(1), 115–124. https://doi.org/10.1016/j.colegn.2019.07.006

Health Workforce Australia. (2012). *Health workforce 2025: Doctors, nurses and midwives* (Vol. 1). https://www.hwa.gov.au/sites/uploads/FinalReport_Volume1_FINAL-20120424.pdf

Health Workforce Australia. (2014). *Australia's future health workforce: Nurses overview report*. http://www.health.gov.au/internet/main/publishing.nsf/Content/australias-future-health-workforce-nurses.

Hunt, C., & Marini, Z. A. (2012). Incivility in the practice environment: A perspective from clinical nursing teachers. *Nurse Education Practice*, *12*(6), 366–370. https://doi.org/10.1016/j.nepr.2012.05.001

International Council of Nurses. (2015). *Faculty migration*. http://www.icn.ch/news/whats-new-archives/salaries-demand-and-career-opportunities-contribute-to-globalnursing-faculty-migration-1178.html

Jackson, D., & Haigh, C. (2010). Nursing workforce and workplaces: Contemporary concerns and challenges. *Contemporary Nurse*, *36*(1–2), 3–5. https://doi.org/10.1080/10376178.2010.11002464

Kaiser, L., Bartz, S., Neugebauer, E., Pietsch, B., & Pieper, D. (2018). Interprofessional collaboration and patient-reported outcomes in inpatient care: Protocol for a systematic review. *Systematic Reviews*, *7*(1), 126–131. https://doi.org/10.1186/s13643-018-0797-3

Kuziemsky, C. (2016). Decision-making in healthcare as a complex adaptive system. *Healthcare Management Forum*, *29*(1), 4–7. https://doi.org/10.1177/0840470415614842

Laschinger, H. K. S. (2012). Job and career satisfaction and turnover intentions of newly graduated nurses. *Journal of Nursing Management*, *20*(4), 472–484. https://doi.org/10.1111/j.1365-2834.2011.01293.x

Laschinger, H. K. S., & Grau, A. L. (2012). The influence of personal dispositional factors and organizational resources on workplace violence, burnout, and health outcomes in new graduate nurses: A cross-sectional study. *International Journal of Nursing Studies*, *49*(3), 282–291. https://doi.org/10.1016/j.ijnurstu.2011.09.004

Laschinger, H. K. S., Cummings, G., Leiter, M., Wong, C., MacPhee, M., Ritchie, J., Wolff, A., Regan, S., Rhéaume-Brüning, A., Jeffs, L., Young-Ritchie, C., Grinspun, D., Gurnham, M. E., Foster, B., Huckstep, S., Ruffolo, M., Shamian, J., Burkoski, V., Wood, K., & Read, E. (2016). Starting out: A time-lagged study of new graduate nurses' transition to practice. *International Journal of Nursing Studies*, *57*, 82–95. https://doi.org/10.1016/j.ijnurstu.2016.01.005

Laschinger, H. K. S., Finegan, J., & Wilk, P. (2009). New graduate burnout: The impact of professional practice environment, workplace civility, and empowerment. *Nursing Economics*, *27*(6), 377–383.

Lynette, J., Echevarria, I., Sun, E., & Ryan, J. G. (2016). Incivility across the nursing continuum. *Holistic Nursing Practice*, *30*(5), 263–268. https://doi.org/10.1097/hnp.0000000000000167

Martyn, J., Scott, J., van der Westhuyzen, J. H, Spanhake, D., Zanella, S., Martin, A., & Newby, R. (2019). Combining participatory action research and appreciative inquiry to design, deliver and evaluate an interdisciplinary continuing education program for a regional health workforce. *Australian Health Review*, *43*(3), 345–351. https://doi.org/10.1071/AH17124

McCloskey, B., Dar, O., Zumla, A., & Heymann, D. L. (2014). Emerging infectious diseases and pandemic potential: Status quo and reducing risk of global spread. *Lancet Infectious Diseases*, *14*(10), 1001–1010. https://doi.org/10.1016/s1473-3099(14)70846-1

Medical Council of New Zealand. (2019). *The New Zealand medical workforce in 2018*. https://www.mcnz.org.nz/

Ministry of Health. (2014). *About diabetes*. https://www.health.govt.nz/our-work/diseases-and-conditions/diabetes/about-diabetes

Ministry of Health. (2017). *Overview of the health system*. Retrieved January 6, 2020, from https://www.health.govt.nz/new-zealand-health-system/overview-health-system?mega=NZ%20health%20system&title=Overview

Ministry of Health. (2018). *NZ health system: Key health sector organisations and people*. https://www.health.govt.nz/new-zealand-health-system/key-health-sector-organisations-and-people

Ministry of Health. (2019a). *About the health workforce*. Retrieved March 9, 2020 from https://www.health.govt.nz/our-work/health-workforce/about-health-workforce

Ministry of Health. (2019b). *About primary health organisations*. Retrieved January 6, 2020 from https://www.health.govt.nz/our-work/primary-health-care/about-primary-health-organisations

Ministry of Health. (2019c). *NZ health system: Funding*. https://www.health.govt.nz/new-zealand-health-system/overview-health-system/funding

Ministry of Health. (2019d). *Obesity statistics*. https://www.health.govt.nz/nz-health-statistics/health-statistics-and-data-sets/obesity-statistics

Ministry of Health. (2019e). *Obesity*. https://www.health.govt.nz/our-work/diseases-and-conditions/obesity

Ministry of Health. (2019f). *Vote health: The estimates of appropriations 2019/20 – Budget 2019*. https://treasury.govt.nz/sites/default/files/2019-05/est19-v6-health.pdf

Ministry of Health. (2019g). *Wai 2575 Māori health trends report*. https://www.health.govt.nz/publication/wai-2575-maori-health-trends-report

Ministry of Health. (2020a). *Longer, healthier lives: New Zealand's health 1990–2017*. https://www.health.govt.nz/system/files/documents/publications/longer-healthier-lives-new-zealands-health-1990-2017.pdf

Ministry of Health. (2020b). *Primary health care*. https://www.health.govt.nz/our-work/primary-health-care

New Zealand Government. (2018). *Accident compensation corporation*. https://www.acc.co.nz/

New Zealand Government. (2019a). *Pharmaceutical management agency PHARMAC*. Retrieved January 6, 2020 from https://www.pharmac.govt.nz/about/

New Zealand Government. (2019b). *The well-being budget*. Retrieved November 29, 2019 from https://budget.govt.nz/index.htm

Nichols, B. L., Davis, C.R., & Richardson, C. R. (2011). International models of nursing. In Institute of Medicine, *The future of nursing: Leading change, advancing health* (pp. 565–642). National Academy of Sciences, Washington, D.C. http://www.iom.edu/~/media/Files/Activity%20Files/Workforce/Nursing/International%20Models%20of%20Nursing.pdf

Nursing Council of New Zealand. (2019a). *The New Zealand nursing workforce: A profile of nurse practitioners, registered nurses and enrolled nurses 2018–2019*. Nursing Council of New Zealand, Wellington.

Nursing Council of New Zealand. (2019b). *Register of nurses*. Retrieved November 18, 2019 from https://www.nursingcouncil.org.nz/

Parker, V., Giles, M., Lantry, G., & McMillan, M. (2014). New graduate nurses' experiences in their first year of practice. *Nurse Education Today, 34*(1), 150–156. https://doi.org/10.1016/j.nedt.2012.07.003

Productivity Commission. (2015). *Efficiency in health*. (I10, I18). http://www.pc.gov.au/research/completed/efficiency-health/efficiency-health.pdf

Roche, M. A., Duffield, C. M., Homer, C., Buchan, J., & Dimitrelis, S. (2015). The rate and cost of nurse turnover in Australia. *Collegian, 22*(4), 353–358. https://doi.org/10.1016/j.colegn.2014.05.002

Skaria, R., Whitehead, D., Leach, L., & Walshaw, M. (2019). Experiences of overseas nurse educators teaching in New Zealand. *Nurse Education Today, 81*, 7–12. https://doi.org/10.1016/j.nedt.2019.05.032

United Nations, Department of Economic and Social Affairs, Population Division. (2019). *World population prospects 2019: Highlights (ST/ESA/SER.A/423)*. https://population.un.org/wpp/Publications/Files/WPP2019_Highlights.pdf

Viotti, S., Converso, D., Hamblin, L. E., Guidetti, G., & Arnetz, J. E. (2018). Organisational efficiency and co-worker incivility: A cross-national study of nurses in the USA and Italy. *Journal of Nursing Management, 26*(5), 597–604. https://doi.org/10.1111/jonm.12587

Walker, A., Costa, B. M., Foster, A. M., & de Bruin, R. L. (2017). Transition and integration experiences of Australian graduate nurses: A qualitative systematic review. *Collegian, 24*(5), 505–512. https://doi.org/10.1016/j.colegn.2016.10.004

Walker, A., Storey, K. M., Costa, B. M., & Leung, R. K. (2015). Refinement and validation of the Work Readiness Scale for graduate nurses. *Nurse Outlook, 63*(6), 632–638. https://doi.org/10.1016/j.outlook.2015.06.001

World Health Organization. (2010). *Framework for action on interprofessional education and collaborative practice*. www.who.int/hrh/resources/framework_action/en/

World Health Organization. (2019). *Ten threats to global health in 2019*. https://www.who.int/news-room/feature-stories/ten-threats-to-global-health-in-2019

World Health Organization. (2020a). *Digital health*. https://www.who.int/health-topics/digital-health#tab=tab_1

World Health Organization. (2020b). *State of the world's nursing 2020: Investing in education, jobs and leadership*. Geneva.

OXFORD UNIVERSITY PRESS

Chapter 3

Developing a Professional Portfolio

Morgan Smith and Lynette Cusack

Learning Outcomes

Following completion of this chapter, you will be able to:

1. Describe the purpose of a portfolio for a registered nurse.
2. Explain the main components of a professional portfolio.
3. Identify portfolio-related privacy and confidentiality considerations.
4. Compile a portfolio for different purposes.

Key terms

Curriculum vitae

E-portfolio

Evidence

Lifelong learning

Professional portfolio

Quality evidence

Reflection

Introduction

Professional portfolio

An organised collection of evidence that maps and validates an individual's personal and professional learning and development, capabilities and achievements over time.

No doubt in your studies you have been introduced to the **professional portfolio.** It is important that registered nurses keep a portfolio. Andre (2010) describes a professional portfolio as 'a structured argument about an individual's learning or performance that draws upon items of evidence (artefacts) to support the quality and authenticity of the claims made' (p. 122). A portfolio may be developed for certification, employment, promotion or educational purposes and is developed, revised and updated over time. While each portfolio is unique to the registered nurse who develops it, there are principles and practices that apply to all portfolio development. In this chapter you will explore the various purposes of a portfolio and its value to you as a registered nurse. You will learn some approaches to portfolio construction for specific purposes. Throughout the chapter we will provide some examples and options for structuring your portfolio in a way that can best serve your individual professional development and career aspirations.

Case Study 3.1: Introducing Maddy

Maddy went straight to university after leaving school and has enjoyed her nursing degree. At 21, Maddy is in her final year as an undergraduate and is preparing to apply for a graduate nurse program for the coming year. Maddy learnt about professional portfolios and their importance for her nursing career during her studies and has been carefully collecting evidence to populate her portfolio.

Portfolios and the registered nurse

A professional portfolio can serve a range of purposes for a registered nurse. A portfolio can be used to illustrate a nurse's knowledge and skills as well as areas requiring development. It can also provide a road map for achieving career aspirations. All nurses should consider having at least one professional portfolio. Each portfolio is designed to meet a specific goal. A registered nurse may have a basic portfolio that they draw from to create different portfolio presentations for different purposes.

OXFORD UNIVERSITY PRESS

Portfolios are developed over the duration of a career. Ensuring you commence a portfolio at the beginning of your career will support you to make the most of your professional experiences. By regularly documenting your professional experiences in a portfolio you create a comprehensive record of activities, events and learning that you might otherwise forget. You also have material to reflect upon, and therefore the potential to further develop your knowledge and skills. Used wisely, a portfolio can provide the foundation for fast-tracking your career. It can also provide a sense of personal satisfaction when you review your career development over time. Nursing is a dynamic profession. There is always more to explore, learn and achieve. You will never reach a point in your career when you think you know enough or have learnt enough. There will always be more to learn, and so more potential material for inclusion in your portfolio. Registering as a nurse is just the beginning of a **lifelong learning** journey.

When designing a portfolio, it is important to identify its intended audience. Shaping your portfolio to the intended audience is essential if you are to communicate your chosen messages effectively. As a registered nurse your audience could be, for example, auditors, line managers, promotion committees or employment panels. All will require a slightly different portfolio presentation.

A portfolio may take different forms. Many nurses have an **e-portfolio**. This can be structured around a specifically designed e-portfolio platform, such as 'Mahara' (Mahara, 2019), but doing so is not essential. When using a commercial portfolio platform, check the privacy policy and terms and conditions carefully (Stewart, 2017). Students who have used a particular e-portfolio platform may be able to continue using this platform after graduation, if they wish, as some undergraduate education providers facilitate this process. A basic e-portfolio, however, can be created using word-processed or scanned pdf documents and a series of electronic folders. It is also possible to have a portfolio based on hard copy materials. Hard copy portfolios are more difficult to share but can often be transferred into a basic digital format if and when required. Digital formats tend to offer greater flexibility and convenience, but the best portfolio format is the one that suits your needs and wishes.

A portfolio must be fit for purpose. A portfolio can be irrelevant if not developed appropriately (Andre, 2010). Simply accruing a large number of materials without considering their quality is problematic (Andre, 2010). Volume is not a substitute for quality. Quality requires that the materials demonstrate

Lifelong learning

Self-directed deliberate pursuit of education that promotes ongoing personal and/or professional learning and development.

E-portfolio

A digital approach to the structure, storage and presentation of materials that demonstrate an individual's knowledge, skills and experiences.

contemporary standards for nursing practice and reflect ethical and professional practice. The relevance of items of evidence must be considered in relation to the portfolio's purpose. Being clear about the purpose of a portfolio is central to achieving a product of worth.

 ### Portfolio Activity: Making the transition

Do you already have a professional portfolio? What form does it take? If you don't have a portfolio, consider how you might structure and compile it. Explore different options for e-portfolios on the internet and decide which approach is best for you.

Throughout this text you will be encouraged to 'stop, reflect and think' about what you are reading and how it applies to you. A number of other activities will help you to make the transition to the professional role. We recommend you capture your responses to these activities in your professional portfolio to enhance your learning and showcase your professional development.

Components of a professional portfolio

While a portfolio can take different forms depending on its purpose and target audience, all portfolios must be constructed using some specific principles if they are to be fit for purpose. When constructing a portfolio, it is necessary to include personal reflections on your practice/profession, and quality evidence of any abilities, courses and activities undertaken that demonstrate that you possess specific knowledge and skills, or that learning goals have been achieved. Reflection and quality evidence will now be explored in relation to portfolio construction for the registered nurse.

Reflection

An organised, deliberate process of thinking that examines past experiences to understand what happened, gain insight and develop a range of new or different actions for a specific situation.

Reflection

All portfolios should demonstrate evidence of personal **reflection**. The extent of this varies depending on the purpose of the portfolio, but all portfolios require evidence of reflection. Reflection is described as a thoughtful process;

one that involves cognitive processes to examine experiences and generate new perspectives and understandings of a situation. In the context of health, Asselin et al. (2013) define reflection as 'a deliberate process of thinking about a clinical situation which leads to insight and a subsequent change in practice' (p. 905).

Reflection is the foundation of reflective learning, reflective practice and professional development planning including career planning (Cusack & Smith, 2020). The process of systematically undertaking reflection has clear implications for enhancing nursing practice. Reflective practice involves the individual examining their own actions, thoughts, feelings and knowledge in order to enhance professional practice (Dubé & Ducharme, 2015). Reflection is central to a well-thought-through and logically constructed portfolio.

Reflection can occur in different ways, but in a portfolio it is mostly demonstrated through writing. Some people enjoy writing and find reflecting through writing cathartic and enlightening. Others do not. Demonstrating reflection through writing is not something everyone is comfortable doing. Some find it time-consuming and challenging, and doubt its benefits. That said, documenting reflections can become easier with practice. It is also unavoidable in a portfolio, so if you find yourself procrastinating just sit down and start writing. No doubt at the end you won't be happy with what you have written, but that doesn't matter. You can go back and edit what you have written, delete material that you perceive to be less relevant and add any new ideas. You can craft your work over time. Your ability to reflect in writing will develop with time and practice.

Reflection is necessary for ensuring a portfolio develops in richness and depth over time. A portfolio should demonstrate how you have extended your expertise and depth and breadth of knowledge over time. A portfolio that records the same information repeatedly does not demonstrate new learning. For example, a portfolio that only demonstrates that the annual competencies required by your employer have been completed year after year, does not demonstrate that you have extended your understanding of the breadth and depth of your nursing role from a personal perspective. Specific competency demonstration may be a requirement of your employer, and a condition of employment, but it does not necessarily demonstrate growth in your professional practice as an individual. To be in a position to learn what is required to demonstrate personal growth, reflection is required. Reflection enables you to look at yourself objectively, identify your strengths and weaknesses and plan professional development that is unique to you.

Reflection is required as part of the continuing professional development cycle. Often, reflection on an issue will reveal areas where greater knowledge or skill is required. Learning through reflection is ongoing. There is always more to learn – hence the term 'lifelong learning'. We are never finished with learning! Reflection is necessary if an effective learning plan is to be developed, to address the identified gaps arising from reflection.

Similarly, in order to effectively showcase professional expertise, reflection must occur. The analytical aspects of reflection are necessary for constructing an argument in your portfolio in support of existing knowledge and skills. Reflection requires that you create links between your professional role or position description, and the artefact you are using as evidence in support of your personal abilities. Each piece of evidence must be linked through reflection to the role you are showcasing. Jointly, your reflections and pieces of evidence support the argument you create to validate your professional experience, knowledge and skills.

Evidence

Evidence

Artefact used to substantiate a claim of knowledge, skill or experience.

A professional portfolio must include **evidence** that supports the claims of knowledge, skills and experience being made. It is insufficient to simply state that you have a particular knowledge and skill set in your portfolio. You must provide evidence to support the claims; a statement alone is insufficient. Evidence is often in the form of a written document but may also be an audio, video or image (Stewart, 2013). Some examples of evidence are certificates of completion with notes and learning outcomes, certificates of attendance, evidence of on-the-job training, publications read with review notes and practice-related implications for yourself (Cope & Murray, 2018).

Different forms of evidence serve different purposes. Items of evidence within a portfolio provide the basis for your argument in relation to achievement. Several items of evidence, or only one, may be required to argue a case for achievement. The case being made determines the amount and type of evidence required. For example, certificates awarded for a training course or higher education program can be used to support knowledge claims in specific areas, but other items of evidence may be required if claims are being made in relation to abilities, or improvements in specific skills, or procedures. Such a claim might be supported by a clinical evaluation report, for example.

Portfolio Activity 3.1: Stop, reflect and think

Consider your intended area of future practice. Do you plan to move into a specialised area after you graduate? What evidence do you have, or will need to acquire, to demonstrate your suitability to work in your preferred area of practice?

Evidence provided in a portfolio may be primary or secondary. Primary evidence is an item or artefact that is developed by the practitioner; that is, by you (Jasper et al., 2013). An example of primary evidence could be a health information brochure you designed or an assignment you wrote on a particular issue. Secondary evidence already exists (Jasper et al., 2013), and originates from sources other than the portfolio creator. Examples of secondary sources include certificates of achievement or letters of recommendation. Both primary and secondary sources of evidence are desirable as they increase the strength of a claim.

Your portfolio should include current evidence. As you know, best practice changes over time as a result of research. Research findings inform evidence-based practice and therefore nursing practice. As you move through your career you will accumulate considerable evidence in support of your knowledge and skills. With time, there will be recent pieces of evidence that supersede existing items. You need to move these older items of evidence to a different storage site, or delete them. Demonstrating that your practice is contemporary can be supported in your portfolio by web links to best practice evidence. Your portfolio should reflect contemporary nursing practice and highlight your most recent achievements.

The evidence in your portfolio should be **quality evidence**. Quality evidence is *tangible*, *suitable* and *relevant* (Cusack & Smith, 2020). Quality evidence that is *tangible* is in a form that can be evaluated by another person. An example is a certified academic transcript. The certification ensures it is legitimate. The contents of the transcript can be evaluated independently by another person. Quality evidence is also *suitable*. Where possible, it should reflect evidence-based practice. A practice that is considered 'tried and true' but lacks a theoretical basis cannot be considered suitable evidence of quality. Quality evidence must also be *relevant*, aligning with the claim being made. An item of evidence may be

Quality evidence

Evidence for a portfolio that is tangible, suitable, relevant to purpose and from a range of sources.

tangible and suitable but if it does not support the claim being made it cannot be considered relevant. Finally, quality evidence should come from a *range of sources* if possible, either primary and/or secondary. When evaluating the quality of evidence, check how it meets the above criteria to determine its worth.

As discussed earlier, remember that your portfolio must argue a case for how your chosen evidence supports your knowledge claims. These claims explain why your evidence is reliable, suitable and appropriate for inclusion in your portfolio. It is necessary to explain the purpose of including the evidence. It is also necessary to explain what standard, learning outcome or employment criterion the item of evidence supports. You may also use the literature to support your claims, including best practice protocols, standards, professional guidelines, journal articles or any other quality sources.

Case Study 3.2: Quality evidence

Since the beginning of her nursing career in year 1, Maddy has collected evidence for her portfolio. Categorise each of the following as primary and secondary evidence then create a list that represents quality evidence.

- Assignments and class activities.

- Clinical placement assessments and performance reviews.

- Examples of clinical tasks completed on placement (e.g. discharge summaries, patient reports, medication charts).

- Thank-you cards from patients.

- A prize for a first-year nursing philosophy presentation.

- Certificate of achievement as a student mentor.

Evidence is central to a portfolio. A portfolio without evidence is not a portfolio, so store your evidence securely, using a system that will enable you to retrieve items easily. Evidence that clearly supports your knowledge claims will be impressive and very persuasive. However, it must also respect the privacy of others and this can sometimes be unexpectedly problematic. Portfolio-related privacy and confidentiality issues are discussed in the next section.

 Portfolio Activity 3.2: Stop, reflect and think

Think about the evidence you have collected over the duration of your nursing program. Is your evidence tangible, suitable, relevant and from a range of different sources? Is your evidence primary or secondary, and can you link it to your professional standards or competencies? If this evidence is not already contained in your portfolio, can you retrieve it easily?

Privacy and confidentiality

Privacy and confidentiality are important considerations when developing a portfolio. Legal obligations, professional standards and codes of practice include consent and confidentiality requirements and expectations, designed to protect consumers of healthcare. When compiling a portfolio, it is important to familiarise yourself with relevant policies, guidelines and directives from both the nurse regulator (Nursing and Midwifery Board of Australia [NMBA]; Nursing Council of New Zealand [NCNZ]) and your employer. Breaches of privacy and confidentiality can have serious consequences for individual practitioners. If you are unsure whether a personal reflection or an item of evidence breaches privacy, consider removing it from your portfolio.

Client confidentiality must be maintained at all times. Information that is collected from patients/clients as part of their healthcare must be used only for that purpose. Using client information for other purposes, such as in a personal portfolio, can be problematic. This also applies to de-identified information. Written consent is always required when a portfolio includes the words or images of other people (Cusack & Smith, 2020). For example, difficulties may arise in relation to photographs. Most staff have access to a smart phone with a camera. Photos, however, cannot be taken without the consent of the person(s) being photographed. In addition, some organisations ban photography in specific, or sometimes all, situations.

Employers have confidentiality-related requirements that nurses should be aware of when preparing portfolio items. Organisational policies aim to protect not only the consumers of healthcare but also the reputation of the organisation. Organisations usually prohibit the removal of healthcare-related information.

For example, it would be inappropriate to copy a discharge summary you have written for a client, for your portfolio, even if you de-identify it. Such an item should not be included in a portfolio without the permission of the employing organisation.

Using social media to explore professional issues within an e-portfolio is fraught with difficulties. Some e-portfolio platforms support the use of public online spaces for professional collaboration (Stewart, 2013). This is potentially very risky. The NMBA (2019) provides general advice on the use of social media in the nursing and midwifery context, as does the NCNZ (2012). There are also practical issues around making comments in a public space. Your comments may be incorrectly interpreted, or interpreted in ways you did not anticipate (Stewart, 2013). It is also possible that over time your perspectives and opinions will change but the past view of your ideas will remain online if you are unable to delete or change it. Many e-portfolios, representing a range of different professions, can be located online for public view. These are often for the purpose of promoting the individual to the world at large. They are not generally the profiles of people who work in the health professions. They do not reflect those professions, such as nursing, that undertake work that is largely confidential. To avoid potential difficulties, it is recommended that e-portfolios remain private and be shared with others on a need-to-know basis.

While an e-portfolio may be private, once it is shared with someone there is a risk it will be shared more widely. One of the issues with digital items is that they can be shared readily. The speed with which items can spread across social media platforms shows what is possible. There is also an issue with privacy settings. If they are not sufficiently robust, materials may be viewed by people other than the intended audience. Therefore, revealing personal or professional information without sufficient caution can be risky (Andre, 2010). It is recommended that, as a general principle, only artefacts suitable for the public domain be included in your portfolio.

One of the benefits of an e-portfolio is the capacity to collaborate and/or share reflections, ideas and artefacts with others. However, while sharing offers opportunities to contribute and learn, it also has potential privacy and confidentiality implications. Many profession-specific social media sites are private and protected from non-members (Ventola, 2014). While sites may be private, any given individual has little control over where their materials and posts are shared by others. It is important to be mindful of confidentiality not only of clients but also of colleagues. For example, a collaboratively constructed document should only be shared with the consent of other contributors and/or the chair of the committee or group.

Portfolio presentations must meet privacy and confidentiality expectations. While one of the strengths of an e-portfolio is the ability to share, collaborate and receive feedback from others, the privacy of others must always be maintained. Striking the right balance is often challenging. When compiling a portfolio, it is vital to ensure that privacy and confidentiality requirements are met.

Case Study 3.3: Privacy and confidentiality

Maddy shared her portfolio with her lecturer, Dr Hobson. Dr Hobson expressed concern about the inclusion of discharge summaries, patient reports, medication charts and thank-you notes and cards from patients. How might Maddy deal with the potential breaches in privacy and confidentiality that these may present?

Compiling a portfolio

A portfolio may be compiled for a number of reasons. It can be used to demonstrate that a registered nurse is addressing their professional responsibilities around lifelong learning and development. It is also useful for showcasing professional expertise and achievements for career progression and changes in career direction. While there are other purposes for a portfolio, these two are the most common ones. The next section explores how to construct a portfolio for continuing professional development, followed by a showcase portfolio.

Creating a continuing professional development portfolio

A portfolio can be used to demonstrate continuing professional development (CPD). The NMBA suggests that creating a professional portfolio is one way that registered nurses can demonstrate that they have met CPD expectations

(NMBA, 2016b). CPD is a registration standard for registered nurses. It ensures nurses maintain and develop their knowledge and expertise in order to provide effective, safe and ethical care (NMBA, 2016b). To remain competent, nurses must stay up to date in their practice and connected to the profession. Penalties apply for nurses who cannot demonstrate that they meet CPD requirements. The NMBA guidelines state that evidence of CPD should be kept for five years (NMBA, 2016b). Similarly, the NCNZ requires all nurses to maintain and provide evidence of their continuing competence to practise. To meet this requirement, nurses must complete 60 days (450 hours) of practice and 60 hours of professional development in the last three years, and meet the competencies of their scope of practice (NCNZ, 2020). Records of CPD may be stored in a portfolio and should include evidence of reflection, planning and evaluation of achievements.

Reflection for CPD

Reflection on your current level of knowledge and skills is necessary before you can plan any learning opportunities for CPD. As a soon-to-be graduate you probably believe there is still an enormous amount for you to learn. This, of course, is true but throughout your career there will always be new knowledge and skills that you will identify that you need to develop. As a graduate, when reflecting for CPD purposes it is probably best to focus on your current role and position description. Nurses have diverse roles, so what might be the most appropriate area of development for one nurse will be different from that of another. As a graduate, it will be best for you to reflect on your current nursing role or position description and identify the areas where you perceive you are sufficiently skilled, as well as the areas where you think you need to develop. If you have a performance review session with your supervisor, this is an opportunity to discuss your reflections, development needs and learning opportunities. An important part of reflection is to identify learning needs that, if addressed, will enable you to move from your present position of understanding and skill to master new, but related, areas of knowledge and skill. Identifying gaps in knowledge is an important part of the process of professional development. It enables you to then move ahead and systematically plan new learning opportunities.

When reflecting, and recording your reflections, in your portfolio, it is important that the reflective component links to a specific standard or criterion. As the purpose of the portfolio is to demonstrate CPD, then the reflective component and the evidence provided should be linked to the registered nurse standards or competencies for practice (NMBA, 2016a; NCNZ, 2020). For example, when you graduate and start work as a registered nurse, you may find the experience so stressful that it impacts on your ability to fulfil your role. You will probably find that other recent graduates feel the same. You may decide to investigate additional strategies you and your colleagues can use to better manage this stress. Your reflections about the stress you are experiencing and the need to develop increased knowledge around stress management can be linked to RN practice standard 3 ('Maintains the capability for practice') and more specifically 3.1 ('Considers and responds in a timely manner to the health and well-being of self and others in relation to the capability for practice') (NMBA, 2016a). In New Zealand, this would relate to Domain 2, competency 2.8 ('Maintains professional development') (NCNZ, 2007). Another example is you might be reflecting on your experience caring for people impacted by bushfires. You may decide you need to learn more about how people experience bushfires and the various community resources available to support them in their recovery. Your learning goal could be related to RN practice standard 2 ('Engages in therapeutic and professional relationships'), specifically 2.3 ('Recognises that people are the experts in the experience of their life'). Linking reflections to standards ensures the professional development you undertake, and the evidence you use to support your learning outcomes, sits firmly within the domain of the registered nurse role.

Planning CPD

Once you have identified a gap in your learning, it is useful to identify some learning outcomes. These should align to a practice standard. Identifying learning outcomes can assist you to ensure that what you aim to achieve is manageable in the established timeframe. It is better to have learning goals that are incremental over time, to avoid potentially becoming overwhelmed. You may remember that at the beginning of a semester you worked out all you had to achieve by the end. There would have been moments when you felt the requirements were impossible to meet. Presumably you coped with this by planning how to meet all course and program requirements over the semester. The same applies to a CPD plan – identify small incremental steps that will get you where you want to go over time. Acker (2020) suggests the use of SMART learning outcomes for CPD – outcomes that are specific, measurable, attainable, results-focused and time-focused. A specific learning outcome is one that states clearly what you need to learn. It is also the easiest to evaluate. A measurable learning outcome is one where you can easily identify its completion. An attainable learning outcome is one that poses a sufficient degree of challenge but is not impossible. Results-focused means the outcome is relevant to your role description. Finally, time-focused requires you to specify a date for completion of the required learning. It is worth setting a timeframe as it focuses your attention on when you need to complete your learning. You can always extend the completion date if your learning is not accomplished on time, but having a due date can act as a motivator.

When you have reflected on your learning needs and set some objectives, you need to develop a learning plan. The learning plan is very important. It involves you identifying what you can do to fill your knowledge or skill gap. Learning activities may be formal, such as attending a workshop or short course, or completing an online activity. They may also be less formal, such as a self-directed review of the literature. You may want to identify a support person or mentor who can advise and guide you; for example, your workplace supervisor or a preceptor. As part of the performance review cycle, you will get the chance to discuss how your learning needs can be addressed. Your supervisor can offer advice and may even be able to facilitate opportunities that will enable you to learn specifically what you require. Each learning outcome requires a plan of action. Do not set yourself too many goals or activities that are clearly not feasible to meet.

Employers often require nursing staff to undertake mandatory staff development training as part of CPD. For example, an employer may require you to complete an online course on a specific topic. The employer may provide access to the course. On completion, the certificate can be downloaded or printed and included in your portfolio as evidence of professional development. Similarly, an employer may require you to attend staff development, whether annually or more often. Evidence of attendance is usually provided by the employer. There can be considerable staff development requirements. Healthcare is a rapidly changing area and there is much to learn to keep abreast of change. It is important to remember that each nurse has unique learning needs and career aspirations, so thinking beyond employer-mandated staff development is important. We recommend a combination of self-directed learning activities and mandated ones. This will enable you to meet employer expectations and to address your unique areas of knowledge deficit.

 ## Portfolio Activity 3.3: Stop, reflect and think

Reflect on your clinical placement experiences. What opportunities for CPD were offered to staff? Which of these did you participate in? If they are not already part of your portfolio, consider how you may include evidence of them.

In your portfolio, it is important to document the number of hours you spend on CPD activities. As noted previously in this chapter, maintaining CPD is a registration requirement. For example, registered nurses in Australia must demonstrate that they have accomplished at least 20 hours of learning each year (NMBA, 2016b). Many nurses will do much more, but keeping this in mind may help you to develop a plan that is feasible for you. You need to indicate the number of hours spent on each learning activity so that it is clear how your annual total CPD hours have been calculated.

Engaging in CPD

Your learning plan must be actioned if you are to learn new knowledge and skills. Sometimes your plan will need adjusting – opportunities you anticipated would be available may not be after all, or may not provide the learning you had anticipated. When a learning activity is complete, include in your portfolio the evidence required to support your claim. When identifying how you can gain the knowledge and skills you need, it is important to also identify the evidence you will require to demonstrate your increased understanding, as discussed earlier in this chapter.

Evaluation of learning related to CPD

Once a learning activity has been completed, a thoughtful evaluation of what has been learnt is important for understanding what has been achieved and what a future learning goal might be. The evaluation of learning should be documented in the portfolio as part of the CPD process. Learning is not always as effective or as relevant as we would like. Sometimes we can be disappointed with our learning. Whatever the outcome, an honest account of the learning is required if future learning is to be successfully planned and achieved.

Action for further CPD

As you document your CPD in your professional portfolio you will inevitably identify further gaps in your learning. From your learning you will identify knowledge, skills and other areas of expertise that you need to address to enhance your professional capabilities. These gaps in knowledge become the basis of future learning outcomes.

To assist with record-keeping, professional and industrial nursing bodies may provide electronic or hard copy templates for CPD for members. Some employers may also provide CPD templates or structures for staff. The NMBA has developed a self-directed CPD record (NMBA, 2016b). The template is an example only. There is no requirement to use it; however, it is recommended and is a useful method of documenting CPD. The template shown in Appendix 3 is adapted from the NMBA's self-directed CPD record and covers the essential areas of documentation, with additional space to reflect on learning achieved. Coupled with the learning plan template (Appendix 1) and supported with quality evidence where required, these become excellent methods for demonstrating your learning and development over time and hence your competence for practice.

Developing a portfolio for CPD purposes is not onerous. It simply requires you to be systematic in thinking about, and identifying, your personal learning needs, then securely storing the evidence that supports your learning achievements. For example, if you receive a certificate of attainment for a workshop, short course or study day, store it where you can find it easily and document your reflections as soon as possible after the learning experience. Update your CPD summary as you go – don't wait until the end of the yearly cycle then try to remember what you have done. That approach will probably result in you omitting to document some key learning experiences and thus will reduce the quality of your portfolio.

Portfolio Activity: Making the transition

Review the CPD template and guidelines provided in Appendix 3.

- Consider activities (not including your degree studies) that you have undertaken in the last 12 months that you would identify as CPD.
- Using these examples, complete the CPD template (Appendix 3).
- Evaluate how these activities align with the criteria for CPD used by the registering authority in your country.

Include the CPD summary template in your portfolio. As you encounter further CPD opportunities, update the template to include them.

It is worth remembering that learning occurs all the time in the work environment, and not all of it can or should be recorded for CPD purposes. There is always more that could or should be learnt. As part of your day-to-day work you will come across issues that you need to know about to successfully carry out your role. Sometimes this learning occurs through asking a more experienced colleague. Sometimes you need to read about an issue when it arises or, if safe to do so, afterwards when you get home. Nursing involves complex knowledge and skills. The environment is constantly changing and expectations of nurses are high. There will always be something new to learn – you will be able to capture some of this learning in your portfolio, but almost certainly not all of it.

Case Study 3.4: A portfolio for practice readiness

Maddy has secured a position in a graduate year program, but it doesn't start until four months after she completes the requirements for registration. How might Maddy utilise her professional portfolio to develop, maintain and showcase her readiness for practice?

Creating a showcase portfolio

Another type of nursing portfolio is broadly known as a showcase portfolio. A showcase portfolio illustrates the breadth and depth of your knowledge and expertise. It should be designed in such a way that it illustrates your abilities at their highest level of achievement, to make the best impression on those who view it. The designing of a showcase portfolio requires creativity. It will be unique to the person who owns it.

A showcase portfolio is always a work in progress and should be updated as your knowledge and skills develop. Therefore, when you develop new knowledge and/or skills, update your portfolio so you showcase that which best demonstrates your capability at any moment in time. A showcase portfolio may need to be adjusted to address different audiences and purposes, similar to a **Curriculum Vitae** (CV). For example, a showcase portfolio designed for a performance review will be different from one designed for a promotion application. As a student, your education provider may require all students to use a similar format and features when constructing their portfolio. As a registered nurse, you will have more freedom to choose your own approach and demonstrate greater creativity.

While showcase portfolios are unique to the person who develops them, there are some general guidelines you can consider when structuring one. Burns (2018) suggests the components shown in Table 3.1 as the basis of a showcase portfolio.

Curriculum Vitae

A detailed, comprehensive summary of an individual's experiences, capabilities and achievements over time.

Table 3.1 Components of a showcase portfolio (Burns, 2018)

• Demographic data (personal details) on a cover page
• Table of contents
• Educational qualifications with certified transcripts
• Registration certificate
• Positions held • Professional experiences
• Teaching roles
• Professional memberships • Awards
• Consultations, grants
• Publications and conference presentations • Other scholarly work
• Professional development activities
• Professional references
• Evaluations, performance reviews • Letters of commendation

The list is neither comprehensive nor a list of expectations for all nurses. Most nurses would not have evidence that addressed all the components, and a nurse further into their career would be more likely to be able to address more components than a nurse early in their career. However, they provide some ideas about what would be acceptable and what might be possible. Having an idea about what to work towards could be helpful for planning learning and career development.

As you construct your showcase portfolio, you may identify gaps in the evidence to support your claims. In fact, you are likely to identify gaps in evidence. Sometimes the gaps are oversights; you can go back and locate the required evidence. Sometimes there may be a gap in your knowledge and skills that you need to address. If so, you need to identify a learning objective, develop a learning plan that will enable you to learn about the required area, undertake the required learning and access the form of evidence that supports your knowledge claim.

Compiling a showcase portfolio requires decision-making around the items of evidence selected. Evidence selection should be based on purpose. Not all items will be required in all portfolio presentations. Keep items of evidence stored securely so they can be accessed when required. Each item should be accompanied by a statement that explains the importance of its inclusion, as discussed earlier.

When compiling the showcase portfolio, it is important to ensure that any reflective component and evidence link to some specific criteria. Do not assume that the viewer will understand the links between reflection, evidence and criteria. Explain it, clearly and concisely. If the purpose of the portfolio is to demonstrate your knowledge and skills to a future employer, then link your reflection and evidence to the position description of the job you are applying for. Addressing each criterion systematically and logically enables the person viewing your portfolio submission to move through it easily and seamlessly.

 Portfolio Activity: Making the transition

Review the application process for graduate year positions in your area. What type of evidence would be appropriate to support your application for a graduate program? Audit your existing portfolio to determine whether it is suitable for this purpose. Where are the gaps? How will you fill these to give you the best chance of success in a competitive environment?

Conclusion

Based on your reading in this chapter, you will now be aware of the benefits and processes associated with keeping a professional portfolio. A professional portfolio is an important way to meet the regulatory requirements of a registered nurse. A carefully constructed portfolio assists you to learn and develop and can enable you to showcase your knowledge and skills to current and future employers. Establishing, developing and maintaining a portfolio does not need to be a complex process and can give you a professional advantage. As you transition into the professional role and beyond, it can guide your learning and ensure that you are prepared for new opportunities and promotions. While one portfolio presentation may not serve all purposes, it can be the basis for others that you may want to develop. A portfolio can provide an overview of how far you have come in your professional development as a nurse –a source of great personal satisfaction and pride. Nurses are skilful, creative people and the reality of this can be revealed through a portfolio. Start your personal portfolio today if you have not already done so.

Key summary points

- It is important that all registered nurses maintain a professional portfolio throughout their career.
- A portfolio must demonstrate reflection on self and link to evidence-based practice.
- A portfolio must include items of evidence that support claims of knowledge, skills and experience.
- Portfolios should not include content that breaches the confidentiality of healthcare consumers or colleagues.
- Portfolios should not include evidence that breaches healthcare organisation policies.
- Portfolios can be compiled for different purposes, including for continuing professional development and for showcasing knowledge and expertise.

OXFORD UNIVERSITY PRESS

Critical thinking questions

1. Think about developing your own professional portfolio. What form will it take? What platform and/or digital resources will you use? Why?

2. Recall a significant nursing-related incident that happened to you recently. Write a description of the incident, your feelings, the positives and negatives of the situation, how or why the situation may have happened and what you could have done differently.

3. In relation to your reflection, document what skills you need to manage similar situations differently in the future. What evidence could you include in your portfolio to demonstrate your enhanced knowledge and skills?

4. When next on placement in a healthcare setting, investigate the organisation's policy on health consumer confidentiality and identify how this will impact on artefacts you can use as evidence in your portfolio.

5. Can you recall the different portfolio-related tools you have used throughout your nursing program? Which one did you prefer and why?

References

Acker, J. (2020). Communicating competence for practice in paramedicine. In L. Cusack & M. Smith (Eds.), *Portfolios for nursing, midwifery and other health professions* (4th ed., pp. 106–109). Elsevier.

Andre, K. (2010). E-portfolios for the aspiring professional. *Collegian, 17*(3), 119–124. https://doi.org/10.1016/j.colegn.2009.10.00

Asselin, M. E., Schwartz-Barcott, D., & Osterman, P. A. (2013). Exploring reflection as a process embedded in experienced nurses' practice: A qualitative study. *Journal of Advanced Nursing, 69*(4), 905–914. https://doi.org/10.1111/j.1365-2648.2012.06082.x

Burns, M. K. (2018). Creating a nursing portfolio. *Ohio Nurses Review, 93*(3), 16–17.

Cope, V., & Murray, M. (2018). Use of professional portfolios in nursing. *Nursing Standard, 32*(30), 55–62. https://doi.org/10.7748/ns.2018.e10985

Cusack, L., & Smith, M. (Eds.) (2020). *Portfolios for nursing, midwifery and other health professions* (4th ed.). Elsevier.

Dubé, V., & Ducharme, F. (2015). Nursing reflective practice: An empirical literature review. *Journal of Nursing Education and Practice, 5*(7), 91–99. https://doi.org/10.5430/jnep.v5n7p91

Jasper, M., Rosser, M., & Mooney, G. P. (2013). *Professional development, reflection and decision-making in nursing and healthcare* (2nd ed.). John Wiley & Sons.

Mahara. (2019). *Open source portfolios*. https://mahara.org/

Nursing and Midwifery Board of Australia. (2016a). *Registered nurses' standards for practice*. https://www.nursingmidwiferyboard.gov.au/Codes-Guidelines-Statements/Professional-standards/registered-nurse-standards-for-practice.aspx

Nursing and Midwifery Board of Australia. (2016b). *Continuing professional development*. https://www.nursingmidwiferyboard.gov.au/Registration-Standards/Continuing-professional-development.aspx

Nursing and Midwifery Board of Australia. (2019). *Social media: How to meet your obligations under the national law*. https://www.nursingmidwiferyboard.gov.au/Codes-Guidelines-Statements/Codes-Guidelines/Social-media-guidance.aspx

Nursing Council of New Zealand. (2007). *Competencies for registered nurses*. https://www.nursingcouncil.org.nz/Public/Nursing/Standards_and_guidelines/NCNZ/nursing-section/Standards_and_guidelines_for_nurses.aspx?hkey=9fc06ae7-a853-4d10-b5fe-992cd44ba3de

Nursing Council of New Zealand. (2012). *Guidelines: Social media and electronic communication*. https://www.nursingcouncil.org.nz/Public/Nursing/Standards_and_guidelines/NCNZ/nursing-section/Standards_and_guidelines_for_nurses.aspx

Nursing Council of New Zealand. (2020). *Standards and guidelines for nurses*. https://www.nursingcouncil.org.nz/Public/Nursing/Standards_and_guidelines/NCNZ/nursing-section/Standards_and_guidelines_for_nurses.aspx

Stewart, S. M. (2013). Making practice transparent through e-portfolio. *Women and Birth*, *26*(4), e117–e121. https://doi.org/10.1016/j.wombi.2013.02.005

Stewart, S. M. (2017). *A new, free e-portfolio for nurses and midwives*. http://sarah-stewart.blogspot.com/2017/

Ventola, C. L. (2014). Social media and health care professionals: Benefits, risks and best practices. *Pharmacy and Therapeutics*, *39*(7), 491–499, 520.

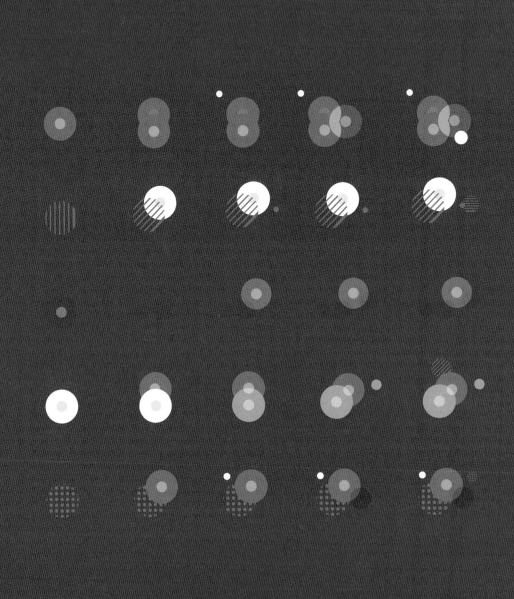

PART II

BECOMING A REGISTERED NURSE

A Development Continuum

I have found this transition best described as a roller coaster. At multiple times you feel excited and relieved to finally have your registration but then a sudden feeling of dread and anxiety that you will now be thrown out of your comfort zone. However, it is with the amount of support from your colleagues and getting stuck in, that being outside that zone isn't so bad after all and actually an amazing experience.

Vanessa, Graduated 2019, New Zealand

Chapter 4

The Experience of Transition

Judy Duchscher and Jayne Hartwig

Learning Outcomes

Following completion of this chapter, you will be able to:

1. Explain the concept of transition.
2. Outline the process and stages of transition for new graduate nurses.
3. Identify strategies to mitigate challenges new graduate nurses can experience with transition.
4. Describe factors that enhance learning and support a positive transition process.

Key terms

Role transition	Transition	Transition shock

Introduction

In this chapter we will explore the experience of transition for new graduate nurses and the challenges it can present. **Role transition**, the process of moving from one role and responsibilities to another, is a significant part of becoming a professional, independent registered nurse. This is a period of change that is known to be simultaneously enriching and challenging. Studies have shown that for new nurses the transition period from student to registered nurse during their first year of practice can be a difficult time that is sometimes overwhelming. With the right preparation, capabilities and support, the transition process is smoother and more rewarding. As a new graduate ready to embark on your career as a nurse, the concept of transition is an important one to understand. We begin this chapter by reviewing the process of transition and how this applies to you as a new nurse. We then draw on this discussion as we explore evidence-based strategies for easing the impact and creating rewarding and exciting transition experiences.

Role transition

The process of moving from one role and responsibilities to another.

Case Study 4.1: Introducing Emma

Emma is a 21-year-old student at a metropolitan university. She secured a position on a graduate program affiliated with her university and has just begun practising as a new registered nurse. She is extremely excited to put the knowledge she has gained into practice; however, she is also nervous about fitting into her new team and is apprehensive about the new responsibilities her role will bring.

Transition

A non-linear evolutionary and transformative journey that features a complex exchange between emotion and intellect, relational dynamics, and context along a continuum.

Transition

Transition is not a new concept or experience for any of us. Defined as something that bridges two environments or states of being (Malouf & West, 2011), transition occurs in the personal and working lives of all human beings and encompasses people's responses during a passage of change. We undergo transition when we need to adapt to a new situation or circumstance and incorporate the change into our life or new way of being (Kralik et al., 2006). Many transitions are inevitable as we grow and develop – think about your development over time and the number of transitions you have made throughout your life. While there are similarities in how and why a transition occurs, all of us respond differently to the experience. The process and outcome rely not on whether we do or don't transition, but rather on how well an individual adapts and manages their responses to assimilate the change. Being able to manage a transition experience depends on our internal and external resources and supports.

As we will discuss in Chapter 5, the transition to become a registered nurse occurs along a continuum, one that began on the day you commenced your nursing program and will continue to the end of your first year of practice as a registered nurse (Harrison et al., 2020). Therefore, whether you have realised this or not, each year, as you have learnt and experienced more about being a nurse, you have been transitioning to the professional role. In this chapter, we focus on the final stage of your transition as you enter your first year of practice as a new graduate nurse. There is a significant amount of research and discussion about this transition period – you will have heard or read about it and will be familiar with what we will discuss. Given that we have all experienced transition periods, some of the information will likely resonate with you. Drawing on this information can help you understand the process more comprehensively and discover ways to move seamlessly through the transition process. The insights you glean in this chapter will be useful to carry forward into your graduate year.

Portfolio Activity 4.1: Stop, reflect and think

Reflect on your personal and professional development over your life. Can you recognise different transitions you might have experienced? Think about the factors that helped your transition. Were they personal internal resources like your resilience, knowledge and how you think about things, or external factors such as your family and friends?

The experience of transition

There is ample evidence describing the transition period for new nurses. As the most significant stage of the transition is the first year of practice, much of the existing evidence focuses on this period of time. Moving from the familiar role of nursing student to the relatively less familiar role of registered nurse can be both transformational and turbulent, influenced by personal, professional and environmental factors (Hawkins et al., 2019). Evidence suggests that when this transition is understood and managed effectively, the process is smoother and more positive – new graduates adapt and assimilate into their role more effortlessly (Graf et al., 2020; Murray et al., 2019).

Transition: A reality shock

The 1974 seminal work by Marlene Kramer (1974) provided our first real insight into the experience of nurses entering the workforce after a period of study. Kramer (1974) coined the term 'reality shock' to explain that on entry to practice for the first time, the professional values and expectations of being a nurse, as held by the nurse educated at school, clashed with the values and expectations of the practice context, causing a 'reality shock' that results in a series of physical, socio-cultural and emotional responses. Reality shock is described as having four phases that new nurses progress through during the process of transition: the honeymoon phase, the shock phase, the recovery phase and finally to resolution (Graf et al., 2020).

The *honeymoon phase* is when new graduates first commence their role, and there a period of excitement and optimism about the new role. The *shock phase* follows – as new nurses experience the reality of their new role, they realise that their ideas and expectations about the role are inconsistent with the reality of clinical practice and their new role. This phase usually occurs in the first three to four months of practice and is known to be the most challenging phase due to the values conflict and subsequent frustration, disillusionment and stress new nurses can experience (Graf et al., 2020). As new nurses become more familiar, accepting and confident with their role and responsibilities, these challenges turn to opportunities for professional development.

This signals the beginning of the *recovery phase* where, when equipped with internal and external supports, new nurses begin to see a new perspective, cope with the day-to-day work and develop creative solutions to their challenges that help them learn and grow as a nurse. This brings them to the final *resolution phase* – the new nurses adapt and assimilate the changes and become confident, competent registered nurses (Wakefield, 2018).

Importantly, each nurse may have a different experience of reality shock – not all nurses will pass through every phase or spend the same amount of time in each phase. Further, it can be cyclic – new nurses may move back and forth between shock and recovery with each new experience they face (Graf et al., 2020).

The process of transitioning

More than 40 years after reality shock was identified, Kramer's ideas continue to inform our understanding and research on new graduates' experiences of transition (Graf et al., 2020). Duchscher's stages of transition theory (2008, 2009) is a particularly pertinent model as it captures the experience of new graduates transitioning from university directly to the workplace. According to Duchscher (2008, 2009), a new graduate's transition is a 12-month non-linear process in which the new graduate evolves through a series of stages of 'doing, being, and knowing' to become a competent registered nurse (p. 443). Duchscher's 20-year program of research built on Kramer's original assertion that the main challenge for new graduate nurses rests in their ability to reconcile the values conflict and construct a new professional identify that blends the ideals of being a nurse established during their education with the realities of the practice context (Duchscher, 2001, 2008, 2009).

The transition shock model (Figure 4.1) and stages of transition theory (Figure 4.3) (Duchscher, 2008, 2009) provide well-defined frameworks to explain the role transition of new graduate nurses and, consequently, the means by which targeted solutions can be utilised to ease some of the more turbulent aspects associated with it (Graf et al., 2020). These frameworks present the experience of transition as a non-linear journey that features a complex, dynamic exchange between emotion and intellect, relational dynamics, and the impact of unfamiliar or complex practice situations introduced during a new graduate's transition continuum. Overall, the experience is 'evolutionary and ultimately transformative' (Duchscher, 2008, p. 444).

In the next section we will explore transition shock and the stages of transition described by Duchscher (2008, 2009) and provide suggestions that can help optimise a more seamless transition to the professional role. As a new graduate, this information can help you understand and hence respond more effectively to some of the more challenging experiences you might encounter during your first year of practice.

Transition: A shock to the system

Transition shock

A new nurse's response to the acute and turbulent relationship between the roles, responsibilities, relationships and knowledge required of a new nurse.

'**Transition shock**' is the term Duchscher (2009) coined to embody the new graduate nurse's initial experience on entry to the workplace, usually within two months after orientation. Similar to Kramer's reality shock, transition shock emerges as the new graduate moves from their familiar student role to the less known role of a registered nurse and begins to reconcile what they expected to encounter with the reality of what they actually encounter in the workplace.

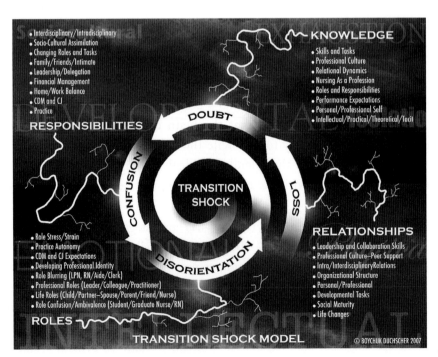

Figure 4.1 The transition shock model (Duchscher, 2007. Reproduced with permission)

Often characterised by feelings of insecurity, doubt, fear and disillusionment (Duchscher, 2009), the intensity and duration of the experience is mediated by the relationship between aspects of the new graduate's role, responsibilities, relationships and knowledge. The depth of disparity between what the new nurse expects or anticipates for the role and the levels of responsibility and accountability expected from the workplace is one factor. How much insight a new nurse is given into these expectations during their education can also mediate the experience – the more prepared the nurse is, the less acute the experience becomes. Other aspects that mediate this experience is how quickly and frequently new nurses are asked to take on increasingly complex and risk-intensive situations, and the support they are given to reconcile challenges during this time (Duchscher, 2009; Graf et al., 2020; Wakefield, 2018).

Further factors related to new graduates have been found to correlate with the duration and intensity of a new graduate's transition shock. These include the following.

1. Being 'accepted' as a competent practitioner and 'fitting in' is important. New nurses want their workplace colleagues to respect and embrace what they have to offer.

2. Securing and keeping a job is a high priority. Over the years of education, new nurses can accumulate financial, physical, emotional and relational stressors.

3. New nurses' experience with socio-cultural aspects of the workplace is limited. The socio-cultural aspects of the workplace environment have an important influence on how well a new nurse integrates and copes with their transition. Navigating their new social structure can intensify feelings of not belonging and professional competence.

4. Confidence levels fluctuate and are often fragile during the initial months of transition – it can take up six months for a new nurse to feel a balanced level of confidence.

5. The theory learnt intellectually about the ways human illness or wellness expresses itself does not always translate easily into practice.

6. New nurses are very focused on ensuring their practice is safe, and practise according to what they were taught. An inability to do so is often perceived as a personal failure and/or as a failure of their education to adequately prepare them for practice. Nurse education programs and

healthcare services attempt to capture and replicate the reality of working as a registered nurse in a dynamic healthcare environment; however, this is difficult while in a student role. Hence the depth and breadth of the experience cannot be realised until new nurses enter the workplace.

In summary, there are two critical points that underscore the experience of transition shock. The first point is that developing professional practice is not as straightforward as the application of theory to textbook-clinical events. Rather, the development of proficient practice results from a number of different factors.

- The subtle integration of theory into diverse practice experiences;

- Maturation of an individual's political, economic, organisational, cultural and socio-developmental insight;

- Know-how that comes with collaboratively consulting with nursing peers and other healthcare professionals throughout the course of a day; and

- Expertise that is established as an individual observes and participates in practice over time.

The second point related to transition shock is that it is not isolated just to your professional experience; it is also a deeply personal experience. While it is commonly accepted that there will be an adjustment when making such a significant change, what is often underestimated is the pervasiveness of this experience. The response to a major change like the initial integration into a professional role affects the whole person: it is an intellectual, physical, social, cultural, developmental, spiritual, emotional and economic change (Duchscher, 2008). This initial transition can impact on your personal energy and time, and your evolving professional identity. Figure 4.1 provides insight into the breadth of the impact some individuals can experience with transition shock. While you may not experience all of these responses, how your transition plays out can alter the way you view yourself as a professional. Therefore, it is good to know about the responses so you understand what is happening and can work with it more effectively.

Portfolio Activity 4.2: Stop, reflect and think

Reflect on your development as you progressed through your nursing degree. Can you relate to any of the concepts discussed here about transition shock? Have you experienced some of the feelings and emotions described?

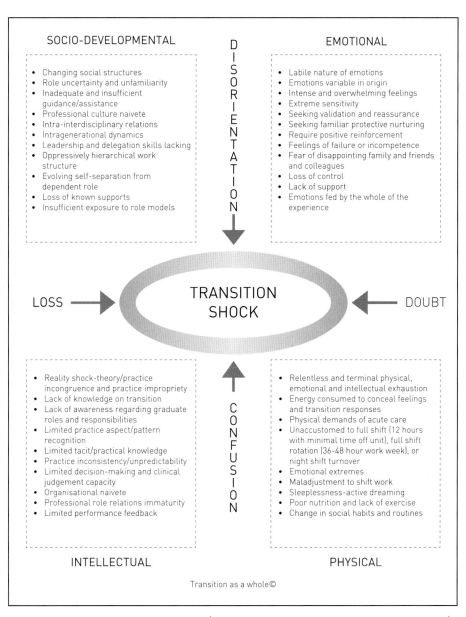

Figure 4.2   Effects of transition shock (Duchscher, 2008. Reproduced with permission)

Case Study 4.2: Preparing for transition

Emma has been working part-time at an aged care facility while studying for her nursing degree, and her mother was a nurse. She feels confident that she will not experience the transition shock that most new graduate nurses experience. Emma feels prepared and has high expectations of herself – she wants to fit in, make a good impression and learn as much as she can as soon as possible.

- Consider how Emma is feeling. Given her background and experience, are these normal expectations for a new registered nurse? Are these realistic expectations for a new registered nurse?

- Why might Emma's work in the aged care facility make her feel more confident and support her transition to practice?

- How do you feel about starting your first role as a registered nurse? Is it the same as or different from Emma's? Why do you think your feelings are similar/different?

Transition: A series of stages

The process of transition and becoming a registered nurse is described as occurring gradually in three stages during a new graduate's first year of practice as a registered nurse. These occur at different timepoints:

- *Stage 1: Doing* – usually occurs over the first three to four months;

- *Stage 2: Being* – falls during the next four to six months of a new graduate nurse's first year; and

- *Stage 3: Knowing* – occurs over the final six to 12 months of practice.

As noted earlier, progress through these stages will vary according to the length and quality of the new graduate nurse's orientation, their employer's transition and integration programs, and the level of support available from experienced colleagues. In this next section we will explore these in more detail and discuss some useful strategies to manage each of the stages.

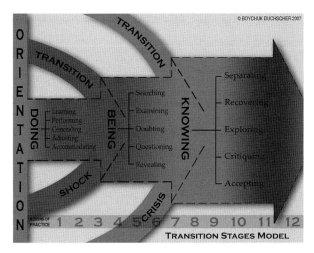

Figure 4.3   Stages of transition model (Duchscher, 2007. Reproduced with permission)

Stage 1: Doing

Stage 1 usually occurs over the first three to four months of practice after orientation or introduction into the workplace, and encompasses transition shock. The doing stage is dominated by changes and physical adjustments as you learn the role of registered nurse first-hand, and what it means. For most new graduate nurses, this is a most exciting yet vulnerable and critical timeframe as it correlates with your first shift on your own, managing a full clinical workload and adjusting to a new workplace, which can affect your confidence. During these initial few months of practice, the focus will be on what you need to 'do'. It is characterised by five different processes (Duchscher, 2009, 2012).

1. *Adjusting* – to new roles, responsibilities (including shift work), relationships (personal and professional) and the expectation that you will apply the knowledge from your formal education, while also learning new knowledge from working as a registered nurse.

2. *Accommodating* – new routines for practice that may have prescribed timelines and policy guidelines that are different from what you knew as a student. While you have options and choices related to the practices you adopt, there will be some practices, policies and procedures specific to an area that you will need to accept as part of the way things are done in that area.

3. *Learning* – new skills, roles, responsibilities and clinical knowledge that relate to the registered nurse role and/or specific area of practice.

4. *Performing* – skills, tasks and procedures that you may have performed competently as a nursing student can take on a different level of complexity when you are practising them as a fully responsible and accountable professional.

5. *Concealing* – normal feelings of insecurity, anxiety and inadequacy. It is normal to experience these emotions and normal to want to conceal them from your experienced colleagues so that you appear competent.

Case Study 4.3: Stage 1

Emma has been working for about two months now and is really tired. The shift work and the busyness of the ward have been exhausting. She did not think it would be this hard, and is finding it difficult to manage her workload. Despite being taught many skills and having knowledge, the reality of practice just seems different.

- Explain what you think is happening to Emma at this point in her transition.

- How could Emma improve her situation? Think about what you did during experiences when you might have felt like this – what did you do to adapt and adjust to new situations?

As indicated, there is a lot happening in this initial stage and consequently it can be very tiring. More than at any other time during the transition process, this is the stage when new nurses are more likely to feel physically, emotionally, intellectually and spiritually exhausted. As a result, you might feel depleted of energy, and experience some of the following.

- Feeling tired despite prolonged sleeping periods.

- Poor quality sleep due to dreaming about work.

- Disengaging with friends and family.

- Forgetting appointments or commitments.

- Losing interest in social activities.

- Gaining or losing weight (too tired to exercise or eat).

- Feeling short tempered, unusually anxious, angry or detached.

- Experiencing a sense of loss or grief.

OXFORD UNIVERSITY PRESS

Box 4.1 presents simple strategies drawn from the experiences of previous new graduates, that you can use to help you through this stage of your transition. Keep in mind that each person experiences these stages differently, so find out what works for you and adjust the strategies as needed.

Box 4.1   Stage 1 strategies

---

1. Seek support

- Ask to have a consistent preceptor during the initial four months of your employment, preferably one who has volunteered and had some preparation for the role.
- Find a coach or mentor who can offer regular support and encouragement. If you are not sure who would be suitable, ask your manager or educator. Sometimes a senior nurse in your workplace, with whom you feel comfortable, can be a good source of support. In Chapter 11 we talk more about clinical coaches and preceptors within a transition program, and in Chapter 12 about seeking a coach or mentor to support your career development.
- Arrange to meet with your support person regularly after a set of shifts at least for the first two months, then monthly for eight months, then as needed. This regular discussion creates productive reflections that can help you express concerns and learn from your experiences.
- After difficult shifts, have a discussion or debrief with a trusted peer, mentor or coach.
- Talk to other new graduates or your university peers who are going through the same thing.

2. Create stability, consistency and structure

- If possible, ask for a more predictable roster. This extra structure and consistency can help you plan and balance your work and personal commitments, and learn the practices of a consistent team member and clinical care related to the patient population.
- If you are required to float (moving from one unit to another), limit this to two or three areas only.
- Advance your skills gradually. Ask your team leader to assign you less complex patients when possible for at least the first two to three months.
- Set yourself some learning goals – simple yet achievable goals (SMART goals) – that can give you a sense of accomplishment and increase your confidence.
- Celebrate your achievements.

3. Balance your professional and personal commitments

- Give family and friends your roster. Plan time to socialise, be alone, and do personal errands.
- Organise your meals the day before a shift.
- Work limited overtime, as it can deplete your energy.
- Create time to relax. Avoid planning activities the day directly after a set of shifts: sleep in, wind down and find a way to work off your stress (sports, meditation, exercise, hobbies).
- Keep a journal of what went well went during a shift. Aim to reflect on the positive feedback from peers or patients and how you can improve.

 ## Portfolio Activity: Making the transition

When navigating the **doing** stage of transition, it is important to have clear learning objectives about what you want to achieve. Consider the following questions and see if you can develop three learning goals for Stage 1 of your transition.

- What do you need and want to achieve? Make a list or concept map these ideas.
- How can you achieve your objectives? List some key strategies you can employ to achieve your goals.

- Who/what can help you to do this? Identify key people that you believe you will need to support you in achieving your goals.
- How will you measure achievement of your goals and celebrate these achievements?

Stage 2: Being

The next four to five months of the transition experience are usually marked by a consistent and rapid advance in your knowledge, thinking, competency and confidence. At this point, many new graduate nurses feel that they know what they are doing and, despite some anxiety, are more confident and independent: challenges still exist, but they find they cope with them better. The focus in this stage is not so much on the physical, emotional and intellectual adjustments experienced in Stage 1 but more on adjusting the culture of the profession and workplace environment – the socio-cultural elements of the workplace. During this stage your energy is focused on the social aspects of working with others (establishing relationships with colleagues, adjusting to individual personalities in the workplace, and reconfiguring a personal life while being a working professional), cultural aspects of life as a nurse (understanding how power and influence are exercised in the workplace and who the formal and informal leaders are), and political aspects that influence healthcare (determining what control you have over your practice and how you can use that to meet the needs of those under your care) (Duchscher, 2009). The need to coexist in multiple spheres of your life (physical, emotional, intellectual, social, cultural and political) accounts for the majority of adjustments associated with this stage. You may well begin to challenge your undergraduate notions of nursing, noticing contradictions and shortcomings in the healthcare system. This can disrupt your impressions of nursing. This critique amounts to an awakening of sorts, with a goal of restoring a sense of equilibrium. It motivates an increased awareness of yourself professionally. The stage is marked by five processes:

1. *Searching* – looking for more insight into the role of the nurse relative to the roles of other healthcare professionals. You may find yourself wanting to understand the influence of the nurse within the larger system or context of practice.
2. *Questioning* – with a greater level of overall comfort and familiarity with your work and role expectations, you have time and energy to ask questions about your transition and new role:

OXFORD UNIVERSITY PRESS

a. Why did I go into nursing?

b. Can I reach the level of expertise I see in my experienced colleagues?

c. Will I ever experience the professional respect that I feel I deserve?

d. Will my life ever be well balanced?

e. Who am I as a nurse?

3. *Doubting* – doubting your competency is natural at this point as you are required to perform new skills, act in unfamiliar roles, take on complex responsibilities and apply specific clinical knowledge. These challenges can stimulate doubt and add to your anxiety. You may begin to wonder why you went into nursing, or question whether you are capable of reaching the level of competence you have set for yourself.

4. *Examining* – looking at the distinctions and differences between what you thought nursing was and what it actually is. Seeing things as they are can be disconcerting to the idealist, but is critical to your evolving professional self.

5. *Revealing* – this is connected to examining the realities you face as a professional nurse. Sometimes we see our circumstances through rose-coloured lenses that both motivate and protect our values and expectations. When reality hits, we can feel betrayed or disillusioned. It becomes important to discover others who have found the balance between the ideal and the real to assist in finding the middle ground – holding the profession to a high standard while recognising and accepting its limitations.

Throughout this stage you will still experience feelings of energy drain, and at times really notice a level of exhaustion. This is normal and a healthy part of the process of finding that equilibrium – the middle ground. The exhaustion forces you to make separations and, in doing so, allows you to take in the multiple and complex dimensions of your new life. To cope with the drain on your energy, you may want some distance from work and seek refuge in your personal life. As a result, you might refuse overtime, call in sick to avoid having to face the workplace, or put distance between yourself and your colleagues by avoiding staff functions or isolating yourself during breaks. This act of pulling away is temporary, but necessary and healthy. Remember that the goal of Stage 2 is to come to terms with the changes in your life and work, and to re-engage in your career. Pulling away can help you reassess and recharge. Once you have found your equilibrium, you will return with more energy, engaging in your work and relating to your colleagues on your terms.

Portfolio Activity 4.3: Stop, reflect and think

Reflect on your professional experience placements. Have there been situations where you have questioned inconsistencies and inadequacies in the healthcare contexts you have worked? Have you ever questioned your professional choices? What did you do, and could you use those strategies to support your transition process?

It is during Stage 2 that, at times, you may want to leave. Keep in mind that this is a temporary feeling, and find strategies to help you work through the process. Being able to find your equilibrium and move forward is worth it. While it is not recommended that you remain in a work environment that is unsafe or unsupportive, staying the course for eight to 12 months of your first year will lead to fulfilling and rewarding outcomes. Box 4.2 provides some strategies to help support you during Stage 2.

Case Study 4.4: Stage 2

Last week Emma worked a series of night shifts. While she completed single night duty shifts as a student, she had never worked night duty full-time doing a consecutive number of night duty shifts. She has noticed that at the beginning of her days off she often feels exhausted, and that when she starts to feel better it is already time to return to work. She is also frustrated that her lack of energy means she hasn't been able to catch up with friends for a few weeks and she doesn't feel like going to the gym. She is beginning to wonder if she will ever become accustomed to shift work, if it will ever feel easier.

- What advice would you give Emma at this stage of her transition to help her feel more energised and motivated?

- As night duty will be part of your role as a registered nurse, how can you prepare for this? How will you manage the physical changes that accompany working night shift, and ensure you get plenty of quality sleep?

OXFORD UNIVERSITY PRESS

Box 4.2   Stage 2 strategies

---

1. **Reduce work-related stress**
   - Limit your overtime. While it is enticing to earn more money or experience, the additional work exposes you to the very things that you need less of – work and stress.
   - Leadership roles. You might want or be asked to take on a leadership role such as an in charge, or team leader. If you take it, ensure that you have adequate support and formal orientation. Being in a formal leadership position is a big responsibility and will require support.
   - Connect with a mentor. If you weren't able to do this in Stage 1, now is a great time to do it. In this stage, lead some of the conversation to ensure you address your concerns. For example:
     a. Have you ever felt frustrated by what you see going on in the workplace?
     b. How did you cope with your frustrations?
     c. How do you deal with negative people at work?
     d. What do you love most about nursing?
     e. How do you balance work with the rest of your life?
   - Find a buddy. Similar to Stage 1, find someone that you can debrief with after shifts, particularly the difficult ones. This could be a trusted peer, mentor or coach. Keep the conversation positive and constructive. Focus on what happened, why it happened, what you might do differently, and how you can learn from the situation.
   - If at any time you do feel overwhelmed, seek the support of someone you trust. Employee assistance programs are available in most organisations and provide confidential support.

2. **Establish external focuses**
   - Find something enjoyable outside of work that brings out a different side of you. We are multifaceted human beings and we do best when exposed to a variety of stimuli. Challenge yourself in ways other than work to help find your balance.
   - Spend time with family and friends. At this point, it is refreshing to spend time with people who talk about something other than nursing. Putting yourself in situations that do not allow you to think about work, give your mind a reprieve from the constant debriefing that is characteristic of a new graduate's thinking processes.

Stage 3: Knowing

Having moved through Stages 1 and 2, your mid-year transition, you have arrived at the final stage of your initial transition journey. This final stage occurs six to 12 months into your transition year. It is a period of stabilisation and deeper reflection, where the new graduate nurse is integrating and evolving their new identity as a professional registered nurse. One of the main objectives is to establish the new identity that moves beyond the status of nursing student and graduate nurse. By the full 12 months, new graduate nurses are generally well rounded and able to manage and cope with their responsibilities. This is a terrific stage – your confidence will stabilise and you will have a solid understanding and level of competence in your role as a registered nurse. Similar to Stages 1 and 2, five processes characterise Stage 3:

1. *Exploring* – at this point, you may find a renewed interest in where you are going in your career and how the capabilities you have developed over the past 12 months have advanced your level of competence. You might find yourself taking a deeper dive into understanding (or questioning) the inconsistencies you have found within the healthcare system and the nursing profession.

While this can lead to some disenchantment or disillusionment, your ability to reconcile it is more effective. Monitor this carefully, with a solution focus rather than a problem focus.

2. *Separating* – who you are as a professional from your colleagues, characterises this development period. The boundaries that frame your standards and ethics will be refined, and you make decisions (whether you are aware of them or not) about what you are willing to accept as ways of being, doing and knowing in nursing. You may want to consider more advanced practice experiences and request more complex clinical scenarios, take a leadership position or explore other areas of practice.

3. *Critiquing* – your primary objective and comparing the values, aspirations and expectations you initially had for your work and workplace with what you have come to know. This may include deconstructing some of your colleagues' clinical practices, with the intent to understand why they do things the way they do.

4. *Recovering* – some of the energy, motivation and passion you had when you graduated. In this final stage you will work to stabilise and balance your work and personal lives.

5. *Accepting* – professional practice standards exist on a continuum. Perfect practice may not exist but safe high-quality practice does. Learning to accept the realities of practice while striving to improve both the standard and the environment within which that practice is enacted, becomes a focus in Stage 3 of transition.

During this final stage, you will continue the recovery you started during Stage 2; however, this time you will be engaging in more future-oriented priorities. A relative detachment from work, and sometimes from life around you, continues through the early months of Stage 3. You might spend more time critiquing your professional landscape and taking stock of the more unsettling aspects of your socio-professional, cultural and political work environment. Stress during this stage can vary considerably, but the contributing factors are now focused on the system at large (the workplace, institution or healthcare in general). You may take more notice of your position of power and authority relative to others (how nurses relate to physicians or other healthcare providers in the workplace). If you have experienced or witnessed professional devaluing

OXFORD UNIVERSITY PRESS

during your initial months, this can motivate discontent and another, albeit less dramatic, reduction in your energy and enthusiasm for work. However, a benefit of this is that it can motivate a search for professional fulfilment in a different role beyond clinical practice at the point of care. At this point of your transition, there is often a shift in your primary support relationships, from friends and family members to co-workers and experienced nursing colleagues, extending your professional network. Your new network can help you in circumstances such as these. Box 4.3 presents some strategies to help you through Stage 3 of your transition. Again, find what works for you.

Box 4.3 Stage 3 strategies

---

1. **Establish professional development opportunities**
   - Connect with an experienced manager or educator and revisit your career pathway to ensure you are moving in your desired professional direction. In Chapter 12 we discuss the different career pathways for nurses, and strategies to help determine the direction you might want to take. These are also helpful at this stage of your transitional year.
   - Engage in continuing educational opportunities that expand your competency portfolio and, if you feel ready, find opportunities to begin preparation for a more senior or advanced role such as an educator, manager, specialist or advanced practice nurse.
   - If you want to take on a leadership or management role such as team leader, shift in charge or project manager, this is a good time to explore your options. Most institutions have programs that can help you develop the role. Try not to get pulled into taking on a role just because they need someone. A formal leadership position is a professional career decision, so make your decisions about this carefully.
   - Consider volunteering to work on a professional committee in your place of work, community, profession or state. Ask your manager or mentor how you might find an organisation that could be suitable.

2. **Manage your concerns effectively**
   - Continue sessions with your mentor to work through practice concerns or issues that may have surfaced for you. Consider some of the following questions.
     a. What made them choose their career path? How did it unfold?
     b. What do they think are your greatest strengths?
     c. Where do they think your strengths would best be utilised?
     d. How do they deal with their frustrations and disappointments as a professional?
     e. Have they ever been burnt out? How did they cope with it?
   - Continue to find ways to share your experiences and concerns. Meet regularly with a good friend, university colleague or trusted peer, or write in your journal.

3. **Maintain a balance between your personal and professional commitments**
   - Take frequent outings and book leave regularly to shift your focus from work, have a break and recharge.
   - Pick up a hobby that you want to do or return to one that you enjoyed.
   - Engage with family and friends to keep perspective.

Achieving healthy transition

As noted earlier, by 12 months most new graduate nurses reach a stable level of comfort and confidence with their role, responsibilities and professional relationships. The stability is influenced by the level of consistency, familiarity and predictability associated with a new graduate's development. Overall, the healthiest transition experiences are facilitated when you:

- have stable and supportive personal and professional relationships;

- receive consistent workplace support and constructive feedback;

- are provided with positive reinforcement and reassurance about your progress, which is evidenced by a strengthening of your knowledge and care outcomes;

- are familiar with, and successful in enacting, evolving expectations around care delivery and skill performance;

- are provided opportunities to consult and collaborate with experienced nurses about increasingly complex clinical decisions and judgments;

- are repeatedly successful in responding accurately to practice scenarios; and

- are supported in your workplace to deliver quality care and influence policy related to care and practice standards.

It should be acknowledged that conflicts do occur as you work through the process of reconciling your expectations of the role with what you find in the real world. We strongly encourage you to find a mentor, and talk with your clinical coach, nursing unit manager, educator or experienced colleagues about what you are thinking and feeling. They can help you steer yourself away from thinking about all the practice or work incompatibilities. Talking with others who have been down this path will allow you to recognise if an incompatibility exists, determine what steps can and need to be taken and then, if possible, resolve it. Resolution may mean that the issue that concerns you cannot be altered to your satisfaction; it may require that you change your perception.

In the rare situation where your transition experience has not been favourable, you may feel a sense of discouragement or disappointment from which you struggle to recover. If this is the case, seek help from your organisation's Employee Assistance Program or the counselling service within your workplace – a service where you can openly discuss your feelings and experiences. Remember that there are many experienced nurses who have successfully found their way back from career disappointments, so access them as often as you need to. They will have strategies that can assist you to process and make sense of your experience.

In summary, it is important to emphasise that the transition process is not linear and that each individual will have a unique transition experience. Not all new nurses go through every stage, nor do so in the same timeframe. While organisations put support structures and strategies in place, most often through transition programs, no one size fits all. As your experience will be different from those of your peers, it is important to find strategies that work effectively for you. This highlights the need for you to be self-aware and self-directed in seeking support during your transition period. In Chapter 5 we discuss the capabilities that will help you prepare effectively for your first year of practice as a registered nurse. Focusing on developing these capabilities will support you during your transition and allow you to cultivate fulfilling and rewarding learning experiences.

Case Study 4.5: Stage 3

Emma has been working as a registered nurse for nearly 11 months. She clearly recognises how the transition period affected her whole self and found she experienced varying degrees of emotions, thoughts and physical changes as she adjusted to her new role. She feels she has learnt more than she thought she ever would, and feels satisfied, confident and capable in her professional role. Today, the nursing unit manager asked if she might consider doing more in charge shifts as she thinks Emma would be a good manager. She even offered to send Emma to the organisation's leadership course. Emma, however, is not sure – she was thinking she might prefer to wait a while, and take a rest from studying. She has more interest in education than in management.

- Should Emma take this role? It is a great opportunity. Explain your answer.

- What could Emma do in this situation to ensure she makes an informed choice that suits her interests and makes the most of the opportunity?

Portfolio Activity: Making the transition

Consider your professional development over the last year. Reflect on your clinical placements and what you learnt while on placement.

- Have you experienced workplaces with the strategies and conditions described in the chapter that help new graduate nurses achieve a healthy transition?
- Have you identified a mentor who can continue to support you in the next stage of your career?
- What would you like to learn as you move into the next stage of your early career?
- Could you support newly graduated nurses by sharing your own transition experiences and tips?

Conclusion

The experience of transitioning to a new role involves a range of emotions, professional and personal changes, socio-developmental, intellectual and physical characteristics. While starting a new professional role is exciting, individuals will also experience a degree of shock as they become accustomed to their new role and environment, gain new knowledge and develop new relationships. Having an understanding of each stage of transition will allow you to navigate your personal emotions and professional experiences. A successful transition process requires support from colleagues, and a range of educational and professional strategies. In Chapters 11 and 12 we describe in detail the strategies that accompany new graduate transition programs. Surrounding yourself with support and allowing yourself to excel personally and professionally will lead to enjoyable and productive growth and development.

OXFORD UNIVERSITY PRESS

Key summary points

- Transitioning to a new professional role includes elements of personal, professional, socio-developmental, intellectual and physical characteristics.

- Every new graduate nurse will experience the transition process differently in terms of the intensity and duration of each stage.

- Each stage of the transition process is mediated by a new graduate's personal and professional capability and experiences.

- Understanding the stages of transition is essential for new graduate nurses to adequately prepare for the range of physical, emotional and cognitive reactions they will experience.

- Most new graduate nurses will experience a period of shock within the first two to four months of practice as they realise that what they have thought of as the role of the professional nurse is different from what they experience in practice.

- Support is essential during the transition experience. It includes help and encouragement from colleagues, peers and family, and strategies that meet the new graduate's individual needs.

Critical thinking questions

1. What can you do to prepare and support yourself in the DOING stage?

2. When navigating the BEING stage of transition, it is important to recognise and take time to celebrate your achievements. Why is this important?

3. Describe the cognitive, emotional and physical benefits of reflecting on and celebrating achievements throughout your transition.

4. Now that you are aware of some of the emotional and physical changes you might experience throughout your transition, what can you do to minimise the transition shock, in particular the sense of fatigue?

5. What self-care practices would you advise your future self to implement to support yourself?

6. Who are the people in your life who can support your transition to practice?

JUDY DUCHSCHER AND JAYNE HARTWIG

119

7. Murray is feeling more confident despite sometimes questioning his choice about being a nurse. He has found a number of inconsistences in the practices of nurses on the ward where he is working, and feels he needs to discuss these. What stage of transition do you think Murray is likely experiencing, and why?

8. If a new graduate nurse reached the end of their transition year and was still experiencing discontentment and a lack of confidence, what do you think happened during their transitional year and what can be done about it?

References

Boamah, S. A., & Laschinger, H. K. S. (2016). The influence of areas of work-life fit and work-life interference on burnout and turnover intentions among new graduate nurses. *Journal of Nursing Management, 24*(2), e164–e174. https://doi.org/10.1111/jonm.12318

Duchscher, J. B., & Windey, M. (2018). Stages of transition and transition shock. *Journal for Nurses in Professional Development, 34*(4), 228–232. https://doi.org/10.1097/NND.0000000000000461

Duchscher, J. E. B. (2001). Out in the real world: Newly graduated acute-care nurses speak out. *Journal of Nursing Administration, 31*(9), 426–439. https://doi.org/10.1097/00005110-200109000-00009

Duchscher, J. E. B. (2008). A process of becoming: The stages of new nursing graduate professional role transition. *Journal of Continuing Nursing Education, 39*(10), 441–450. https://doi.org/10.3928/00220124-20081001-03

Duchscher, J. E. B. (2009). Transition shock: The initial stage of role adaptation for newly graduated registered nurses. *Journal of Advanced Nursing, 65*(5), 1103–1113. https://doi.org/10.1111/j.1365-2648.2008.04898.x

Duchscher, J. E. B. (2012). *From surviving to thriving: Navigating the first year of professional nursing practice* (2nd ed.). Nursing the Future.

El Haddad, M., Moxham, L., & Broadbent, M. (2017). Graduate nurse practice readiness: A conceptual understanding of an age-old debate. *Collegian, 24*(4), 391–396. https://doi.org/10.1016/j.colegn.2016.08.004

Graf, A. C., Jacob, E., Twigg, D., & Nattabi, B. (2020). Contemporary nursing graduates' transition to practice: A critical review of transition models. *Journal of Clinical Nursing, 29*(15–16), 3097–3107. https://doi.org/10.1111/jocn.15234

Gross, R. (2002). *Socrates' way: Seven master keys to using your mind to the utmost.* Penguin Putnam.

Harrison, H., Birks, M., Franklin, R., & Mills, J. (2020). Fostering graduate nurse practice readiness in context. *Collegian, 27*(1), 115–124. https://doi.org/10.1016/j.colegn.2019.07.006

Hawkins, N., Jeong, S., & Smith, T. (2019). Coming ready or not! An integrative review examining new graduate nurses' transition in acute care. *International Journal of Nursing Practice, 25*(3), e12714. https://doi.org/10.1111/ijn.12714

Kralik, D., Visentin, K., & Van Loon, A. (2006). Transition: A literature review. *Journal of Advanced Nursing, 55*(3), 320–329. https://doi.org/10.1111/j.1365-2648.2006.03899.x

Kramer, M. (1974). *Reality shock: Why nurses leave nursing.* C. V. Mosby.

Laschinger, H. K. S. (2016). New nurses' perceptions of professional practice behaviors, quality of care, job satisfaction and career retention. *Journal of Nursing Management, 25*(4), 656–665. https://doi.org/10.1111/jonm.12370

Malouf, N., & West, S. (2011). Fitting in: A pervasive new graduate nurse need. *Nurse Education Today, 31*(5), 488–493. https://doi.org/10.1016/j.nedt.2010.10.002

Missen, K., McKenna, L., Beauchamp, A., & Larkins, J. A. (2016). Qualified nurses rate new nursing graduates as lacking skills in key clinical areas. *Journal of Clinical Nursing, 25*(15–16), 2134–2143. https://doi.org/10.1111/jocn.13316

Murray, M., Sundin, D., & Cope, V. (2019). Benner's model and Duchscher's theory: Providing the framework for understanding new graduate nurses' transition to practice. *Nurse Education in Practice, 34*, 199–203. https://doi.org/10.1016/j.nepr.2018.12.003

Regan, S., Wong, C., Laschinger, H. K., Cummings, G., Leiter, M., MacPhee, M., Rhéaume, A., Ritchie, J. A., Wolff, A. C., Jeffs, L., Young-Ritchie, C., Grinspun, D., Gurnham, M., Foster, B., Huckstep, S., Ruffolo, M., Shamian, J., Burkoski, V., Wood, K., & Read, E. (2017). Starting out: Qualitative perspectives of new graduate nurses and nurse leaders on transition to practice. *Journal of Nursing Management, 25*(4), 246–255. https://doi.org/10.1111/jonm.12456

Wakefield, E. (2018). Is your graduate nurse suffering from transition shock? *Journal of Perioperative Nursing, 31*(1), 47–50. https://doi.org/10.26550/311/47-50

Chapter 5

Readiness for Practice – A Transition Continuum

Vicki Cope and Melanie Murray

Learning Outcomes

Following completion of this chapter, you will be able to:

1. Define the concept of practice readiness.
2. Explain the importance of practice readiness in nursing and healthcare.
3. Describe the essential capabilities of practice readiness.
4. Explain how practice readiness develops on a continuum.
5. Identify levels of practice readiness.

Key terms

Clinical readiness	Level of practice readiness	Reflective practice
Critical thinking	Personal readiness	Transition continuum
Evidence-based practice	Practice readiness	
Industry readiness	Professional readiness	

Introduction

Being ready to practise as a registered nurse is the end goal of completing an undergraduate nursing program. But what does it mean to be practice ready? This chapter will define practice readiness and introduce the essential capabilities and processes associated with practice readiness. New graduate registered nurses are expected to be educated and prepared with the capability to practise according to the standards outlined by the profession. Healthcare organisations need competent registered nurses who are able to adapt, assimilate and practise efficiently on entry to practice. Both healthcare organisations and educational institutions know, however, that nursing graduates need further development and support when they first commence practice (Boamah et al., 2016; Missen et al., 2016; Murray et al., 2020; Regan et al., 2017). As discussed in Chapter 4, the transition from the cocoon of the university environment to the reality of registered nursing in the 21st century involves a degree of transition shock – new nurses enter an often-chaotic working environment, which for many may be overwhelming and challenging. Determining what you need to be practice ready is the focus of this chapter.

Case Study 5.1: Introducing Harry

Harry is a 26-year-old nursing student in his final semester of study. Prior to enrolling in his nursing degree, Harry studied three years of medicine but left that program for personal reasons. He is popular with his peers and is always happy to help them understand complex concepts and procedures.

Practice readiness

The necessary capabilities to work as a novice–beginner registered nurse in a healthcare environment and provide a basic level of safe, competent and efficient healthcare in a complex and dynamic environment.

Practice readiness defined

Being practice ready is much more than just being competent in a set of clinical knowledge and skills (Graf et al., 2020; Harrison et al., 2020a; Murray et al., 2019b; Walker et al., 2015). **Practice readiness**, sometimes referred to as work readiness or fitness for practice, is a multidimensional concept, consisting of four domains of readiness capabilities that are interrelated and evolve over time – personal readiness, professional readiness, clinical readiness and industry readiness (Figure 5.1). These domains are interdependent and articulate together in practice to exemplify what it means to be practice ready (Harrison et al., 2020a).

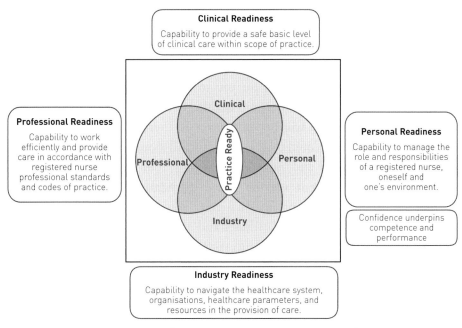

Figure 5.1   Practice readiness (adapted from Harrison et al., 2020a)

Being practice ready means that, upon graduation from your nursing degree, you have a basic level of capability in all four domains and are able to perform competently as a beginning practitioner. Therefore, you have the capability to maintain a safe standard of care; manage and be accountable for your nursing responsibilities within your work role and context; be organised with time and task management; have empathy and place patients at the centre of care; possess the ability to respond to many and varied episodes of client care and clinical situations; and acknowledge the diversity of patients and their individualistic needs (Harrison et al., 2020a). In the following section we will describe each of the four domains of readiness and the capabilities (knowledge, abilities and attributes) associated with each. In Chapters 6, 7, 8 and 9, we will delve deeper into these domains and capabilities to ensure you have the necessary understanding of what it means to be practice ready and how this can be demonstrated in your nursing practice.

Domains of readiness

Personal readiness

The capability to manage the roles and responsibilities of a registered nurse, oneself and one's environment.

Personal readiness incorporates many aspects of practice preparedness. Of all the domains, personal readiness has the most significant influence on practice readiness. It emphasises the need for you to be able to adapt to change and manage a workload within a dynamic healthcare setting. For many graduates, your registered nurse role will be your first job. There is a lot of mental and emotional preparation required to cope with full-time shift work as well as working with acutely ill and vulnerable patients. Your compassion, tolerance, resilience and commitment will be tested, particularly in the early stages of your transition to your professional role. You will need to display self-management in respect of your attitudes and abilities. Establishing respectful, effective professional relationships with your new colleagues, maintaining your personal relationships outside of work, and continuing to learn and build on the foundational skills you established as a student will be key to your success. As indicated in Figure 5.1, practice readiness is underpinned by confidence. It is important that you maintain a balanced level of confidence that ensures that you are not so over-confident that you will not seek help when needed, nor so lacking in confidence that you will not act or intervene when necessary. Finding that balance of confidence can at times be difficult; however, being positive, keen, open and approachable will support you toward developing your confidence as a registered nurse. Capabilities associated with personal readiness are examined in detail in Chapter 6.

Portfolio Activity 5.1: Stop, reflect and think

How much of the personal domain of practice readiness relies on an individual's personality and character? Which of the skills can be taught and which are simply inherent characteristics?

Professional readiness links directly to the requirements for practice according to the standards that govern the profession and the healthcare context in which you will work. As a nursing student you are aiming for registration and therefore you are required to achieve and adhere to the professional standards that regulate and govern nursing practice. This involves understanding and functioning within your scope of practice, using **critical thinking** and **reflective practice** to inform your practice, and engaging in continuing professional development to ensure that your approach to practice remains relevant. As a professional nurse you are expected to act with integrity, demonstrate accountability, be honest and trustworthy and display professionalism in all contexts in which you engage. Given the extremely complex environments in which you will work, you will need to effectively manage the resources available to you to ensure high-quality, safe and efficient practice. These capabilities are those associated with professional readiness and we examine them further in Chapter 7.

Clinical readiness relates to your ability to provide a safe level of clinical care according to your scope of practice. As a new graduate nurse, you may feel that your knowledge and skill set are limited and that getting all the 'tasks' done in your shift is your focus. Looking beyond 'doing obs' and the 'med round' can be difficult (Murray et al., 2019c). Getting 'tasks' done is *not* the focus of your practice, nor can clinical readiness be quantitatively defined. Providing safe, quality patient care must be your priority. With prevention of harm uppermost in your mind, recognising a change in a patient's condition, and the knowledge that you as a nurse need to keep the patient safe, will underpin your approach to care (Murray et al., 2019b). Your undergraduate education is designed to equip you with basic, broad, general knowledge and skills that allow you to provide safe and effective patient care. This knowledge and these skills have prepared you with evidence-based foundations that are fundamental to your clinical knowledge. **Evidence-based practice** will continue to be a significant contributor to your ability to provide safe and effective nursing care. However, a comprehensive knowledge base and the ability to perform skills do not in themselves ensure clinical readiness. Rather, you need to be able to pull it all together by translating your knowledge and skills into practice. Chapter 8 presents a discussion on how this can be achieved.

Professional readiness

The capability to work efficiently and provide care in accordance with registered nurse standards and codes of practice.

Critical thinking

The structured approach to analysis and interpretation of information as a basis for understanding and responding to a range of simple to complex situations.

Reflective practice

The formal or informal process of reviewing and evaluating events for the purpose of improving future outcomes.

Clinical readiness

The capability to provide a safe, basic level of clinical care within one's scope of practice.

Evidence-based practice

The use of available, reliable and current evidence to support the delivery of nursing care.

Case Study 5.2: Personal readiness

Harry believes that the knowledge and skills he acquired as a medical student give him an edge over his fellow nursing students. He is a high achieving student in the theoretical elements of his studies, in particular the professional studies subject and science subjects. Harry is strong in clinical skills performance but has been told by clinical supervisors over the course of his studies that he needs to work on improving the quality of his personal interactions. Harry is very confident and doesn't feel the need to take this advice.

- What are the potential pitfalls for Harry if he fails to develop his personal readiness skills?

- Given the extent to which domains of readiness overlap, what can Harry draw from his strengths in respect of professional and clinical readiness to improve his personal readiness?

Industry readiness

The capability to navigate the healthcare system, organisations, healthcare parameters and resources in the provision of care.

Industry readiness describes the capabilities that will support you to work efficiently and effectively in the healthcare system. As you are aware, the healthcare system is multifaceted and constantly evolving. Knowing how to navigate this dynamic context will help you practise safely and efficiently. During clinical placements as a nursing student, you would have encountered different aspects of the healthcare system and different organisations providing care to a variety of patients, clients and residents. This knowledge of different contexts of nursing practice provides basic industry readiness for employment as a nurse, able to apply your knowledge and abilities as a novice practitioner or advanced beginner. Given the complex nature of the healthcare system, knowing how and where to access relevant resources will save you time and make you more effective at providing a safe standard of care. Nursing practice within different organisational environments requires new employees to abide by prevailing regulations. Organisational policy gives guidance on what is expected of you in your new nursing environment. As with clinical readiness, however, simply possessing broad basic knowledge and skills does not ensure industry readiness. There is an expectation that the personal, professional and clinical capabilities you possess will translate into appropriate workplace behaviour as you adapt to the realities of practice. Chapter 9 explores the industry readiness capabilities that will enable you to identify, develop and maintain your readiness for practice in this domain.

 Portfolio Activity: Making the transition

In the coming chapters you will have an opportunity to reflect on your level of practice readiness in these four domains. To this point in your studies, have you focused on one domain at the expense of others? How might this affect your transition to practice? In Part III of this book (Chapters 6–9), you will have the opportunity to explore strategies for addressing any of your limitations in respect of the domains of readiness.

The importance of practice readiness

As you know from your professional experience placements, healthcare systems are complex and unpredictable. Multifaceted and characterised by constant change, healthcare is an exciting context in which to work, but it is also one that can be hectic and demanding. Healthcare organisations need graduate nurses to be practice ready so that they can manage the complexity and dynamism inherent in healthcare organisations. In these contexts, a safe level of quality care is imperative. New graduate nurses who are practice ready are more capable of providing a safe level of care. As we discussed in Chapter 4, the transition experience of new graduate nurses during their first year of practice presents a period of steep learning and adjustment that can produce a range of physical, intellectual, emotional, developmental and socio-cultural responses (Duchscher & Windey, 2018). During this time, challenges associated with feeling overwhelmed and stressed can interfere with your professional development. The ability to practise to the required level can be hampered by your limited experience in the role of a registered nurse and your fluctuating levels of confidence. Being practice ready can help mitigate these types of experiences so that you feel more confident and capable to apply your knowledge and skills in practice and to access experiences, individuals and other resources that progress your development.

The transition continuum

Transition continuum

Practice readiness develops over a period of time, commencing on the first day of nursing studies and continuing through to the end of the first year of practice.

A nursing student does not suddenly transform into a practice ready registered nurse overnight. As Harrison et al. (2020b) discuss, there is a **transition** process that occurs as a **continuum**, beginning when a student commences their nursing studies and continues through to the end of their first year of practice as a registered nurse. Figure 5.2 illustrates this continuum, assuming a three-year pre-registration program followed by a graduate year.

The concept of a continuum of practice readiness reflects Benner's (1984) adaptation of the Dreyfus and Dreyfus model of skill acquisition (1980). Benner's novice to expert model (1984) (Figure 5.3) indicates that skill acquisition occurs over time, through exposure to certain experiences. Your undergraduate years place you in the 'novice' category. As you grow as a professional, you continue to learn

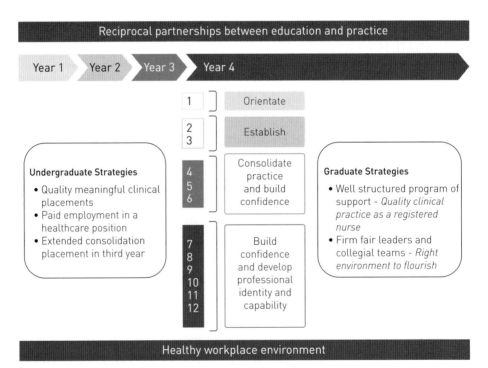

Figure 5.2 Developing practice readiness – a transition continuum (Harrison et al., 2020b, p. 119)

and hone your skills and will eventually become 'expert' in your chosen area of practice. Thus, learning occurs on a continuum, as does your transition to becoming practice ready. During your undergraduate degree you are supported to acquire the knowledge, skills and attributes necessary to become a registered nurse. Nursing programs scaffold your development to gradually build your capability. Each stage of a nursing program builds on the preceding stages, so you will assimilate new capabilities each year. This, augmented with clinical experiences, is designed to help you consolidate and acquire relevant industry and nursing knowledge to further extend your development as a nurse. Knowledge is entrenched in expertise, and expertise develops with practice and exposure to clinical situations (Benner, 1984; Benner & Wrubel, 1982). Thus, everything you learn throughout each year of your nursing program works together to prepare you with the capabilities to practise as a registered nurse at a novice and advanced beginner level.

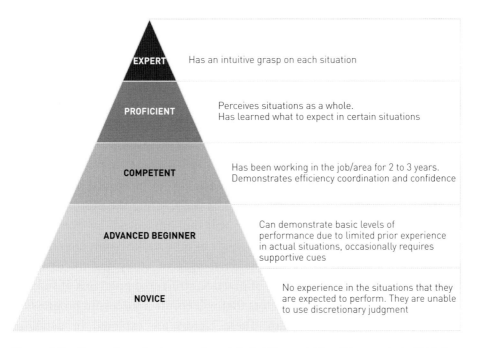

Figure 5.3   Benner's novice to expert model of skill acquisition (Murray et al., 2019a)

During your first year of practice, you can expect some common milestones as you consolidate your practice readiness. As discussed in Chapter 4, the first month is a period of orientation when you become familiar with your new environment. Up until the third month, like all graduates you will be establishing yourself as a healthcare professional and adapting to the workplace environment. You will be introduced to the unpredictable complexities of clinical practice as a registered nurse; complexities that were not encountered during your pre-registration education. Your confidence and performance may be challenged during this time, as you are concurrently learning about and coping with responsibilities and workplace demands. With focused support, however, you can use this time to establish the foundations of your ongoing clinical practice and learning. With this foundation in place, you will develop the ability to work more independently, build capability and function more effectively as a registered nurse in different contexts of practice.

Between four and six months into your first year of practice, your confidence will be growing and you will feel more comfortable in your new role. You will begin to practise more independently and manage your responsibilities comfortably. From this point until the end of your first year of practice, you will be functioning at the level expected of a competent registered nurse. While there will still be challenges, you will be able to draw on your personal, professional, clinical and industry readiness capabilities to manage them appropriately.

How the transition continuum progresses for an individual will depend on numerous factors, as indicated in Figure 5.2. During the pre-registration nursing program, practice readiness will be influenced by the quality of clinical placements, the opportunity to undertake paid employment and an extended placement in the final year of study (as discussed in Chapter 10). During the first year of practice, structured programs of support and leadership are among the factors that will ensure a successful progression along the transition continuum. These factors are explored in detail in Chapter 11.

OXFORD UNIVERSITY PRESS

Case Study 5.3: Transition continuum

As Harry approaches the end of his nursing program, he has received offers of entry to two graduate programs in his local area. The health services in which these programs are delivered are both large complex organisations that will offer Harry a breadth of experiences. One of the programs offers four three-month rotations between different departments. The other offers two six-month rotations.

- Which graduate program would offer greater opportunity to develop Harry's practice readiness? Why?

- Harry is very confident and feels that he would succeed in either program. What advice would you give him?

- Which graduate program would you select if you were Harry?

Levels of practice readiness

Thus far in this chapter we have discussed the concept of practice readiness, described the essential capabilities of practice readiness and explained that practice readiness develops along a continuum, influenced by various factors. The differing experiences and contexts of practice encountered by individuals along the transition continuum will result in them having variations in their **levels of practice readiness** as they enter their first year of practice (Harrison et al., 2020a). You will have experienced performing at a different level from that of your fellow students throughout your nursing studies. Safeguards are in place in educational institutions to ensure that students demonstrate a minimum level of performance prior to undertaking any clinical placement. Ensuring that students are safe for placement does not mean that all students perform at the same standard, however, it simply means that they meet a *minimum* standard.

This variation in levels of performance is not confined to nursing students. The requirement that nurses meet a minimum standard for registration does not determine equality in practice readiness of graduates. It is expected, however, that by the end of the first year of practice, registered nurses are able

Level of practice readiness

The extent to which a graduate nurse is prepared and ready for the professional role in personal, professional, clinical and industry domains.

to demonstrate practice readiness in all domains. Again, Benner's (1984) novice to expert framework is a useful model for understanding level of performance in newly qualified nurses. The stages of this framework relevant to the graduate nurse are presented in Table 5.1. New graduate nurses are at the beginning of their learning as a registered nurse and will grow progressively more competent throughout their first year of practice. They are therefore generally considered to be at the novice or advanced beginner level of practice, with fluctuations between the two stages (Harrison et al., 2020a).

Table 5.1 Levels of performance (adapted from Benner, 1984)

Novice	Advanced beginner	Competent
No experience in the situations in which they are expected to perform. Rule-governed and dependent on a level of direction and supervision where clinical development gradually progresses as confidence improves. Clinical practice may take longer and using clinical judgment may be difficult.	After gaining experience and being involved in adequate real-world situations, the individual grows in knowledge and the ability to independently apply it to practice. Clinical practice may still take longer. While there is still a focus on rules and guidelines, the nurse has more flexibility in thinking and uses discretionary judgment. Support and guidance from a senior colleague is still needed to set priorities and make some decisions. Constructive feedback is essential to improve performance.	After 12 months of clinical practice, the nurse performs independently and confidently, knows what to expect, thinks more critically, decides more accurately and manages their responsibilities more efficiently. The nurse has had time and experience in the setting and the role, working with other nurses to live and learn to be a nurse. The nurse has assimilated the expectations of the profession and the workplace.

As a novice commencing your first year of practice, you will be expected to possess a basic level of competence, requiring some direction and supervision. At a minimum, you need to demonstrate the multidimensional capabilities for practice readiness described in this text. We encourage you to aim to improve your proficiency to perform at an advance beginner level (Benner, 1984) as soon as possible. As we will discuss in Chapter 10 and later in Chapter 12, you should seek opportunities that will propel your development during both your nursing program and your first year of practice. As you progress through your first year of practice, you will find that you have moved to the competent stage (Benner, 1984, pp. 25–27).

In reality, nurses will display variations in level of practice readiness on commencing their first year of practice. While some of this can be attributed to differences in how higher education institutions design and deliver their nursing programs, much relates to the individual and the influence of the healthcare context. Throughout their first year of practice, most new graduate nurses move within their employer organisation and advance in stages. Thus, they may demonstrate high levels of practice readiness when they are familiar with an environment, yet display low levels once moved to an unfamiliar work context.

Portfolio Activity 5.2: Stop, reflect and think

Thinking back on your clinical placement experiences, how important were the orientation sessions in preparing you for a new environment? Did you find that returning to a different ward or unit in a familiar health service was easier than adjusting to a totally new environment, or were there similar challenges?

A graduate nurse demonstrating low levels of practice readiness lacks confidence, struggles with the role and has poor time and workload management. Being overconfident and refusing help also indicates lower levels of practice readiness. In the workplace, nurses with low levels of practice readiness can be easily overwhelmed and struggle to finish their work on time. They may have gaps in their clinical practice, appear disorganised, withdrawn or quiet, and not open to learning opportunities (Harrison et al., 2020b). Nurses displaying low levels of practice readiness require closer, more intensive one-on-one educational support and often require a longer period of support or working in a supernumerary capacity. This need for additional supervision increases the workload of other team members. As there are many factors that influence a new graduate's level of practice readiness, demonstrating a low level of readiness does not mean that you are a poor practitioner or that you cannot improve. It is therefore important that you seek help and support if you feel your level of practice readiness is insufficient for the context in which you are working. Knowing your limitations and seeking help where necessary demonstrates your level of maturity as a reflective practitioner.

Case Study 5.4: Low level of practice readiness

Harry commences his graduate year and is struggling with his role. His difficulty in communicating effectively with the team, along with his belief that he doesn't need help, have resulted in him making a number of mistakes, including a medication error. However, Harry believes he is adapting to his new role just fine, and thinks his friends are experiencing the same adjustment issues. You are working in the same surgical unit as Harry and know that he is struggling more than others in your graduating group.

- What could you say to Harry to help him develop insight into his limitations?

- How should his preceptor approach the problem?

- What are the potential risks if Harry fails to acknowledge his low level of practice readiness?

Graduate nurses demonstrating higher levels of practice readiness are organised and time-efficient, and therefore successfully navigate the workplace environment. These nurses manage a normal patient load while competently providing basic nursing care. They are effective communicators and develop relationships easily. Graduate nurses with high levels of practice readiness know the standard and scope of their practice, readily recognise their limitations and know when and how to escalate issues and ask for help. Practice ready graduate nurses adapt well to fluctuating workloads and change, are decisive and able to function with minimal support from colleagues in the workplace. As a result, they are reliable, helpful team members who are resourceful in the provision of care. While they are still supervised as a novice practitioner, they do not require intensive one-on-one support and therefore do not add to the workload of the healthcare team nor disrupt the workflow (Harrison et al., 2020b).

As with all professions, the transition to practice is challenging yet rewarding. You will encounter difficult and exciting times as you develop practice readiness and become a competent registered nurse. You may have low levels of practice readiness in some domains, and high levels in others. As we reinforce throughout this book, you must develop skills in critical thinking and reflection to acknowledge your limitations, know when to seek help, and support and celebrate your achievements along the way.

Portfolio Activity: Making the transition

After completing this chapter, use the worksheet in Appendix 5 to list the top five capabilities you think will support you to practise confidently and safely as you transition within a dynamic, complex healthcare system. When you have finished your lists, write a short reflection about why you think these capabilities are the most important. As you move into Part III of this book, compare your list with your self-rated practice readiness capabilities.

Conclusion

New graduate registered nurses play a vital role in the current and future health workforce. Nursing education does not aim to graduate expert nurses; rather, it aims to produce novice to advanced beginners who are able to grow and develop into their role. With appropriate support and guidance, new graduates are the fresh eyes of the healthcare system, able to see things with new vitality and able to place patient safety at the forefront of their care. While practice readiness develops on a continuum from day one of your nursing study, you will continue to demonstrate various levels of practice readiness throughout your career in the various roles and nursing contexts in which you will work. By working towards being personally, clinically, professionally and industry ready, you will set a solid foundation to continue developing your confidence and competence as you transition to the role of registered nurse.

Key summary points

- Upon graduating from their nursing degree, nurses are expected to function at the level of novice to advanced beginner registered nurse.

- Practice readiness is the capability to manage the roles and responsibilities of a registered nurse in a complex and dynamic environment.

- Practice readiness is multidimensional, consisting of four domains of readiness capabilities (personal, professional, clinical and industry) that intersect to represent practice readiness.

- Personal readiness is reflected in the graduate's ability to manage the roles and responsibilities of a registered nurse, themselves personally, and the work environment.

- Professional readiness encompasses the ability to work efficiently and provide care in accordance with registered nurse standards and codes of practice.

- Clinical readiness is demonstrated in capabilities that enable the graduate to provide a safe, basic level of clinical care within their scope of practice.

- Industry readiness refers to the ability to navigate the healthcare system, organisations, healthcare parameters and resources in the provision of care.

- Practice readiness develops as a continuum that commences when a nursing student commences their nursing program through to the end of first year of practice.

- The differing experiences and contexts of practice encountered by individuals along the transition continuum will result in variations in levels of practice readiness

Critical thinking questions

1. Consider the four domains of practice readiness. Which domain do you think has the most influence on practice readiness for new graduate nurses, and why?

2. What factors in the education and healthcare context do you think have the greatest influence on an individual's level of practice readiness, and why?

3. The domains of readiness are described as multidimensional and interdependent. What do you think this means, and why?

4. Do you think it is reasonable that nurses, on entering their first year of practice, function as advanced beginners? How does this align with expectations as outlined in the codes and standards for practice for registered nurses?

5. Referring back to Chapter 2, what challenges do you think you might face in your graduate year in respect of each domain of readiness?

6. What advice would you give a first-year nursing student about developing practice readiness?

References

Benner, P. (1982). From novice to expert. *American Journal of Nursing, 82*(3), 402. https://doi.org/10.2307/3462928

Benner, P. (1984). *From novice to expert: Excellence and power in clinical nursing practice.* Addison-Wesley.

Benner, P., & Wrubel, J. (1982). Skilled clinical knowledge: The value of perceptual awareness. *Nurse Educator, 7*(3), 11–17. https://doi.org/10.1097/00006223-198205000-00003

Boamah, S., Read, E., & Laschinger, H. K. S. (2016). Factors influencing new graduate nurse burnout development, job satisfaction and patient care quality: A time-lagged study. *Journal of Advanced Nursing, 73*(5), 1182–1195. https://doi.org/10.1111/jan.13215

Dreyfus, S., & Dreyfus, H. L. (1980). *A five-stage model of the mental activities involved in directed skill acquisition*. Operations Research Center, Berkeley University. https://shortdoi.org/scribd

Duchscher, J. (2009). Transition shock: The initial stage of role adaptation for newly graduated registered nurses. *Journal of Advanced Nursing, 65*(5), 1103–1113. https://doi.org/10.1111/j.1365-2648.2008.04898.x

Duchscher, J. B., & Windey, M. (2018). Stages of transition and transition shock. *Journal for Nurses in Professional Development, 34*(4), 228–232. https://doi.org/10.1097/NND.0000000000000461

El Haddad, M., Moxham, L., & Broadbent, M. (2017). Graduate nurse practice readiness: A conceptual understanding of an age-old debate. *Collegian, 24*(4), 391–396. https://doi.org/10.1016/j.colegn.2016.08.004

Graf, A. C., Jacob, E., Twigg, D., & Nattabi, B. (2020). Contemporary nursing graduates' transition to practice: A critical review of transition models. *Journal of Clinical Nursing, 29*(15–16), 3097–3107. https://doi.org/10.1111/jocn.15234

Harrison, H., Birks, M., Franklin, R., & Mills, J. (2020a). An assessment continuum: How healthcare professionals define and determine practice readiness of newly graduated registered nurses. *Collegian, 27*(2), 198–206. https://doi.org/10.1016/j.colegn.2019.07.003

Harrison, H., Birks, M., Franklin, R., & Mills, J. (2020b). Fostering graduate nurse practice readiness in context. *Collegian, 27*(1), 115–124. https://doi.org/10.1016/j.colegn.2019.07.006

Missen, K., McKenna, L., Beauchamp, A., & Larkins, J. (2016). Qualified nurses' perceptions of nursing graduates' abilities vary according to specific demographic and clinical characteristics: A descriptive quantitative study. *Nurse Education Today, 45*, 108–113. https://doi.org/10.1016/j.nedt.2016.07.001

Murray, M., Sundin, D., & Cope, V. (2019a). Benner's model and Duchscher's theory: Providing the framework for understanding new graduate nurses' transition to practice. *Nurse Education in Practice*, *34*, 199–203. https://doi.org/10.1016/j.nepr.2018.12.003

Murray, M., Sundin, D., & Cope, V. (2019b). A mixed-methods study on patient safety insights of new graduate registered nurses. *Journal of Nursing Care Quality*, *35*(3), 258-264. https://doi.org/10.1097/ncq.0000000000000443

Murray, M., Sundin, D., & Cope, V. (2019c). New graduate nurses' understanding and attitudes about patient safety upon transition to practice. *Journal of Clinical Nursing*, *28*(13–14), 2543–2552. https://doi.org/10.1111/jocn.14839

Murray, M., Sundin, D., & Cope, V. (2020). Supporting new graduate registered nurse transition for safety: A literature review update. *Collegian*, *27*(1), 125–134. https://doi.org/10.1016/j.colegn.2019.04.007

Regan, S., Wong, C., Laschinger, H., Cummings, G., Leiter, M., & MacPhee, M., Rhéaume, A., Ritchie, J. A., Wolff, A. C., Jeffs, L., Young-Ritchie, C., Grinspun, D., Gurnham, M. E., Foster, B., Huckstep, S., Ruffolo, M., Shamian, J., Burkoski, V., Wood, K., & Read, E. (2017). Starting out: Qualitative perspectives of new graduate nurses and nurse leaders on transition to practice. *Journal of Nursing Management*, *25*(4), 246–255. https://doi.org/10.1111/jonm.12456

Walker, A., Storey, K. M., Costa, B. M., & Leung, R. K. (2015). Refinement and validation of the Work Readiness Scale for graduate nurses. *Nurse Outlook*, *63*(6), 632–638. https://doi.org/10.1016/j.outlook.2015.06.00

OXFORD UNIVERSITY PRESS

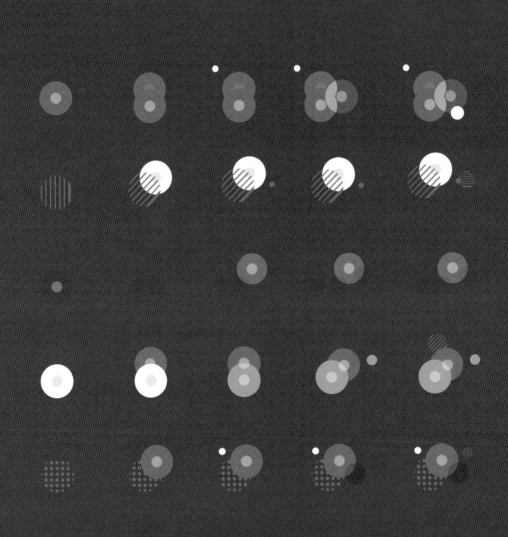

PART III

BEING PRACTICE READY

The Essential Capabilities

Being personally ready to transition as an RN was difficult. The feeling of being an impostor in your work environment was a mindset I struggled with. Clinically you were competent to complete the tasks which you had studied for but impostor syndrome took over. Regular reflection and evaluation helped ease this feeling.

Sean, Graduated 2019, Australia

Chapter 6

Personal Readiness

Melanie Birks, Helena Harrison and Jane Mills

Learning Outcomes

Following completion of this chapter, you will be able to:

1. Define the term 'personal readiness' in respect of nursing practice.

2. Explain the importance of personal readiness in nursing.

3. Describe the capabilities associated with personal readiness.

4. Reflect on your own personal readiness.

5. Formulate a plan for developing and maintaining personal readiness in practice.

Key terms

Attitude	Emotional intelligence	Self-management
Attribute	Personal readiness	Tolerance
Commitment	Resilience	
Confidence	Self-efficacy	

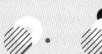

Introduction

As you have worked through your studies you have developed a raft of knowledge and a range of skills to prepare you for an exciting and rewarding career. We know from previous chapters, however, that being prepared and ready for the role of a registered nurse requires more than just cognitive ability and psychomotor skills. Successful preparation and transition involve the integration and application of learned capabilities in practice and the ability to manage the responsibilities of a registered nurse. As discussed in Chapter 5, practice readiness is multidimensional and encompasses four domains: personal, clinical, professional and industry readiness. In this chapter we will explore personal readiness – the key capabilities associated with personal readiness, and why personal readiness is identified as the most critical area that new nurses need to develop for a successful transition to their professional role.

> ## Case Study 6.1: Introducing Ally
>
> Ally is a 28-year-old single mother of two young children. Ally has wanted to become a nurse for as long as she can remember and is proud of her success over the previous years of study. She is looking forward to completing her degree this year. Ally feels she has a solid understanding of the professional nursing role and has no concerns about making the transition to registered nurse.

Personal readiness defined

As discussed in Chapter 5, personal readiness is about personal preparedness: having the capability to manage the role and responsibilities of a registered nurse, yourself and your environment. Personal readiness incorporates the mental and emotional preparation required to cope with a new way of working, managing your emotions and your professional development while simultaneously caring for vulnerable individuals who are experiencing changes in their health and well-being. Personal readiness capabilities also support you in maintaining a balanced level of confidence – the type of confidence that enables you to know your limitations, ask for help, accept feedback, keep patients safe and intervene on their behalf.

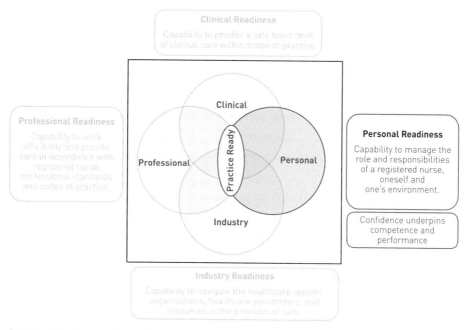

Figure 6.1 Personal readiness

Personal readiness has a significant influence on a new nurse's ability to move seamlessly into professional practice and continue to grow and develop as a registered nurse. In Chapter 2, we read about the complexity of the healthcare system and the challenges new nurses can experience during their transition from student to registered nurse. How well a new nurse is prepared with the capabilities to cope with change and manage workloads within dynamic complex healthcare settings will influence how well they are able to adapt to their new role. These capabilities are those encompassed within personal readiness, and overlap all the domains of readiness (Figure 6.1). As such, they underpin a graduate nurse's ability to function competently. A well-developed level of personal readiness is associated with safe professional practice and quality patient outcomes (Altmiller & Hopkins-Pepe, 2019; Amer, 2013; Cronenwett et al., 2007). Thus, these capabilities are emphasised above all others as essential to the work of a registered nurse in all contexts of practice (Harrison et al., 2020a).

Personal readiness

The capability to manage the roles and responsibilities of a registered nurse, oneself and one's environment.

The importance of personal readiness

Barnett (2012) contends that all graduates need to be prepared with generic skills for an 'unknown future' (p. 65). Learning for the future is goal-driven yet needs to accommodate future practice that remains unknown (Barnett, 2012). Barnett (2012) argues that our current world is characterised by uncertainty and complexity. This uncertainty and complexity include unknowable events, where resources – including our personal resources – are constantly expanded and unbalanced, creating stress. Acquiring a level of human development that cultivates the attitudes and skills necessary to cope and learn in this uncertain world is needed (Barnett, 2012).

The COVID-19 pandemic is a stark example of the type of situation Barnett (2012) is referring to, where health and human resources required swift adaptation and expansion in limited time to address an unprecedented and unexpected health crisis. Preparing new nurses with personal qualities to respond promptly, yet appropriately, means they not only function effectively and safely within a complex world but are able to respond and flourish within it. Uncertainty has been found to boost learning where unpredictability and volatility stimulate cognition for learning (Massi et al., 2018). In their study about practice readiness, Wolff et al. (2010) advocate that new nurses need to be prepared to adapt to the new and constant evolution that accompanies healthcare and nursing to ensure clients receive safe, contemporary and relevant healthcare.

Similarly, Harrison et al. (2020a) indicate that personal readiness enables new nurses to not only cope with the unpredictable change that pervades healthcare contexts, but also to manage the diverse relationships that create the workplace environment. As a new nurse you will engage in a range of situations and relationships that can often expose you to pressure, conflict or hostility (D'Ambra & Andrews, 2014; Hartin et al., 2018). Perhaps you have encountered this as a student. Negative interactions with others can be intimidating and undermine your confidence and performance (Harrison et al., 2020b). These factors can cause significant stress, interrupt learning and alter your perception of the workplace. Heightened anxiety, stress and burnout are known to perpetuate nurse attrition (D'Ambra & Andrews, 2014). It is therefore important to have the personal readiness capabilities to minimise, mitigate and manage these situations.

OXFORD UNIVERSITY PRESS

Your personal readiness also contributes to your ability to continually learn and develop and practise safely within interprofessional teams. The workplace environment and the people within it offer a range of exciting opportunities to develop and extend your nursing practice. Being able to confidently seek out others, ask questions, accept feedback on your performance and build supportive relationships will help you optimise these opportunities. This relies on your personal readiness, particularly your communication skills and confidence. In emergency situations or when you are unsure about your nursing care and need help, speaking up and seeking assistance is not only necessary for patient safety but is welcomed – your peers and colleagues want you to ask questions and ask for help (Harrison et al., 2020a). Well-developed personal readiness will support you to feel comfortable and safe to convey concerns clearly and seek appropriate and necessary support. It will also strengthen your relationships within the team, extend your support network and, again, develop your nursing practice.

Personal readiness capabilities

The capabilities associated with personal readiness are the qualities that represent who we are as individuals and our ability to manage our thoughts, emotions and behaviours when we undertake our role and interact with others. A number of capabilities are associated with personal readiness, all of which are underpinned by the foundational knowledge acquired during your nursing studies. For convenience, we will discuss these capabilities in terms of personal readiness attributes and personal readiness skills (Table 6.1).

Table 6.1 Capabilities associated with personal readiness

Personal readiness attributes	Personal readiness skills
• Positive attitude • Commitment • Resilience • Compassion • Tolerance • Confidence	• Respectful communication • Effective interaction • Relationship management • Emotional intelligence • Self-management

Personal readiness attributes

Attribute

Inherent characteristics or qualities of a person.

Attitude

A person's disposition or state of mind, how they carry themselves and respond to an object, issue, situation or other people.

An **attribute** refers to the inherent characteristics or qualities of a person. Commonly described as personality traits, attributes characterise and guide how an individual manages themselves, their interactions with others and their day-to-day activities.

Personal readiness is conveyed in a positive attitude. An **attitude** is a person's disposition or state of mind, how they carry themselves and respond toward objects, issues, situations or other people. It can be described as an enduring way of thinking and feeling about something or someone that is commonly reflected in their behaviour. A person's attitude is underpinned by their values and beliefs. It is formed over time, as they encounter and evaluate different stimuli. Through our experiences, our thoughts and emotions come together as attitudes, and affect our behaviour. A person's attitude can permeate their surroundings and influence how individuals respond to and interact with each other.

A positive attitude can be described in many different ways. Often it is reflected in the level of motivation that an individual expresses towards their circumstances. Someone who is keen to be at work and happy to take on any challenge, for example, will be displaying a positive attitude. When an individual has a positive attitude, they view the world more favourably – and often they are viewed more favourably by others. A positive attitude aligns with optimism and can make it easier to manage situations more constructively and reduce stress and anxiety. A positive attitude can help a person to focus on opportunities and solutions rather than on challenges, problems or failures, and therefore cope more easily with day-to-day activities. Someone who is positive interacts with others respectfully, is more open to new experiences, has a willingness to do things differently and seeks opportunities. When you demonstrate enthusiasm for your new situation and embrace opportunities to learn, you attract positive interactions and support, accomplish tasks more readily and feel more confident and fulfilled with what you are doing.

Portfolio Activity 6.1: Stop, reflect and think

What are the characteristics of a positive attitude? Think about someone you would describe as having a positive attitude. What is it about the way that they communicate, behave, interact or carry themselves that reflects a positive attitude?

As nurses, our attitude can be conveyed in our composure, communication and teamwork, thus it can influence how we respond to others and provide nursing care. The healthcare environment can be challenging and demanding; having team members with a positive attitude potentiates a positive environment and progressive, solution-focused approaches to healthcare. As we will discuss in Chapter 11, a positive workplace environment is one where everyone, including patients, can flourish. Each individual contributes to the atmosphere in the workplace environment, and a positive attitude augments a flourishing environment.

New nurses with a positive attitude are those who are keen, motivated and committed to their work. Being positive attracts positive interactions that engender good relationships with staff and patients. Members of a healthcare team are more willing to assist colleagues who are keen and enthusiastic, and to provide them with opportunities to support their personal and professional development. In this section, we discuss attributes in terms of commitment, resilience, compassion, tolerance and confidence.

Personal readiness involves **commitment** to fulfilling the inherent obligations of the professional role. It reflects being open and enthusiastic, with a desire to learn and grow. Nurses who are committed take the initiative and actively seek opportunities to engage in work and learn more. These individuals ask questions and listen to the responses of others. This behaviour is motivating for others, and people want to share information with them. Attitudes affect how a person receives and responds to feedback. Constructive feedback is necessary to improve performance, and novice nurses with a high level of commitment are keen to improve and are therefore open to feedback and able to use it productively. As we shall discuss in the next chapter, this commitment extends beyond what is personally beneficial for the individual nurse to others they interact with.

Commitment

Acceptance of the obligations inherent in the professional role.

Personal readiness requires **resilience**. This enables new graduate nurses to respond to and perform effectively in any situation. While the definition of resilience varies, common descriptions explain it as the capacity or ability to respond to and recover from adverse, difficult and/or challenging circumstances (Aburn et al., 2016). Characteristics of resilience commonly include being adaptable, flexible and having an optimistic, can-do attitude that enables the individual to overcome adversity (Aburn et al., 2016). Nurses

Resilience

The ability to respond and adapt to changing and challenging situations.

that demonstrate resilience simultaneously manage their day-to-day activities and respond positively to different challenges in the workplace. They are able to bounce back under pressure and approach challenges positively in undertaking their work.

Adapting and assimilating to new environments can be significant sources of stress. New graduates with resilience are able to handle this stress and accommodate the constant fluctuations that are common in the workplace. They are flexible in their thinking, accepting differences in clinical practice and reprioritising work commitments with ease. Through the enhanced critical thinking and time management that accompanies well developed resilience, they become resourceful and able to work more independently. As a result, nurses with a positive attitude do not add to the workloads of others, but help the team to be efficient in meeting patient needs.

Personal readiness includes having a highly developed sense of compassion. It may seem redundant to discuss attributes such as kindness, compassion and empathy as being characteristic of nurses; however, these qualities cannot be taken for granted. These traits enable nurses to translate the essence of 'care' during clinical practice. While many individuals are attracted to the profession of nursing because they have well developed empathetic and compassionate traits, nursing is a complex, technical and highly skilled profession. The traits of kindness, compassion and empathy combine with the technical, scientific aspects of nursing to enhance the quality and safety of patient care. Compassionate nurses use empathy to listen and understand an individual's situation and hence build rapport – they facilitate person-centred care, which demonstrates respect and helps to ensure an individual's rights and needs are included in the provision of care (McCormack et al., 2013).

As you will have gleaned through reading this text and your studies so far, developing readiness for practice is a challenging process that occurs over a number of years, from when you first enrolled in your course through to your initial years of practice. During this time, your definitions of kindness, caring, empathy and compassion will be challenged as you develop as a professional. This is to be expected and embraced, as you transition to your role as a professional nurse. Over time these traits will become a seamless part of your nursing care.

OXFORD UNIVERSITY PRESS

Portfolio Activity 6.2: Stop, reflect and think

Reflect on your reasons for choosing a career in nursing. To what extent did your natural attributes feature in your decision? How have these traits developed over your years of study?

The personal qualities discussed in this chapter are critical to effective practice, as they ensure that nurses develop tolerance. Tolerance is the ability to accept the values, beliefs and practices of others without judgment. Tolerance is key to the quality of a nurse's relationship with patients and healthcare colleagues. Nurses who are tolerant recognise their role as part of a team, and are accepting of others and their diverse backgrounds and perspectives.

Tolerance requires a commitment to person-centredness. Nurses use a person-centred approach when they embrace individual differences and seek an inclusive approach to their practice. Being person-centred is not reserved for working with patients. It extends to patients' families, significant others and all members of the healthcare team (Santana et al., 2018). Through a person-centred approach, trust and respect are established (Shepherd & Biedermann, 2020), cultivating a positive environment that is critical to improving healthcare structures, functions and outcomes (Santana et al., 2018).

Tolerance

The ability to accept the values, beliefs and practices of others without judgment.

Case Study 6.2: Positive attitude

Ally is completing her final consolidation placement at a local health service. She is assigned to work with Jimmy, a nurse who qualified overseas. Jimmy is highly skilled and a good teacher, but he makes it clear that he feels that Ally should be at home looking after her children, rather than pursuing a qualification in nursing. Ally recognises that Jimmy has a cultural background that is very different from hers.

• How might Ally maintain a positive attitude in this potentially difficult situation?

• What personal traits can she draw on to respond appropriately in her interactions with Jimmy?

Finally, the most important personal readiness attribute for a nurse to develop is confidence. As can be seen from Figure 6.1, confidence underpins competence and therefore performance. Confidence develops with time, experience and practice. Confidence is defined as an attitude or feeling of trust, belief and assurance in yourself or in other people. A confident person feels competent from the inside out and is sure of their abilities and qualities; they trust and have faith in their capabilities.

Confidence reflects a person's self-efficacy. **Self-efficacy** is a person's belief in their abilities to succeed in a situation or accomplish a task, and to exert control over their own motivation, behaviour and social environment (Bandura 1977, 1997). Self-efficacy is an essential part of an individual's self-system. According to Bandura (1978), a self-system comprises a person's attitudes, abilities and cognitive skills. It plays a major role in how we perceive and respond to different situations. Individuals with a robust sense of self-efficacy approach challenges as opportunities to learn and grow, problems to solve and master. They identify, commit to and have an interest in the goals and activities they undertake. Further, those with high self-efficacy tend to have more resilience and bounce back more swiftly from disappointments or setbacks (Bandura, 1997). As a new nurse you will be faced with a range of new responsibilities that you have never undertaken and fulfilled independently. As a nursing student you may have undertaken, encountered or observed these responsibilities during your professional experiences; however, they will take on new meaning in your professional capacity as a registered nurse. A strong self-efficacy will support you to approach this new situation with a belief that you have the capability (knowledge, attributes and skills) to learn and perform your role well. Even though at times you may feel overwhelmed or challenged, you will perceive this positively and take useful actions to manage the situation, including seeking help and instituting self-management strategies to support yourself. We will discuss these in the next section, where we talk about personal readiness skills.

Newly qualified nurses generally build their confidence to the required level during the first three to six months of practice as a registered nurse. You may find when you begin practice that you feel confident in your knowledge and skills; however, you may not have the confidence to apply these to practice and

Confidence

An attitude or feeling of trust, belief and assurance in yourself, in others and/or in plans for the future.

Self-efficacy

A person's belief in their abilities to succeed in a situation or accomplish a task, and to exert control over their own motivation, behaviour and social environment.

OXFORD UNIVERSITY PRESS

fulfil all the responsibilities of a registered nurse. As described in Chapter 4, when faced with the reality of the new role and the level of responsibility, many new nurses feel overwhelmed and begin to lose confidence. The more you practise and gain experience, however, the more confident you will feel. It is important to ask questions and seek support during this time.

Keeping a balanced level of confidence will help you to successfully accomplish a number of different responsibilities. A balanced level of confidence is about having a belief and level of certainty in what you are doing, and communicating your concerns when you need to – this is essential. In doing so, you demonstrate that you have a safe level of independent practice in managing your responsibilities and those you work with, that you have confidence in your capabilities and that you will seek support if needed. When you convey confidence in your clinical practice, patients will feel more secure and comfortable in your care and believe that you will keep them safe from harm. You will be more likely to escalate concerns and respond to challenges more effectively.

Conversely, being under- or overconfident can negatively impact your performance. A new nurse who is overconfident or underconfident may not ask questions or reveal their limitations, and this can raise safety concerns for those working with them. Peers and supervisors worry that the new nurse will practise outside their limitations, which could lead to mistakes or omitting care that could place patients in danger (Harrison et al., 2020a). Your peers want to be sure that you do know what you are doing and that you are not overcompensating to hide any insecurity, fear or incompetence. As discussed, when you ask questions or confirm actions you are unsure about, you give your peers confidence that you will practise safely. Therefore, it is very important that you seek support and ask questions when needed. Don't be afraid to ask questions or avoid doing something if you think it might compromise either yourself or your patients when you are providing care. Figure 6.2 shows the relationship between confidence and performance.

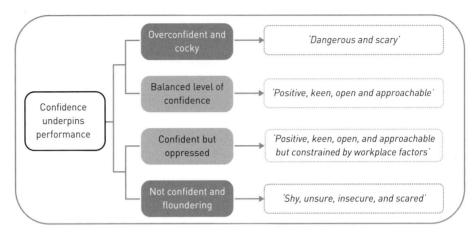

Figure 6.2 Confidence and performance (Harrison et al., 2020a, p. 4)

 Portfolio Activity: Making the transition

Review Figure 6.2. What level of confidence do you think you have? What aspects of your confidence do you need to work on to be ready for practice as a registered nurse?

Acquiring a balanced level of confidence can take three to six months of practice and experience. It is important that you work toward building your confidence and having a belief that the capabilities you have developed over the course of your nursing degree will support you to undertake your new responsibilities. Factors that can influence your confidence include developing your knowledge of the workplace environment in which you will begin your practice as a registered nurse, and understanding the expectations of your performance.

Understanding and acknowledging areas of practice in which you feel you need to develop, or perhaps do not feel confident in, is also important. Seek feedback and affirmation on your performance and for practices that you are unfamiliar or unsure about – take the opportunity to master the skill. Each time you master a new skill you build your self-efficacy and confidence in your abilities (Bandura, 1997). Set a goal, research and review the skill, and ask a senior colleague for the opportunity to practise and support you while performing the skill. Observe the performance of others you identify as confident, capable nurses – look at how they behave, practise and interact with others.

Importantly, pay attention to what you are thinking and feeling. Thoughts and emotions play a key role in how you 'warm up' before a difficult event or task when you are feeling nervous, and how you process the outcomes. If you are feeling anxious or fearful, try to find ways to ease your stress before you begin. Look for opportunities to process your disappointments or setbacks positively, rather than dwelling on the negative aspects of the outcomes. In the next section we discus personal readiness skills. Developing robust personal readiness skills will support you in building the balanced level of confidence you need for a comfortable transition to practice.

Case Study 6.3: Overconfidence

Ally believes that she has had great opportunities and excellent teachers while on placement in the clinical environment. She feels particularly confident in her ability to transition to the professional role. She tells fellow students that she feels this final placement is a waste of time because she isn't learning anything new.

- What are the potential pitfalls for Ally in having this attitude?

- What should she be doing to ensure she uses her final placement as preparation for her role as a registered nurse?

Personal readiness skills

As a nursing student, you have spent a considerable amount of time mastering the psychomotor skills that are necessary for your work as a health professional. You have spent a similar amount of time developing the soft or psychosocial skills that are fundamental to competent performance as a registered nurse. These are the interpersonal skills that help individuals understand each other and enable them to work together in harmony. In this section we discuss them in terms of respectful communication, effective interaction, relationship management, emotional intelligence and self-management.

People with well-developed psychosocial skills foster cooperative and collaborative relationships and support individuals to develop a positive workplace culture and adapt to change (Albrecht, 2006; Goleman, 2006). Central to this outcome is the use of respectful communication. This is one of the most important skills that a nurse possesses. Nurses who are skilled in respectful communication strategies have the tools they need to succeed in their chosen profession.

Respectful communication involves the ability to convey information to others, and listen and respond in a manner that is appropriate to their emotional and development state. Communication is respectful when it reflects all the elements of a positive attitude that we discussed in the first section of this chapter and commitment, resilience, compassion, tolerance and confidence. Respectful communication is both professional and therapeutic in nature (Birks et al., 2020). It may be easy to assume that professional communication is that which occurs between members of the healthcare team, and therapeutic communication is that which occurs between nurses and recipients of their care. In practice, however, respectful communication in the healthcare setting requires that the nurse draws on both professional and therapeutic elements, regardless of who is party to the exchange.

Unfortunately, even with the best intentions, respectful communication does not always occur. We have all experienced well-meaning people who are poor communicators – whose commitment is mistaken for ambition, whose resilience is mistaken for being hard-hearted, who show compassion in ways that appear as pity, whose tolerance is poorly articulated and whose confidence can be perceived as cockiness. Respectful communication helps ensure that the intention of what has been communicated is conveyed clearly and accurately, so that healthcare is safe and miscommunications that can contribute to difficult relationships, misunderstandings or unsafe practice can be avoided.

 Portfolio Activity 6.3: Stop, reflect and think

Consider how you interacted with others during your professional experience placements. Think about the communication skills you use to interact with the healthcare team. In what ways were these the same as or different from the communication skills you used to interact with patients?

OXFORD UNIVERSITY PRESS

Nurses are expected to interact with a range of different people in the workplace for varied reasons. Communicating respectfully involves adapting our communication to ensure that it is appropriate to the individual and the context. Culture and other forms of diversity impact on how communication is constructed and interpreted. Whether it be with supervisors, colleagues or recipients of care, it is impossible to communicate respectfully with those from backgrounds that are different from our own without having awareness of our own values, biases and beliefs (Lim et al., 2020).

Well-developed psychosocial skills are essential. These skills go beyond fundamental communication processes and enable us to engage in effective interaction with others. They enable nurses, particularly new graduates, to ask questions, raise concerns and convey information clearly. As a result, information is received, understood and acted on appropriately. Being able to cooperate effectively with others, hold difficult conversations, negotiate, and resolve conflict relies on effective interactions. Nurses who engage with others in this way are approachable and confident in their interactions. These behaviours cultivate relationships that support you as a novice nurse to learn and, importantly, keep patients safe from harm.

Healthcare is a team activity, wherein effective teamwork relies on positive, mutually beneficial relationships. Communicating respectfully and interacting effectively are the foundations of a new graduate's ability to contribute to positive relationship management. Skills in relationship management enable a graduate who is new to the healthcare team to socially integrate and become an effective team member. These nurses are aware of the roles of others in the team and conscious of what is happening in the environment. The productive and positive relationships that result contribute to a safe standard of person-centred healthcare.

Working in difficult environments and faced with the development of a multitude of new skills, new graduate nurses often feel overwhelmed. Having well-developed **emotional intelligence** and clear thinking skills helps them to develop coping strategies (Mellor et al., 2017). Emotional intelligence is 'the awareness of one's own emotions and those of others [which] includes having the aptitude to manage these emotions to enhance interactions with others' (Shepherd & Beidermann, 2020, p. 49). Competency in emotional intelligence therefore requires a high level of self-awareness,

Emotional intelligence

A high level of self-awareness of your own and others' emotions and the ability to manage these emotions to enhance interpersonal relationships.

being mindful of your own emotions and those of others, and how these may impact decision-making and actions, particularly in stressful situations. There will be situations that affect you and trigger different types of feelings and emotions – this is normal. What is important is what you do with your feelings and emotions – how you manage and express them in your thoughts and behaviours. When we have a high level of emotional intelligence, we manage our feelings well and behave appropriately in a situation, with a level of professional composure. You will be more likely to think clearly and respond to situations in your nursing practice with appropriate actions that keep both you and your patients safe.

Developing your emotional intelligence relies on taking the time to understand yourself and the things in your environment that stress, motivate, challenge and excite you, and being able to regulate and relate these effectively. Pay attention to your emotions, thoughts and behaviours during different events, reflect on them and consider why you responded to a certain event in a particular way. This self-awareness is a key element of emotional intelligence and is essential for effective **self-management**. We define self-management as the ability to manage aspects of ourselves and our lives that promote our own well-being and that of our relationships. Nurses, particularly those starting out in their careers, are often highly focused on managing every aspect of their professional role – managing their time, managing their patient's pain, managing others. Often this is considered an expectation – that the role of nurse involves a degree of sacrifice and that, in putting ourselves last, we are fulfilling the requirements of our role. In reality, failing to care for ourselves has significant consequences. Becoming physically, mentally and emotionally overwhelmed positions us to interact poorly with others, react to situations inappropriately, and fail to take actions that are self-protective.

Self-care and self-compassion are critical to effective nursing practice. This requirement pertains to all aspects of your life, not just your professional role. It is dependent on routine daily activities that reduce stress and prevent burnout (Shepherd & Biedermann, 2020).

Self-management

The ability to manage aspects of ourselves and our lives that promote our own well-being and that of our relationships.

OXFORD UNIVERSITY PRESS

Portfolio Activity 6.4: Stop, reflect and think

Consider your transition to the professional nursing role. Are you prepared for the challenges (and rewards) this will bring? What strategies do you currently practise that can be considered self-management? How will you ensure that you maintain or develop self-management strategies as a professional registered nurse?

 Portfolio Activity: Making the transition

Using the worksheet in Appendix 6, rate your personal readiness capabilities. Are there areas you think you need to improve to enhance your transition to practice? Drawing on what you have learnt in this chapter, formulate a plan for developing and maintaining your personal readiness for practice.

Conclusion

In this chapter we explored and described personal readiness and the capabilities that will support you as a new nurse, to successfully transition, adapt and competently fulfil the responsibilities associated with your new professional role. Personal readiness underscores the efficacy of the capabilities in the other three domains of readiness: professional, clinical and industry readiness, which we will explore in the next three chapters. Therefore, developing a solid level of personal readiness and a balanced level of confidence will help you function safely, efficiently and effectively in unpredictable and complex healthcare systems, those that you will enter as you begin your exciting and rewarding new career as a registered nurse.

Key summary points

- Personal readiness is a graduate's capability to manage the roles and responsibilities of a registered nurse, themselves personally and the work environment.

- Personal readiness supports new nurses to cope with changes experienced during their transition and growth as a registered nurse, and continue to learn and develop during periods of uncertainty.

- Being personally ready involves having the attitude and skills to cope and adapt to change and work effectively with others in the provision of a safe standard of care.

- Personal readiness attitudes include commitment, resilience, compassion, tolerance and confidence.

- Personal readiness skills include respectful communication, effective interaction, relationship management, emotional intelligence and self-management.

Critical thinking questions

1. What would you consider as the important aspects of personal readiness, and why?

2. What does having a 'balanced level of confidence' mean, and how does this contribute to safe nursing care?

3. What is resilience, and how does it contribute to a new nurse's ability to manage the responsibilities of the registered nurse role?

4. Why do you think that it is important for new nurses to be able to be collaborative, tolerant and compassionate?

5. As a new nurse, describe how being personally ready will support you during your transition to practice as a registered nurse.

References

Aburn, G., Gott, M., & Hoare, K. (2016). What is resilience? An integrative review of the empirical literature. *Journal of Advanced Nursing, 72*(5), 980–1000. https://doi.org/10.1111/jan.12888

Albrecht, K. (2006). *Social intelligence: The new science of success*. Jossey-Bass.

Altmiller, G., & Hopkins-Pepe, L. (2019). Why quality and safety education for nurses (QSEN) matters in practice. *Journal of Continuing Education in Nursing, 50*(5), 199–200. https://doi.org/10.3928/00220124-20190416-04

OXFORD UNIVERSITY PRESS

Amer, K. (2013). *Quality and safety for transformational nursing: Core competencies.* Pearson Education.

Bandura, A. (1977). Self-efficacy: Toward a unifying theory of behavioral change. *Psychological Review, 84*(2), 191–215. https://doi.org/10.1037/0033-295X.84.2.191

Bandura, A. (1978). The self system in reciprocal determinism. *American Psychologist, 33*(4), 344–358. https://doi.org/10.1037/0003-066X.33.4.344

Bandura, A. (1997). *Self-efficacy: The exercise of control.* W. H. Freeman.

Barnett, R. (2012). Learning for an unknown future. *Higher Education Research & Development, 31*(1), 65–77. https://doi.org/10.1080/07294360.2012.642841

Birks, M., Chapman, Y., & Davis, J. (2020). An introduction to professional and therapeutic communication. In M. Birks, J. Davis & Y. Chapman (Eds.), *Professional and therapeutic communication* (2nd ed., pp. 3–17). Oxford University Press.

Cronenwett, L., Sherwood, G., Barnsteiner, J., Disch, J., Johnson, J., Mitchell, P., Sullivan, D. T., & Warren, J. (2007). Quality and safety education for nurses. *Nursing Outlook, 55*(3), 122–131. https://doi.org/10.1016/j.outlook.2007.02.006

D'Ambra, A. M., & Andrews, D. R. (2014). Incivility, retention and new graduate nurses: An integrated review of the literature. *Journal of Nursing Management, 22*(6), 735–742. https://doi.org/10.1111/jonm.12060

Goleman, D. (2006). *Social intelligence: The new science of human relationships.* Bantam Books.

Harrison, H., Birks, M., Franklin, R., & Mills, J. (2020a). An assessment continuum: How healthcare professionals define and determine practice readiness of newly graduated registered nurses. *Collegian, 27*(2), 198–206. https://doi.org/10.1016/j.colegn.2019.07.003

Harrison, H., Birks, M., Franklin, R., & Mills, J. (2020b) Fostering graduate nurse practice readiness in context. *Collegian, 27*(1), 115–124. https://doi.org/10.1016/j.colegn.2019.07.006

Hartin, P., Birks, M., & Lindsay, D. (2018). Bullying and the nursing profession in Australia: An integrative review of the literature. *Collegian, 25*(6), 613–619. https://doi.org/10.1016/j.colegn.2018.06.004

Lim, S., Mortensen, A., & Carbines, M. (2020). Communicating in culturally diverse contexts. In M. Birks, J. Davis & Y. Chapman (Eds.), *Professional and therapeutic communication* (2nd ed., pp. 105–133). Oxford University Press.

Massi, B., Donahue, C. H., & Lee, D. (2018). Volatility facilitates value updating in the prefrontal cortex. *Neuron, 99*(3), 598–608. https://doi.org/10.1016/j.neuron.2018.06.033

McCormack, B., Manley, K., & Tichen, A. (Eds.) (2013). *Practice development in nursing and healthcare* (2nd ed.). Wiley-Blackwell.

Mellor, P., Gregoric, C., & Gillham, D. (2017). Strategies new graduate registered nurses require to care and advocate for themselves: A literature review. *Contemporary Nurse, 53*(3), 390–405. https://doi.org/10.1080/10376178.2017.1348903

Santana, M. J., Manalili, K., Jolley, R. J., Zelinsky, S., Quan, H., & Lu, M. (2018). How to practice person-centred care: A conceptual framework. *Health Expectations, 21*(2), 429–440. https://doi.org/10.1111/hex.1264

Shepherd, J., & Biedermann, N. (2020). Communication and self. In M. Birks, J. Davis & Y. Chapman (Eds.), *Professional and therapeutic communication* (2nd ed., pp. 45–60). Oxford University Press.

Wolff, A. C., Regan, S., Pesut, B., & Black, J. (2010). Ready for what? An exploration of the meaning of new graduate nurses' readiness for practice. *International Journal of Nursing Education and Scholarship, 7*(1), 1–14. https://doi.org/10.2202/1548-923X.1827

Chapter 7

Professional Readiness

Lisa McKenna

Learning Outcomes

On completion of this chapter, you should be able to:

1. Define the term 'professional readiness' in respect of nursing practice.

2. Explain the importance of professional readiness in nursing.

3. Describe the capabilities associated with professional readiness.

4. Reflect on your own professional readiness.

5. Formulate a plan for developing and maintaining professional readiness in practice.

Key terms

Continuing professional development

Critical thinking

Delegation

Prioritisation

Professional accountability

Professional readiness

Reflective practice

Scope of practice

Supervision

Introduction

Securing registration as a nurse is a remarkable achievement. It marks the beginning of an exciting, diverse career. It can, however, be a little daunting from a professional perspective. As a student, you were sheltered to a degree by the support of registered nurses and other health professionals while coming to understand the professional expectations that would later be required of you. This chapter introduces the requirements for being professionally ready to make the transition from student to registered nurse. It examines what it means to be a professional and why it is important. The chapter then discusses the nature of professional readiness in nursing by exploring capabilities relevant to this domain. As is the case with all forms of practice readiness, professional readiness relies on the graduate's ability to integrate capabilities from all other readiness domains.

Case Study 7.1: Introducing Jake

Jake is 21 years old and in the final year of his nursing degree. Jake is keen to get plenty of experience as a nurse before going overseas to work in some of the outreach programs run in developing countries by his local church. Jake is a strong student and has done particularly well in all theory aspects of his program. He is, however, a little naïve and so has experienced some uncomfortable interactions with others while on placement.

Professional readiness defined

Professional readiness

The capability to work efficiently and provide care in accordance with registered nurse standards and codes of practice.

Professional readiness has been described as the 'capability that graduate nurses require to work efficiently and provide care in accordance with registered nurse standards and codes of practice' (Harrison et al., 2020, p. 200). The concept of being professionally ready involves a number of key attributes, including adhering to professional standards, establishing and maintaining your professional identify, and being able to manage time, tasks and resources. In this chapter, we examine each of these aspects in detail (Figure 7.1).

OXFORD UNIVERSITY PRESS

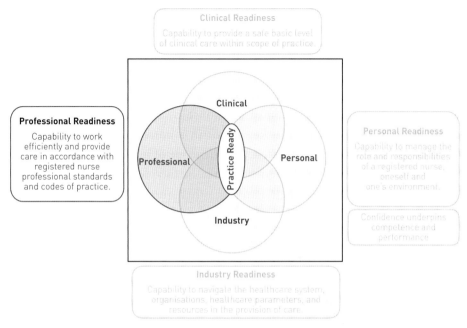

Figure 7.1   Professional readiness

The importance of professional readiness

Nursing is not just an occupation; rather, it has long been recognised across the community as a profession with highly skilled and caring practitioners who uphold strong standards. As you might recall from Chapter 1, a profession is characterised by certain features. According to Perez (2019, p. 212), the three key features are:

1. Specialised education or training of its members;
2. Standards for practice that describe the professional practice expectations; and
3. Commitment to delivering a service that is not limited to the sole interests of the individual professional.

Nursing meets the criteria to be a profession as it is underpinned by specialist education, has standards that regulate practice and requires commitment that extends beyond the individual and indeed the profession itself. In addition, nursing possesses unique attributes that distinguish it from other professions. Many of these were discussed in Chapter 6, where we presented the capabilities associated with personal readiness and described how they permeate all other types of readiness for practice. In particular, the capabilities relating to communication, interaction and relationship management carry great importance in nursing. Blevins and Millen (2016) describe nursing as 'a profession of relationships' (p. 194). Hence, building and nurturing relationships is a key factor in a nurse's professional success. These relationships are multifaceted, and the scope of interactions can be quite daunting at first for the new graduate. They include local relationships such as those with patients and their families, other nurses, health professionals, doctors, hospital managers and clinical educators, as well as relationships more broadly within the profession.

Professional readiness is also essential to practise safely and efficiently. As you are aware, the nursing profession has standards, codes and guidelines that frame and guide nursing practice. Adhering to these standards ensures that, as nurses, we provide nursing care that meets these standards and consequently the level of care expected by the public. As our standards outline, safe practice encompasses the abilities to make informed decisions and to know and address our limitations. Further, given the rapid pace of change and the dynamism that characterises healthcare environments, nurses need to be efficient, which means organising care and resources to ensure we have time to provide an appropriate standard of care and keep patients safe. Well-developed professional readiness will support you to meet these requirements, emulate the characteristics of a professional registered nurse and be a role model for the nursing profession.

Portfolio Activity 7.1: Stop, reflect and think

Prior to commencing nursing studies, did you consider that nursing was a profession? How is nursing regarded by your friends and family? Has your experience as a student influenced their perceptions?

Capabilities associated with professional readiness

Making the transition from nursing student to registered nurse requires you to possess the necessary capabilities associated with professional readiness. These can be categorised under the headings of adherence to professional standards, professional identity and effective resource management (Table 7.1). Elements that make up these capabilities are discussed in the following sections.

Table 7.1 Capabilities associated with professional readiness

Adherence to professional standards	Professional identity	Effective resource management
<ul><li>Scope of practice</li><li>Critical thinking</li><li>Reflective practice</li><li>Continuing professional development</li></ul>	<ul><li>Accountability</li><li>Honesty and integrity</li><li>Professional presence</li><li>e-professionalism</li></ul>	<ul><li>Time management</li><li>Prioritisation</li><li>Leadership</li><li>Supervision and delegation</li></ul>

Adherence to professional standards

In Chapter 1 we discussed the various professional standards, codes and guidelines that regulate and frame nursing practice. Throughout your pre-registration nursing program, your education (both theory and clinical) was aimed at ensuring that you were competent to practise according to these professional codes and standards. To be eligible to register as a nurse, you need to be able to satisfactorily demonstrate each of the required standards, as well as your adherence to professional codes around conduct and ethics. They are used by your university to assess your readiness for registration, but they do not cease to be relevant once you have graduated and registered. On the contrary, professional practice standards provide the *minimum* standards at which you are expected to practise all of the time. It is against these standards that your performance will continue to be measured. Ensure that you stay familiar with them, use them to inform your practice and continue to evaluate your own performance against them. Regardless of where you work, adherence to professional standards involves functioning within your scope of practice, critical thinking, reflective practice and continuing professional development.

As a registered nurse, you hold a protected title and registration with the regulating authority in your country. These are key considerations in recognising your role, responsibilities and expectations as a nurse within the community – they cannot be taken lightly. This recognition of your role encompasses understanding and functioning within your **scope of practice**. Scope of practice is determined by your registration status, organisational role and context of employment (Birks et al., 2016).

Nurses at all levels, not just those entering practice, are required to understand their limitations and practise within the constraints of their level of competency. Functioning within scope of practice is not just a professional requirement, it is also a legal one. Unfortunately, things sometimes go wrong in the healthcare context, resulting in legal or coronial action. When this happens, attention will be paid to whether a nurse functioned in accordance with the expectations inherent in their role. Accepted scope of practice, relevant to the specific context and the educational and experiential levels of the nurse, is the standard applied in such circumstances. It is critical that you understand your scope of practice to ensure that you do not practise beyond what is acceptable. It also ensures that you contribute to the full extent of your professional capacity to achieve positive patient outcomes, regardless of the context.

Critical thinking is a professional capability that is essential for nurses at all levels of experience, in order to perform competently in the professional nursing role. Critical thinking is the structured approach to analysis and the interpretation of information as a basis for understanding and responding to a range of simple to complex situations. It is inherent in all standards for practice, regardless of where you work. Critical thinking underpins most aspects of nursing practice – from time management and the performance of nursing interventions, through to the application of knowledge and the impact of personal values on practice. Sound clinical reasoning and the ability to make informed decisions rely on critical thinking (LeMone et al., 2017). Critical thinking therefore enables psychomotor, cognitive and affective skills to be applied in ways that positively serve independent practice, decision-making, resourcefulness, leadership, advocacy and relationships. It can, however, be one of the most difficult skills for novice nurses to master. The workload of a nurse can be large and fast-paced, often requiring quick thinking and fast but appropriate responses. The critical thinking skills that you learnt in your undergraduate nursing studies are quickly put to the test as a new graduate, sometimes in environments that have the potential to cloud professional judgments.

Scope of practice

The range of responsibilities and activities that nurses are educated, competent and permitted by law to undertake.

Critical thinking

The structured approach to analysis and interpretation of information as a basis for understanding and responding to a range of simple to complex situations.

Therefore, it is important to seek opportunities that help you develop your critical thinking capability. Be aware, however, that critical thinking is achieved over time and with increasing confidence and experience. We often speak about a nurse's 'intuition' associated with thinking and decision-making. This intuition is the result of experience, combined with education and the ability to see beyond what is initially evident. Keep in mind that all nurses commence their nursing careers as novice critical thinkers. With time and practice they were able to develop this skill – so will you, as your experience and confidence grows.

Reflection is an extension of critical thinking in that it enables the necessary examination of a situation from varying perspectives. **Reflective practice** is identified as a key element in professional nursing standards in both Australia and New Zealand. Undertaking reflection can be challenging and its value is therefore often overlooked; however, it is vital to take time to reflect on your practice, your interactions with others and the care you deliver. Reflection is a learned skill and one of the most important in your development as a professional (Francis & Salmon, 2020). The process of reflection can be formal, through mechanisms such as keeping a journal, or informal, such as thinking over your day on the commute home. Regardless of whether you engage in reflection formally or informally, this practice is a key element of the professional nursing role. Your approach to reflection will vary depending on the situation, but it should encompass such aspects as the physical task, the feelings of those involved and the need for further learning.

Reflective practice

The formal or informal process of reviewing and evaluating events for the purpose of improving future outcomes.

🏃 Portfolio Activity 7.2: Stop, reflect and think

Think about a recent experience while on placement that raised concerns for you. Use the following questions to reflect on the experience.

- What did I do? Why did I do it that way? Was it the best way?
- How was I feeling?
- What worked and what did not?
- If it happened again, what would I do differently?
- What was the patient's/colleague's reaction?
- What things do I need to better understand?
- What areas do I need to develop further?

After working through these questions, has your perspective on the experience changed?

Reflecting on your day-to-day activities will help you to identify your ongoing learning needs (Coward, 2018). Healthcare is a field of rapid change with new and continually changing technologies, medications and treatments. Within your area of practice, it is essential that you continue to update your knowledge and skills so that your care is current, best practice and evidence-based. For this reason, and to maintain your annual registration, you are required to undertake **continuing professional development** (CPD) activities. In Australia, this is 20 hours annually and in New Zealand it is 60 hours over the past three years. CPD activities can take many forms such as formal education, engagement with professional activities or engagement with professional literature.

Continuing professional development

Engagement in learning activities that ensure currency of practice and promote professional growth.

Disappointingly, many nurses fail to appreciate the importance of CPD. They may choose educational opportunities randomly, or activities that may be poorly aligned with their work, or they may not keep effective records of their learning. The learning can be meaningless if there is little reflection on what has been covered or if it is irrelevant to the practice setting. In such cases, it is unlikely that any learning will be translated into the delivery of patient care. In both Australia and New Zealand, nurses' education records are audited regularly. It is therefore important for you to be familiar with and understand the requirements of your registering authority, and that you maintain rigorous records of your education activity. As discussed in Chapter 3, maintaining a professional portfolio is an essential component of being a registered health professional. Commencing a professional portfolio early in your nursing career (we recommend from day 1 of your nursing program) cultivates professional readiness, and regularly maintaining it supports you to adhere to professional standards throughout your nursing career.

 Portfolio Activity: Making the transition

As a health professional, you will be required to undertake CPD in order to maintain your registration. Visit the website of your regulatory authority to identify the specific requirements that you must meet in respect of CPD when you are working as a registered nurse.

OXFORD UNIVERSITY PRESS

> ## Case Study 7.2: Adherence to standards
>
> Jake is undertaking placement in his final year. He is placed in a medical unit and is assigned to care for a woman with a substance abuse problem who is receiving treatment for a severe infection of her kidneys. Jake believes that the woman's health problems are of her own making and his attitude clearly reflects this position.
>
> - Which professional standards is Jake breaching in this instance?
>
> - How might he use reflection to address his response to this patient?

Professional identity

In order to function effectively, nurses must establish and maintain their professional identity. This identity is characterised by accountability, honesty and integrity, professional presence and e-professionalism. The concept of **professional accountability** is alluded to throughout much of the nursing literature. Krautscheid (2014) provided a specific definition for professional accountability in nursing:

> … taking responsibility for one's nursing judgments, actions, and omissions as they relate to life-long learning, maintaining competency, and upholding both quality patient care outcomes and standards of the profession while being answerable to those who are influenced by one's nursing practice (p. 46).

Hence, nurses are accountable for their actions to a range of key stakeholders, including patients and their families, their employing organisation, other nurses and health professionals, and the nursing profession more broadly. Nurses who display professional accountability assume ownership of their decisions, admit their mistakes and are not afraid to report errors. Nurses who are accountable recognise that these actions are necessary to protect themselves, their colleagues and their patients.

Honesty and integrity are other key components of your professional identify. As a nurse, you occupy a privileged position. The profession places high expectations on you regarding honesty and integrity. What do honesty and

Professional accountability

Taking responsibility for your decisions and actions.

integrity mean in practice? Being honest is to be authentic and to tell the truth. Acting with integrity is based on honesty and means that you can be relied upon to do the right thing, act in accordance with your professional standards and take responsibility for your actions. Honesty and integrity also relate to your ability to acknowledge limitations in your knowledge and practice, and to address these. Thus, honesty and integrity augment professional accountability.

For decades, nurses have been identified as the most trusted professionals. Trust between nurses and patients, between nurses and nurses and between nurses and other members of the healthcare team is essential for safe and effective practice. Patients and their families need to feel safe and that they will not come to any harm, that they are able to confide in you and share personal experiences, knowing that the information they provide will remain confidential and that they will not be judged. This relies on our honesty and integrity.

Central to gaining insight into your practice, and therefore functioning within the boundaries of our professional standards, is reflective practice. As discussed, reflecting on our day-to-day activities can raise our awareness of how we practise, help identify and acknowledge gaps and limitations and, when we are honest and acknowledge these, allow us to take responsible actions to work on them.

Nurses display their professional identity by having a professional presence, which is reflected in their behaviour and presentation. In Chapter 6, we discussed how our professional behaviour is reflected in our attitude. Attitudes play an important role in the work of professionals. Sometimes we hold personal attitudes that may be different from those our professional values require. In such cases, professional standards dictate that we put our personal beliefs aside and respect the wishes of our patients.

Case Study 7.3: Professional presence

Later in his final year placement, Jake is caring for a 72-year-old man who is suffering from terminal cancer. With his healthcare team, this man has decided to cease all active treatment and receive only palliative care. Jake's belief system is based on the sanctity of life principle, and he is conflicted about caring for a man whose death is imminent in spite of treatment options being available that might prolong his life. Jake has asked to be removed from this man's care team.

- If you were the nurse in charge of this unit, how would you respond to this request?

- What factors are important for Jake to explain, to clarify his request?

Presentation is crucial to the image of a nurse and their ability to demonstrate professionalism. Pawlowski et al. (2019) conducted a review of literature to explore patients' perspectives on professional nursing attire. They found that there was a relationship between the appearance of nurses and patients' perceptions of nurses' skills and professionalism. Professional nursing attire varies from workplace to workplace, and is designed to be comfortable but practical. Infection control considerations should underpin how you present yourself; for example, maintaining cleanliness and regularly laundering your uniform to reduce pathogen transfer to vulnerable patients. Jewellery can lead to patient injury, such as skin tears in elderly patients, so should be kept to a minimum.

Throughout your education, you would have identified clinicians who were good or bad role models. Your professional behaviours were developed through observing their practice, even if you were not aware of it. Access to effective clinical role models has been found to be vital for nursing students in developing their own professionalism (Felstead & Springett, 2016), so it is important to be continually aware of the role modelling you are providing to those around you. Recent research suggests that new graduate nurses actually provide teaching, both formal and informal, for a range of groups, including nursing students (McKenna et al., 2018). As a registered nurse, you will become a role model for students and other health professionals. They will watch how you interact with patients, families, other nurses and the healthcare team. Your professional presence – how you behave and how you present yourself – will influence their own development as a professional and consequently the image they present to the public, that represents the nursing profession.

Portfolio Activity: Making the transition

Consider teachers and role models who have made an impact on you throughout your life. What characteristics and behaviours did they display that made them memorable? How will your experience with these role models influence your own approach to formal and informal teaching in your role as a professional registered nurse?

As nurses, we can use social media to keep abreast of health breakthroughs and new research, upcoming conferences and seminars, and political and professional issues relevant to our work, as well as happenings in professional nursing, midwifery and other organisations (McGrath et al., 2019). Recently, the concept of e-professionalism has emerged to describe the expectations of professionals and their use of online communication platforms (McGrath et al., 2019; Ryan et al., 2019). There are important boundaries that professionals must establish around their use of social media platforms. It is important to remember that anyone can see what you post, even if you post to a closed group. It only takes one member of the group to share what you have posted for it to become public. Without even naming a patient or a hospital, what you post could be identifiable and linked directly to you. It is important to remember that even though you may remove a post, it remains in the system and can be accessed by authorities should the need arise. Brookes (2017) suggests that before making any social media post, we must consider 'to post, or not to post' (p. 34). What you post on social media, including your personal posts, says a great deal about you as a professional. Increasingly, employers are examining applicants' social media pages prior to proceeding with interviews and subsequent employment. Hence, it is vital that, as professionals, you take extreme care with everything you post, like and share on social media.

Box 7.1 contains key recommendations developed by Ryan et al. (2019, p. 34) on how nurses could manage their social media activity. In addition to this sage advice, we suggest that you should avoid posting photographs where you are in uniform or where your staff ID badge is visible. Ensure that your posts do not, directly or inadvertently, indicate endorsement or otherwise of products or services where this may constitute a conflict of interest.

Box 7.1 Managing social media activity

- Use appropriate and separate platforms for personal, educational and professional purposes, LinkedIn for professional profiles and Facebook for personal profiles.
- Draw up a custom list of specific friends and family on online social networks such as Facebook so that posts have limited and focused reach.
- Do not have your employer and position listed publicly on personal online social media profiles.
- Every 3–6 months, or when privacy settings are updated, use an internet search engine or online social network search function to view what information the public can see about you online.
- Where the function is available, unlink your online profile from internet search engines.
- Use functions that control who can tag and share your posts, and use the option to review posts to your Facebook timeline to limit unintended consequences, such as other people being able to copy, edit or share a photo in a different context.
- Make sure any information that relates to healthcare or nursing practice you share is up to date and evidence based.
- Think carefully about the profile pictures you use online and photos that are publicly accessible, and whether you want to be identifiable from these.

(Ryan et al., 2019, p. 34)

Effective resource management

Contemporary healthcare systems are complex, with increasingly more acute patients and sophisticated and continually evolving treatments. Inpatient stays are becoming shorter and resources increasingly tight. On any day, nurses face multiple demands on their time, with many conflicting responsibilities. Unexpected events, such as a postoperative patient suddenly deteriorating, can impact on the care delivered to a nurse's allocated patients. When you manage resources effectively, you are better able to manage your responsibilities in stressful situations and reduce the workload of the healthcare team overall. Key skills that can assist you to manage resources strategically and effectively are time management, prioritisation, leadership, supervision and delegation.

Initially, newly qualified nurses are often set a reduced workload to enable them to adapt to their role and work environment. They nonetheless need to be organised and able to prioritise workloads in order to perform to the required level in their role. A basic level of organisational skills is essential for safe, efficient care, particularly in environments that are characterised by unpredictable change and fluctuating workloads. Time management skills are key to working through the daily responsibilities of a graduate nurse, as these ensure an orderly approach to workload management. All clinical care will be completed and nothing will be missed, particularly in peak periods of high demand and rapid change. Effective time management relies on personal readiness capabilities, as discussed in Chapter 6, in particular being resilient, confident and effective in self and relationship management. It also involves critical thinking and knowing how to prioritise care and delegate appropriately.

Prioritisation

Process of ordering work tasks according to their level of importance.

Prioritisation is about examining your workday and setting priorities for getting through what needs to be done, allowing time for unexpected activities that may occur during your shift. To do this, you need to be able to determine the level of importance of your work tasks and order them accordingly. Naturally, focus needs to be placed on the delivery of basic care needs for your allocated patients such as hygiene, vital signs monitoring, wound management, medication administration and so on. Logically, the most urgent and important tasks will be prioritised; however, the order of priority is not always easy to ascertain. Drawing on your critical thinking and problem-solving skills will help determine this, and how you can manage your tasks and resources efficiently. Ask for help! Your peers and colleagues have clinical and practical experience in prioritisation and can help you develop your ability to prioritise clinical demands. Generally, once determined, these can be scheduled into a daily worksheet of activities, largely focusing on the work to be done at the bedside.

Other things also need to be considered, such as including meal breaks for yourself and your team, covering for colleagues when they are on meal breaks, medical rounds, and organisational tasks such as documentation and attending meetings. Think about the less visible components of patient care, such as attending to social, spiritual or emotional needs – these are often left out (Suhonen et al., 2018) and can lead to patient distress. Failure to prioritise these activities because they are considered to be less important than the tangible aspects of bedside care can contribute to detrimental outcomes that negate any perceived benefit of skipping a break or failing to attend to a patient's non-physical needs. What is the best way to organise the many different activities that need to be done? There is no right or wrong answer, and over time you will find what works best for you. As noted earlier, drawing on your peers, thinking critically and gaining experience will help you develop a system that works effectively. Overall, it is important to ensure that the key patient care activities are completed, and there is time available to address unexpected activities.

A key factor in effective resource management is leadership. As a beginning practitioner, you may not consider yourself a leader. The very nature of nursing practice, however, means that nurses at all levels in all workplace settings must demonstrate leadership in order to fulfil their role effectively. Leadership does not require a formal title; rather, it depends on your ability to recognise and respond to situations in a way that instils in others confidence in the outcome. The most significant resource you will deal with as a registered nurse is people. Leadership skills are critical in getting the most and best out of other people. Every interaction in healthcare is a transaction – patients, clients, colleagues and even management are more likely to respond positively when interacting with you, if you demonstrate leadership skills. Leadership skills are a combination of various personal and professional capabilities and qualities. Many of these capabilities are encompassed in the four domains of readiness; for example, a balanced level of confidence, effective communication and relationship management, emotional intelligence and empathy, problem-solving, decision-making and honesty, integrity and professional presentation. All the readiness capabilities together contribute to your ability to lead others. In Chapter 12 we will extend this discussion on leadership and how finding mentors to guide your professional development will enhance your capability to lead and manage healthcare effectively.

 Portfolio Activity 7.3: Stop, reflect and think

Many of us have worked with people who occupy senior positions yet do not command respect as a leader. Conversely, there are individuals who are our peers yet demonstrate clear leadership qualities. Think about a person you have encountered who you would describe as a leader. What characteristics did they display that made them effective in leading others?

Supervision and delegation are other important parts of time, task and resource management. Supervision is oversight of the activities of another person or group of people to ensure they function safely and effectively. It can involve direct teaching or coaching, as well as confirming that any assigned tasks are completed appropriately.

Supervision

Oversight of the activities of another person or group of people to ensure they function safely and effectively.

Delegation

Allocation of prioritised
activities to another
person to ensure timely
completion.

Delegation involves allocating some of your prioritised activities to another person to ensure timely completion. Registered nurses work with key personnel who can assist with achieving tasks required in a day; for example, enrolled nurses, specialist health workers (such as Aboriginal health workers in Australia and Kaiawhina in New Zealand), nursing assistants and students. Many tasks in the delivery of patient care are delegated by registered nurses as part of an effective system of workload and resource management.

It can take time to develop the confidence to effectively delegate to other healthcare workers. Some of the best resources that assist registered nurses to do this safely and effectively are the various standards and guidelines for practice. Examples of these are given in Box 7.2.

Box 7.2   Standards and guidelines to inform delegation

> Australian Nursing and Midwifery Federation. (2018). *Delegation by registered nurses*. http://anf.org.au/documents/policies/G_Delegation_RNs.pdf
>
> Nursing Council of New Zealand. (2012). *Competencies for enrolled nurses*. https://www.nursingcouncil.org.nz/Public/Nursing/Standards_and_guidelines/NCNZ/nursing-section/Standards_and_guidelines_for_nurses.aspx
>
> Nursing Council of New Zealand. (2007). *Competencies for registered nurses*. https://www.nursingcouncil.org.nz/Public/Nursing/Standards_and_guidelines/NCNZ/nursing-section/Standards_and_guidelines_for_nurses.aspx
>
> Nursing Council of New Zealand. (2011). *Guideline: Delegation of care by a registered nurse to a healthcare assistant*. https://www.nursingcouncil.org.nz/Public/Nursing/Standards_and_guidelines/NCNZ/nursing-section/Standards_and_guidelines_for_nurses.aspx
>
> Nursing Council of New Zealand. (2011). *Guideline: Responsibilities for direction and delegation of care to enrolled nurses*. https://www.nursingcouncil.org.nz/Public/Nursing/Standards_and_guidelines/NCNZ/nursing-section/Standards_and_guidelines_for_nurses.aspx
>
> Nursing and Midwifery Board of Australia. (2016). *Enrolled nurse standards for practice*. https://www.nursingmidwiferyboard.gov.au/Codes-Guidelines-Statements/Professional-standards.aspx
>
> Nursing and Midwifery Board of Australia. (2016). *Registered nurse standards for practice*. https://www.nursingmidwiferyboard.gov.au/Codes-Guidelines-Statements/Professional-standards.aspx
>
> Nursing and Midwifery Board of Australia. (2020). *Decision-making framework for nursing and midwifery*. https://www.nursingmidwiferyboard.gov.au/Codes-Guidelines-Statements/Frameworks.aspx

The ability to effectively supervise and delegate tasks takes time and experience to develop. It can be challenging to start delegating activities as a new graduate, especially if delegating to very experienced or older colleagues. It is important to access available resources and be open to learning opportunities that will assist you to develop the required skills, and to regularly seek guidance from experienced colleagues. Whenever possible, try to observe how more experienced colleagues delegate activities, and monitor the outcomes. Try to understand how they choose the tasks to delegate, and who they do and do not delegate to. Remember that overall patient safety must be paramount in deciding who can deliver elements of care and that delegation, in particular, must be in the best interests of the patient.

Case Study 7.4: Delegation

Jake is excited about commencing his final consolidation placement in a busy surgical unit. He is given a larger patient allocation to assist in transitioning to his role as a registered nurse at the end of the year. An enrolled nurse, June, is assigned to work alongside him. June appears to struggle with taking direction from a student, but Jake really needs June to work with him as a team and accept delegated tasks.

- What should Jake do to facilitate this outcome?

- What personal and professional readiness skills can he draw on to be able to effectively delegate tasks to June?

 Portfolio Activity: Making the transition

Using the worksheet in Appendix 7, rate your professional readiness capabilities. Are there areas you think you need to improve to enhance your transition to practice? Drawing on what you have learnt in this chapter, formulate a plan for developing and maintaining your professional readiness for practice.

Conclusion

Nursing is a highly valued profession within society. One of the many aspects of the role that makes nursing such an attractive career is the opportunity to work closely with patients, their families and the community. Nursing registration is a great achievement, but it brings a range of responsibilities and accountabilities. As a new graduate nurse, you will be expected to adhere to the standards that govern nursing practice, including functioning within the scope of that practice, engaging in critical and reflective thinking, and ensuring ongoing professional development. Establishing and maintaining your professional identity is critical to your ability to practise with honesty and integrity and be accountable for your actions. Your ability to maintain a professional presence, including online, further promotes a positive professional identity. Finally, the ability to manage resources – human and physical – will round off your professional readiness for practice as a registered nurse.

Key summary points

- Professional readiness is the capability that graduate nurses require in order to work efficiently and provide care in accordance with registered nurse standards and codes of practice.

- Capabilities in professional readiness are critical for making the transition from student to registered nurse.

- Capabilities for professional readiness include adherence to professional standards, professional identity and effective resource management.

- Graduate nurses demonstrate adherence to standards through functioning within their scope of practice, engaging in critical thinking, practising reflectively and undertaking continuing professional development.

- Professional identity is demonstrated through professional accountability, honesty and integrity and displaying a professional presence including e-professionalism.

- Time management, prioritisation and delegation are necessary skills for effective resource management.

Critical thinking questions

1. What do you consider are the important aspects of professional readiness, and why?

2. Some may argue that professional presentation is not important as long as a nurse is competent in their role. Do you agree with this statement? What would be the opposing perspective?

3. How will being professionally ready support you during your transition to practice as a registered nurse?

4. As you approach completion of your nursing program, consider the distinction between the professional readiness of a nursing student nearing completion, and that of a new graduate nurse. Do you expect the transition to be a smooth extension of your current role, or are you anticipating a significant jump in expectations? How will you prepare, if it is the latter?

OXFORD UNIVERSITY PRESS

References

Australian Nursing and Midwifery Federation. (2018). *Delegation by registered nurses*. http://anf.org.au/documents/policies/G_Delegation_RNs.pdf

Birks, M., Davis, J., Smithson, J., & Cant, R. (2016). Registered nurse scope of practice in Australia: An integrative review of the literature. *Contemporary Nurse, 52*(5), 522–543. https://doi.org/10.1080/10376178.2016.1238773

Blevins, S., & Millen, E. A. (2016). Foundation for new graduate nurse success. *MEDSURG Nursing, 25*(3), 194–201.

Brookes, G. (2017). To post or not to post? Social media and nursing. *Kai Taiki New Zealand, 23*(2), 34.

Coward, M. (2018). Encouraging reflection in professional learning. *Nursing Management, 25*(2), 38–41. https://doi.org/10.7748/nm.2018.e1752

Felstead, I. S., & Springett, K. (2016). An exploration of role model influence on adult nursing students' professional development: A phenomenological research study. *Nurse Education Today, 37*, 66–70. https://doi.org/10.1016/j.nedt.2015.11.014

Francis, M., & Salmon, A. (2020). Reflection and clinical supervision. In M. Birks, J. Davis & Y. Chapman (Eds.), *Professional and therapeutic communication* (2nd ed., pp. 61–74). Oxford University Press.

Harrison, H., Birks, M., Franklin, R., & Mills, J. (2020). An assessment continuum: How healthcare professionals define and determine practice readiness of newly graduated registered nurses. *Collegian, 27*(2), 198–206. https://doi.org/10.1016/j.colegn.2019.07.003

Krautscheid, L. C. (2014). Defining professional nursing accountability: A literature review. *Journal of Professional Nursing, 30*(1), 43–47. https://doi.org/10.1016/j.profnurs.2013.06.008

LeMone, P., Burke, K., Bauldoff, G., Gubrud-Howe, P., Levett-Jones, T., Hales, M., Berry, K., Carville, K., Dwyer, T., Knox, N., Moxham, L., Raymond, D., & Reid-Searl, K. (2017). *Medical-surgical nursing: Critical thinking for person-centred care* (3rd ed.). Pearson.

McGrath, L., Swift, A., Clark, M., & Bradbury-Jones, C. (2019). Understanding the benefits and risks of nursing students engaging with online social media. *Nursing Standard, 34*(1), 45–49. https://doi.org/10.7748/ns.2019.e11362

McKenna, L., Irvine, S., & Williams, B. (2018). 'I didn't expect teaching to be such a huge part of nursing': A follow-up qualitative exploration of new graduates' teaching activities. *Nurse Education in Practice, 32*, 9–13. https://doi.org/10.1016/j.nepr.2018.06.010

Nursing and Midwifery Board of Australia. (2016a). *Enrolled nurse standards for practice*. https://www.nursingmidwiferyboard.gov.au/Codes-Guidelines-Statements/Professional-standards.aspx

Nursing and Midwifery Board of Australia. (2016b). *Registered nurse standards for practice*. https://www.nursingmidwiferyboard.gov.au/Codes-Guidelines-Statements/Professional-standards.aspx

Nursing and Midwifery Board of Australia. (2020). *Decision-making framework for nursing and midwifery*. https://www.nursingmidwiferyboard.gov.au/Codes-Guidelines-Statements/Frameworks.aspx

Nursing Council of New Zealand. (2007). *Competencies for registered nurses*. https://www.nursingcouncil.org.nz/Public/Nursing/Standards_and_guidelines/NCNZ/nursing-section/Standards_and_guidelines_for_nurses.aspx

Nursing Council of New Zealand. (2011a). *Guideline: Delegation of care by a registered nurse to a healthcare assistant*. https://www.nursingcouncil.org.nz/Public/Nursing/Standards_and_guidelines/NCNZ/nursing-section/Standards_and_guidelines_for_nurses.aspx

Nursing Council of New Zealand. (2011b). *Guideline: Responsibilities for direction and delegation of care to enrolled nurses*. https://www.nursingcouncil.org.nz/Public/Nursing/Standards_and_guidelines/NCNZ/nursing-section/Standards_and_guidelines_for_nurses.aspx

Nursing Council of New Zealand. (2012). *Competencies for enrolled nurses*. https://www.nursingcouncil.org.nz/Public/Nursing/Standards_and_guidelines/NCNZ/nursing-section/Standards_and_guidelines_for_nurses.aspx

Pawlowski, P., Mazurek, P., Zych, M., Zun, K., & Dobrowolska, B. (2019). Nursing dress code and perception of a nurse by patients. *Nursing in the 21st Century*, *18*(1), 60–67. https://doi.org/ 10.2478/pielxxiw-2019-0008

Perez, R. (2019). What does it mean to be a professional? *Professional Case Management*, *24*(2), 212. https://doi.org/10.1097/NCM.0000000000000373

Price, B. (2015). Applying critical thinking to nursing. *Nursing Standard*, *29*(51), 49–60. https://doi.org/10.7748/ns.29.51.49.e10005

Ryan, G., Jackson, J., & Cornock, M. (2019). Exploring public perspectives of e-professionalism in nursing. *Nursing Management*, *26*(6), 29–35. https://doi.org/10.7748/nm.2019.e1870

Suhonen, R., Stolt, M., Habermann, M., Hjaltadottir, I., Vryonides, S., Tonnessen, S., Halvorsen, K., Harvey, C., Toffoli, L., & Scott, A. (2018). Ethical elements in priority setting in nursing care: A scoping review. *International Journal of Nursing Studies*, *88*, 25–42. https://doi.org/10.1016/j.ijnurstu.2018.08.006

OXFORD UNIVERSITY PRESS

Chapter 8

Clinical Readiness

Elisabeth Jacob and Hugh Davies

Learning Outcomes

Following completion of this chapter, you will be able to:

1. Define the term 'clinical readiness' in respect of nursing practice.

2. Explain the importance of clinical readiness in nursing.

3. Describe the capabilities associated with clinical readiness.

4. Reflect on your own clinical readiness.

5. Formulate a plan for developing and maintaining clinical readiness in practice.

Key terms

| Clinical readiness | Evidence-based practice | Policies and procedures |

Introduction

If you are like most nursing students, you have chosen to study nursing because you are attracted to the practice-based nature of the profession. You will have undertaken multiple clinical placements and have no doubt found them to be the most challenging and enjoyable part of your studies. Because the nursing program you are studying has been approved by your country's accrediting authority, you can have confidence that the knowledge and skills you have been acquiring are those that enable you to transition to practising safely as a registered nurse. On achieving registration, health services will be expecting you to commence your graduate year with the required degree of clinical readiness. This chapter focuses on what it means to be clinically ready for nursing practice, and discusses the capabilities that ensure that you are ready to function safely in the clinical environment.

> ## Case Study 8.1: Introducing Kelly
>
> Kelly is a 20-year-old student who enrolled in a nursing program immediately after finishing high school. All her life, her family and friends have said that Kelly has the perfect disposition for a caring profession like nursing. She has done particularly well with the theoretical aspects of her studies and has successfully completed all clinical placements since commencing her course.

Clinical readiness defined

Clinical readiness

The capability to provide a safe, basic level of clinical care within one's scope of practice.

A variety of views exist on what it means to be ready for clinical practice. **Clinical readiness** is shaped by individual expectations on what is required to provide safe and effective nursing care (Wolff et al., 2010). These expectations are often defined according to the context from which the views were obtained, particularly when participants are surveyed from different nursing specialties. New nurses commence practice as a registered nurse in a range of different clinical settings and locations and will experience a variety of clinical scenarios. Therefore, it is important that you have sound fundamental, basic clinical capabilities that can be applied in different situations and settings and ensure safe, efficient nursing practice. Clinical readiness supports you to accomplish this. It is defined as having the capability to provide a safe, basic level of clinical care within your scope of practice. As discussed in previous chapters, contemporary healthcare now deals with higher patient acuity and more complex conditions. Registered nurses must be able to identify and manage changes in patients' conditions, and provide the required nursing care. Clinical readiness encompasses the competent use of nursing knowledge and skills to safely care for patients in a dynamic clinical environment. It therefore draws on all other domains of practice readiness, as seen in Figure 8.1.

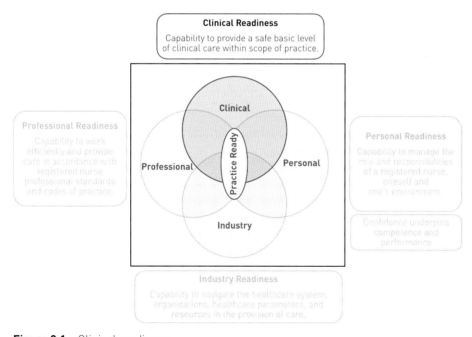

Figure 8.1 Clinical readiness

The importance of clinical readiness

Clinical readiness is one of the most recognisable elements of practice readiness. It is essential that as a graduating registered nurse you are ready for practice in the clinical setting. In Chapter 1 we considered the evolving nature of healthcare and the consequent evolution of nursing roles and practice. In Chapter 2 we considered the growing demand for healthcare in Australia and New Zealand. The complexity of patients with a variety of co-morbidities, changes to healthcare delivery due to political reform, and geographic location of service delivery make clinical practice dynamic and challenging. A well-prepared, clinically competent nursing workforce is critical in addressing these changing needs. The provision of a safe level of care relies on you having a sound level of basic, general clinical knowledge and skills and the ability to bring these together across a range of clinical scenarios.

Possessing a basic level of capability provides a platform for you to build upon, develop and advance your clinical practice. This supports you to manage more clinically complex and/or specialised care and opens options about where you might like to work, thus progressing your career as a nurse. While all forms of readiness discussed in this text are essential for successful transition to the registered nurse role, clinical readiness is the one that most directly impacts patients' physical, mental, emotional and spiritual well-being. Therefore, it is vital that you develop clinical readiness.

As discussed in earlier chapters, industry concerns with respect to clinical readiness tend to be directed at addressing the gap between theory (or knowledge) and practice. This refers to concerns about the difference between practising in an educational context and in a clinical environment. To assist graduates' transition to their new role, many health services provide them with support during their transition year (discussed in Chapter 11). While the transition year is important to consolidate the knowledge, skills and attitudes of new graduates, it is also important to remember that, as discussed in Chapter 5, the process of transition to registered nurse actually commences from the first day of pre-registration study through to completion of the first year of practice (Harrison et al., 2020). Your first year of practice as a registered nurse will be more productive and fulfilling with a sound level of clinical readiness and, with the variety of opportunities open to you during this year, you will continue to hone and develop your clinical readiness capabilities.

Capabilities associated with clinical readiness

Capabilities associated with clinical readiness include the broad range of skills that enable you to function effectively and safely within a variety of healthcare contexts. Clinical readiness requires not only appreciating why clinical activities are performed but knowing how to perform them safely and efficiently in the practice context (Table 8.1). Remember that this book is not intended to revisit the extensive knowledge, skills and advanced nursing concepts learned in your program to this point. The following discussion will instead focus on enabling you to understand how your knowledge and skills (the science of nursing) can be translated into practice (the art of nursing) as you transition to the role of registered nurse. To perform well in your new role, you need to understand the 'why' of your practice, as well as 'how' to perform clinical skills. This has been the focus of your studies to this point. In the final stage of preparation for your role, your focus will shift to integration and consolidation, requiring that you possess an understanding of 'what' needs to be done to function effectively as a registered nurse. Table 8.1 summarises these concepts.

Table 8.1   Capabilities associated with clinical readiness

Appreciating the 'why' of clinical nursing	Knowing 'how' to nurse clinically	Understanding 'what' needs to be done
• Fundamental clinical knowledge • Evidence base for practice	• Basic clinical skills • Safe, quality care within your scope of practice	• Translating knowledge and skills into practice • Pulling it all together

 ## Portfolio Activity 8.1: Stop, reflect and think

Consider the idea that nursing is a science and an art. Is nursing more art than science or is there a balance? Which of these concepts is more important?

Appreciating the 'why' of clinical nursing

Many nursing students commence their studies with great enthusiasm, relishing their time in the simulation laboratories and on placement. You no doubt enjoyed all the opportunities to learn and practise new skills in preparation for your professional role. We often hear students comment that they wish there was more time devoted to the hands-on aspect of their studies. Theoretical understanding is, however, central to appreciating the 'why' of clinical nursing. Appreciating why we perform the skills we do as nurses prevents a focus on performing tasks without understanding the rationale. The ability to think critically is dependent on possessing fundamental clinical knowledge. Note that general nursing knowledge is a fundamental requirement in clinical and professional readiness, but it is in respect of clinical readiness that this knowledge is operationalised.

Broad, basic clinical nursing knowledge that is relevant to all areas of healthcare provides new graduate nurses with a foundation on which to build clinical capabilities. There is no expectation that beginning practitioners will have advanced skills or specialist knowledge, regardless of the area of practice in which they are first employed. Rather, what is required is a fundamental theoretical understanding of the biosciences – anatomy, physiology and pathophysiology. Understanding variations in health and wellness is essential for assessing, diagnosing and managing a range of clinical presentations. A foundation in the sciences includes knowledge of the pharmacological concepts that underpin medication prescribing and administration principles.

In addition to this broad foundation of biological sciences, knowledge of behavioural sciences, including psychology and sociology, is needed in order to understand the relationship between social and psychological factors, health and illness and individual responses to changes in health status. As nurses work in an environment regulated by national, jurisdictional and local legislation and policy, a comprehensive understanding of professional and legal concepts, as well as a thorough understanding of ethical principles, constitutes baseline knowledge for practice.

OXFORD UNIVERSITY PRESS

This fundamental knowledge ensures that graduate nurses have a solid evidence base for practice. **Evidence-based** practice requires the use of available, reliable and current evidence to support the delivery of nursing care. As well as having the technical skills to undertake clinical work, nurses must be able to perform interventions that are grounded in evidence. Being clinically ready demands an ability to use evidence when making clinical judgments about how best to care for your patients. Adherence to standards and codes of practice requires that you are able to access, understand and apply current evidence in the provision of patient care. Evidence may be obtained from reading journal articles, attending conferences or workshops or joining communities of interest. Health services also play a part in enabling nurses to practise from an evidence base by conducting in-service education programs, providing study opportunities, supporting nursing research, and developing evidence-based policies and procedures.

A potential barrier to adopting evidence-based practice is the large amount of healthcare literature that exists. This can be a source of controversy if critical analysis is not applied to the available evidence. Your skill as a critical reader of research findings and their application to clinical practice requires you to make judgments on whether to accept or reject the evidence presented. You will encounter a number of clinical problems in your career – knowing how to find relevant evidence, evaluate that evidence and make a clinical judgment call as to the validity of the study in the context of the circumstances of your clinical problem, reflects clinical readiness. A key resource for practice can be found in the form of evidence summaries that assist in distilling the large amount of evidence available. An example of such resources is clinical practice guidelines. These are:

> … evidence based statements that include recommendations intended to optimise patient care and assist healthcare practitioners to make decisions about appropriate healthcare for specific clinical circumstances. Clinical practice guidelines should assist clinicians and patients in shared decision-making (National Health and Medical Research Council [NHMRC], 2017).

Evidence-based practice

The use of available, reliable and current evidence to support the delivery of nursing care.

Portfolio Activity: Making the transition

Access clinical practice guidelines via the websites below:

- https://www.guidelinecentral.com/summaries/specialties/nursing/
- https://www.clinicalguidelines.gov.au/

  Browse the available guidelines or conduct a specific search on a disease or condition you expect to encounter in your intended area of practice. Were guidelines available? How valuable might clinical guidelines be in ensuring your practice is evidence-based as you make the transition to the professional role?

Knowing 'how' to nurse clinically

You no doubt recognise that, as evidence-based professionals, nurses must possess the ability to utilise a broad set of skills. In most settings, graduate nurses are not expected to demonstrate specialist skills or perform at an expert level. Having a basic level of general clinical capability provides the platform for you to develop proficiency as you practise in the registered nurse role. Consolidating and establishing your basic fundamental clinical capabilities takes three to six months and is a necessary foundation on which you can develop more advanced clinical practice over time. You will, however, be required to commence your professional role with the ability to carry out basic clinical skills.

Basic clinical skills are those that are most commonly performed in the majority of practice settings. The ability to conduct health assessments, plan and evaluate care based on that assessment, assist with activities of daily living (ADLs), wound care, medication administration and documentation are fundamental nursing skills. As healthcare becomes increasingly complex, nurses must be able to operate and keep pace with the growing use of technology in the clinical environment. While we refer to these skills as 'basic', they are nonetheless a specialised component of a unique profession, and competency in the performance of clinical activities is an essential element of clinical readiness.

We have emphasised throughout this text the interrelated nature of the four types of practice readiness. Adherence to standards discussed as a professional capability is also critical for ensuring safe, quality practice. In particular, all professional nurses are expected to practise with reference to their professional framework and to quality and safety standards. Quality and safety standards are designed to support clinicians, protect the public and ensure consistency in the quality of healthcare provision (Australian Commission on Safety and Quality in Health Care [ACSQHC], 2017b; Health, Quality and Safety Commission New Zealand [HQSCNZ], 2020a). For example, medication errors remain a leading cause of death (Sherwood & Nickel, 2017) and the handwashing practices of nurses continue to affect nosocomial infection rates (WHO, 2016). The ability of nurses to recognise and respond to an acute deteriorating patient has become an issue of major concern in recent decades (ACSQHC, 2017a). Even novice nurses must be able to distinguish between normal and deviations from normal, perform basic interventions to promote health, prevent and manage complications and assist with recovery from illness or injury. Both the ACSQHC and the HQSCNZ produce resources to address all of these issues and more (ACSQHC, 2017b; HQSCNZ, 2020b).

In order to function effectively as a registered nurse, you need to be familiar with the quality and safety standards applicable to your jurisdiction. As is the case with scope of practice discussed in Chapters 1 and 7, practising in accordance with quality and safety guidelines contributes to positive patient outcomes. Furthermore, they are the legal yardstick against which your standard of practice will be determined, should a negative outcome in the healthcare setting become a legal matter. For this reason, it is important to know your limitations in respect of clinical readiness, ask for help and escalate concerns where necessary.

The fourth type of practice readiness, industry readiness, is also critical to ensuring the provision of safe, quality care. While on placement in different health industry settings, you will have seen variations in what registered nurses were permitted to do. This is because each organisation uses **policies and procedures** specifically developed for that unique context. While your pre-registration education will provide you with generic skills underpinned by broad principles, your ability to function in a specific environment will be governed by the local policies and procedures. These take the form of a set of instructions used to determine what action is required, or to provide a framework on which to base your clinical reasoning. Following the policies and procedures is compulsory, not optional – as a registered nurse employed in an organisation you will need to ensure compliance with the policies and procedures set by your employer.

Policies and procedures

A set of instructions used to determine what action is required, or to provide a framework on which to base your clinical reasoning.

They provide organisational structure and can assist you in performing skills in a new environment. As the policies and procedures are based on prevailing law and the standards and codes of practice referred to in this and the previous chapter, they protect both patients and staff by promoting quality and safety.

Case Study 8.2: Safe, quality care

Kelly has a strong GPA as she approaches completion of her program. While her ability to perform nursing skills is adequate, she lacks confidence in the simulation laboratories and on placement. This is because a registered nurse who was supervising Kelly on her first placement told her that she is 'all thumbs'.

- What could Kelly do to improve her confidence and ensure she is practising safely?

- What resources (personal, professional and organisational) can she draw on to assess and develop her level of clinical readiness?

Understanding 'what' needs to be done

Clinical skills are developed over time and with practice. You have learnt about the rationale for the performance of skills in your theory classes, then practised the technical aspects of the skills in your clinical laboratories and on placement. These experiences are significant in contributing to development of your clinical readiness. It has been found, however, that when nurses commence their graduate year, they often focus on the tasks that must be achieved in a particular shift in order to manage a full patient load (Fowler et al., 2018). The focus on tasks often occurs as graduates consolidate the skills acquired in an educational setting and learn how to apply them clinically as a registered nurse. While this focus on the 'how' is expected during the first few weeks of a graduate year, it may cause you to neglect the 'why' of your practice. Hence, practising and developing your clinical skills to have confidence in translating knowledge and skills into practice prior to commencing your graduate year is the focus of your nursing education.

OXFORD UNIVERSITY PRESS

The development of clinical readiness is the aim of the educational process; however, as placement experiences differ for each nursing student, the resultant level of practice readiness will vary. It is therefore important for you to reflect on your clinical readiness to practice. As a final year nursing student, you need to identify the skills with which you have become comfortable and those that require improvement, so that they can be your focus during your final simulation and placement activities.

Case Study 8.3: Translating knowledge and skills into practice

Kelly sought support from her lecturers at university and has worked on improving her ability to perform nursing skills correctly and efficiently. She did well in the practical assessments that were conducted in the simulation laboratories prior to commencing her consolidation placement. During the second week of her placement, however, she encounters the registered nurse who criticised her skills ability during her first placement. This nurse makes it clear that she expects Kelly to be slow and clumsy when assisting with a procedure.

- What clinical and professional readiness capabilities can Kelly draw on to manage this situation and maintain her confidence?

Ultimately, as nursing students complete their studies the focus is on pulling it all together. For most nursing students approaching graduation, this is the area of preparedness that concerns them the most. Nursing programs often include consolidation (capstone) subjects in their final year, inclusive of an extended placement, to facilitate this integration of knowledge and skills. Capabilities from the other domains of readiness, in particular commitment, confidence, resilience communication, critical thinking and resource management, feature heavily in this part of the curriculum.

Your new role will be exciting and rewarding, but it will also be challenging. As discussed in Chapters 7 and 11, processes and resources are in place to ensure that graduates are not thrown in at the deep end, but are instead given time to adjust to their new role. In order to contribute at a beginning level, graduates will need to manage a caseload of patients. Many students who are nearing completion of their nursing degree have expressed that lack of confidence in caring for an expected caseload is a major concern when entering the workforce (Woods et al., 2015). While there are many factors that are beyond your control, there are things you can do to build your confidence and increase clinical readiness during your final year of study. For example, prior to commencing in your graduate position, you can undertake research on the type of patients, medical and/or surgical conditions, and medications you are likely to encounter.

Use the time during your extended consolidation placement to become familiar with the day-to-day routines of clinical units and the nurses who work there. We can learn a lot from exploring the typical day of a nurse working in an inpatient facility. Most shifts commence with a patient handover. This handover is fundamental to understanding the caseload of patients you have been allocated to look after. As a nurse working in a unit, you may need to quiz the nurse handing over to you if there are specific aspects of care that require clarification. In facilities where handover is recorded, you may need to seek this clarification from the nurse unit manager. Handover is when you are accepting the responsibility of caring for that patient. You do not want to be left unsure about whether a specific task ordered before your shift commenced was in fact completed by the nurse whose shift has just ended. Your personal readiness capabilities of communication and confidence will support you to do this effectively. Once you have received handover, you will need to employ the time management, prioritisation and delegation skills discussed in Chapter 7 to manage your workload for the shift. The science of priority setting is an area that new graduate nurses can often find difficult to master when given a workload of four to five patients (Kavanagh & Szweda, 2017). A good way to start prioritising nursing care is by making sense of the information given to you during handover. Review each patient's medical record and make a visual inspection at the start of your shift. You are then in a position to use clinical decision-making to determine what needs to be done first and by whom. Tools such as the Nursing and Midwifery Board of Australia (NMBA) decision-making framework for nurses and midwives (DMF) (NMBA, 2020) can be very useful if you are in doubt. The DMF promotes consistent safe, person-centred and evidence-based decision-making by guiding decision-making in relation to scope of practice and delegation (NMBA, 2020). At the end of your shift, you will need to plan carefully how you will handover to your colleagues. Clear, concise and timely communication is a hallmark of clinical readiness.

 Portfolio Activity: Making the transition

Using the worksheet in Appendix 8, rate your clinical readiness capabilities. Are there areas you think you need to improve to enhance your transition to practice? Drawing on what you have learnt in this chapter, formulate a plan for developing and maintaining clinical readiness for your practice.

 Portfolio Activity 8.2: Stop, reflect and think

Different patients require you to use different clinical skills. The following questions are aimed to help you think about how you may prioritise patient care and translate your knowledge and skills to safely and efficiently provide quality nursing care to four patients you have been allocated on a day shift. Handover for these patients is provided using the iSoBAR framework in Tables 8.2, 8.3, 8.4 and 8.5.

- Based on the information you have been given, how would you prioritise the delivery of care for Paul Jones, Adam Hunt, Gillian McCartney and Ian Wilkinson?
- To help you manage your patient load, a nursing assistant has been allocated to work with you. What nursing tasks could you delegate to the nursing assistant, and how could you evaluate their clinical practice?
- What practical measures could you take in helping Paul Jones come to terms with the requirement to make lifestyle changes following his recent diagnosis of diabetes mellitus?
- You are called over by Adam Hunt, who says he feels dizzy. What do you suspect has occurred? Describe your actions to minimise his distress.
- What preparations could you undertake while waiting for a medical review?

Table 8.2 Handover patient 1 – Paul Jones

iSoBAR Handover Patient 1				
Identify	**Name:** **Date:**	**Paul Jones**	**Handover from:** **Handover to:**	
Situation	Day 1 following diagnosis of diabetic ketoacidosis. Transferred from ED with a 2-week history of polyuria and polydipsia accompanied by weight loss. Treated with IV fluids and continuous IV insulin.			
Observation	Temp: 37.2°C	PR: regular 86 beats/min	RR: 12 breaths/min	BP: 120/82mmHg
	SpO$_2$: 96%	BGL: 11mmols/L	Ketones: 0.3mmols/L	K$^+$: 4.1mmols/L
	GCS: 15	UO: last voided 500mL	Pain score: 0	
Background	Newly diagnosed type 2 diabetic. No reported family history of diabetes. His father died of renal failure.			Allergies: Nil known
Assessment	Continue current fluid therapy as charted and continue fluid balance chart. Continue to monitor blood glucose and ketone levels. Refer patient to diabetic educator regarding discharge medication schedule, home glucose monitoring, and dietary advice.			
Read back	A 42-year-old male. Newly diagnosed diabetic admitted with diabetic ketoacidosis. Continue treatment as charted. Needs follow-up by diabetic educator.			

Table 8.3 Handover patient 2 – Adam Hunt

iSoBAR Handover Patient 2				
Identify	**Name:** **Date:**	**Adam Hunt**	**Handover from:** **Handover to:**	
Situation	Day 1 following admission with community-acquired pneumonia. Admitted early hours of the morning with a 4-day history of productive cough. Respiratory examination shows mild tachypnoea. Dullness to percussion over lower-right lung. No crackles or wheezing auscultated. Sputum specimen sent to laboratory for culture and sensitivity. Chest X-ray shows lower-right lobar-type pneumonia.			
Observation	Temp: 37.4°C	PR: regular 92 beats/min	RR: 22 breaths/min	BP: 135/75mmHg
	SpO$_2$: 96% on room air	BSL: Nil	GCS: 15	UO: last voided 250mL
	Pain score: 0			
Background	Relevant history: Hypertension Hypercholesterolemia Cigarette smoker since age of 15 years			Allergies: Nil known allergies
Assessment	Continue 4 hourly observations. Can eat and drink. Mobilise as tolerated. To commence intravenous antibiotics.			
Read back	A 62-year-old man with mild pneumonia. Low-grade temperature, otherwise vital signs within normal limits. To commence antibiotics for suspected bacterial infection.			

Table 8.4 Handover patient 3 – Gillian McCartney

iSoBAR Handover Patient 3					
Identify	Name: Date:	**Gillian McCartney**		Handover from: Handover to:	
Situation	Day 5 following admission following a stroke. Computed tomography scan shows area of infarction in right anterior hemisphere. Left hemiplegia and slurred speech. Commenced rehabilitation program. Needs assistance with activities of daily living. Transfers from bed to chair with one nurse.				
Observation	Temp: 36.8°C	PR: regular 92 beats/ min	RR: 18 breaths/min		BP: 140/85mmHg
	SpO$_2$: 96% on room air	BGL: Nil	GCS: 15		UO: last voided 350mL
	Pain score: 2				
Background	Relevant history: Hypertension (noncompliant with antihypertensive medications)			Allergies: Nil known	
Assessment	Preparations for home visit by occupational therapist and referral to social worker for access to home care packages.				
Read back	A 76-year-old female day 5 admitted following a stroke. Continues on rehabilitation program. Requires assistance with meeting clinical hygiene needs. For referral to OT and social worker.				

Table 8.5 Handover patient 4 – Ian Wilkinson

iSoBAR Handover Patient 4					
Identify	Name: Date:	**Ian Wilkinson**		Handover from: Handover to:	
Situation	Day 3 following admission for acute pulmonary oedema. Bilateral crackles noted on auscultation of lung fields associated with productive cough of bright red frothy sputum. Physical examination showed bilateral swollen legs. Patient had recently stopped taking his fluid pills after medication script had run out.				
Observation	Temp: 36.2°C	PR: regular 62 beats/min	RR: 16 breaths/min		BP: 126/54mmHg
	SpO$_2$: 94% on 2Ls O$_2$ nasal prongs	BSL: Nil	GCS: 15		UO: last voided 150mL
	Pain score:	0			
Background	Ischaemic heart disease Angina			Allergies: Nil known	
Assessment	Fluid restriction 1.5L Administration of medications as documented Maintain 24-hour fluid balance chart Continue supplementary O$_2$ via nasal prongs at 2L per min. Elevate legs to promote venous return.				
Read back	A 72-year-old man admitted with heart failure. Now day 3 following an episode of pulmonary oedema.				

Conclusion

If you are like most nursing students, as you come to the end of your nursing program you are probably most concerned about your ability to perform effectively in the professional role. Your nursing program has prepared you with all the necessary knowledge and skills you need to commence practice as a registered nurse; however, actually being able to translate that knowledge and those skills into practice will be a significant learning curve. Clinical readiness goes beyond performance of tasks and brings in other domains of clinical, professional and industry readiness. Understanding how each of these forms of readiness relates to the others will help you to ensure that you are clinically ready for practice.

Key summary points

- Clinical readiness is the capability to provide a basic level of safe, quality clinical care within a graduate's scope of practice.

- While all forms of readiness are essential for successful transition to the registered nurse role, clinical readiness is the one that most directly impacts patients' physical, mental, emotional and spiritual well-being.

- Clinical readiness involves appreciation of the 'why' of clinical nursing, knowing 'how' to nurse clinically and understanding 'what' needs to be done.

- Appreciating the 'why' of clinical nursing requires fundamental clinical knowledge and the ability to practise using an evidence base.

- Knowing 'how' to nurse clinically requires mastery of basic clinical skills that are employed in the delivery of safe, quality care.

- Understanding 'what' needs to be done involves translating and pulling together knowledge and skills to perform effectively in the clinical environment.

OXFORD UNIVERSITY PRESS

Critical thinking questions

1. What would you consider are the important aspects of clinical readiness, and why?

2. Consider the 'why', 'how' and 'what' of nursing discussed in this chapter. Which do you consider to be the most important?

3. As a new nurse, describe how being clinically ready will support you during your transition to practice as a registered nurse.

4. Many students approaching completion of their studies are most concerned about their ability to pull it all together. Where might you obtain support if you have similar concerns?

References

Australian Commission on Safety and Quality in Health Care. (2017a). *Recognising and responding to acute deterioration standard*. https://www.safetyandquality.gov.au/standards/nsqhs-standards/recognising-and-responding-acute-deterioration-standard

Australian Commission on Safety and Quality in Health Care. (2017b). *National safety and quality health service standards second edition*. https://www.safetyandquality.gov.au/sites/default/files/2019-04/National-Safety-and-Quality-Health-Service-Standards-second-edition.pdf

Fowler, A., Twigg, D., Jacob, E., & Nattabi, B. (2018). An integrative review of rural and remote nursing graduate programmes and experiences of nursing graduates. *Journal of Clinical Nursing, 27*(5–6), e753–e766. https://doi.org/10.1111/jocn.14211

Guideline Central. (2020). *Guideline summaries: Nursing*. https://www.guidelinecentral.com/summaries/specialties/nursing/

Harrison, H., Birks, M., Franklin, R., & Mills, J. (2020). An assessment continuum: How healthcare professionals define and determine practice readiness of newly graduated registered nurses. *Collegian, 27*(2), 198–206. https://doi.org/10.1016/j.colegn.2019.07.003

Health Quality and Safety Commission New Zealand. (2020a). *Mō mātou – About us*. https://www.hqsc.govt.nz/about-us/

Health Quality and Safety Commission New Zealand. (2020b). *Te māwhenga tūroro – Patient deterioration*. https://www.hqsc.govt.nz/our-programmes/patient-deterioration/

Kavanagh, J. M., & Szweda, C. (2017). A crisis in competency: The strategic and ethical imperative to assessing new graduate nurses' clinical reasoning. *Nursing Education Perspectives, 38*(2), 57–62. https://doi.org/10.1097/1001.NEP.0000000000000112

National Health and Medical Research Council. (2017, February 17). *Australian clinical practice guidelines*. https://www.clinicalguidelines.gov.au/portal#:~:text=Clinical%20practice%20guidelines%20are%20evidence,care%20for%20specific%20clinical%20circumstances

Nursing and Midwifery Board of Australia. (2020). *Decision-making framework for nurses and midwives*. https://www.nursingmidwiferyboard.gov.au/Codes-Guidelines-Statements/Frameworks.aspx

Sherwood, G., & Nickel, B. (2017). Integrating quality and safety competencies to improve outcomes. *Journal of Infusion Nursing*, *40*(2), 116–122. https://doi.org/10.1097/NAN.0000000000000210

Wolff, A. C., Regan, S., Pesut, B., & Black, J. (2010). Ready for what? An exploration of the meaning of new graduate nurses' readiness for practice. *International Journal of Nurse Education Scholarship*, *7*(1), 1–14. https://doi.org/10.2202/1548-923X.1827

Woods, C., West, C., Mills, J., Park, T., Southern, J., & Usher, K. (2015). Undergraduate student nurses' self-reported preparedness for practice. *Collegian*, *22*(4), 359–368. https://doi.org/10.1016/j.colegn.2014.05.003

World Health Organization. (2016). *Guidelines on core components of infection prevention and control programmes at the national and acute health care facility level.* https://apps.who.int/iris/bitstream/handle/10665/251730/9789241549929-eng.pdf?sequence=1

Chapter 9

Industry Readiness

Catherine Caballero and Arlene Walker

Learning Outcomes

Upon completion of this chapter you will be able to:

1. Define the term 'industry readiness' in respect of nursing practice.
2. Describe the capabilities associated with industry readiness.
3. Explain the importance of industry readiness in nursing.
4. Reflect on your own industry readiness.
5. Formulate a plan for developing and maintaining industry readiness in practice.

Key terms

Employment awards	Professional workplace	SMART goals
Industry readiness	behaviour	

Introduction

Work readiness, or practice readiness as we refer to it within a nursing context, is a complex and multidimensional construct. Throughout this text we have presented you with information to explain this concept and ways you can develop the necessary level of practice readiness to support your transition to the professional role. Having worked through Chapters 6, 7 and 8 you will have increased your understanding of the first three domains of the multidimensional readiness model (Harrison et al., 2020) – personal readiness, professional readiness and clinical readiness. No doubt, by this time, you will be realising how well your studies in nursing have prepared you for your professional role with capabilities reflected in these domains. This chapter will focus on the fourth capability domain of practice readiness for graduate nurses: that of industry readiness. In this chapter we define and describe the key areas of industry readiness capability that are important for graduate nurses to develop and maintain as healthcare professionals. This chapter will also provide an opportunity for you to critically reflect on your own industry readiness and help to ensure that you are ready to enter practice in the healthcare industry. As the industry in which you will work is healthcare, we would suggest that as you read the chapter, keep in mind what was discussed in Chapter 2 about the healthcare context. This will help you link the capabilities outlined in this chapter to the industry in which you will work.

Case Study 9.1: Introducing Janice

Janice is 39 years old and has recently commenced her graduate year. Janice has been an enrolled nurse for a number of years and has been employed as a graduate nurse by the local health service where she had been working part-time while completing her nursing program. Janice expected that she would have no problem transitioning to her new role based on her experience in the health service; however, she is finding that she is encountering some unexpected issues in adapting to the responsibilities of a registered nurse.

Industry readiness defined

In the preceding chapters, we explored the first three domains of practice readiness – personal, professional and clinical. The fourth domain that nursing graduates need to develop is **industry readiness** (Figure 9.1). For any graduate commencing professional work, effectively navigating the workplace and organisational systems is a crucial aspect of work readiness and a marker of success in the workplace (Caballero et al., 2011; Walker & Campbell, 2013). Commonly, most senior nursing students focus their preparation for practice on the personal, professional and clinical readiness aspects of practice. Industry readiness, however, is a very important domain of readiness that, if not sufficiently developed, can undermine practice in all other domains.

Industry readiness

The capability to navigate the healthcare system, organisations, healthcare parameters and resources in the provision of care.

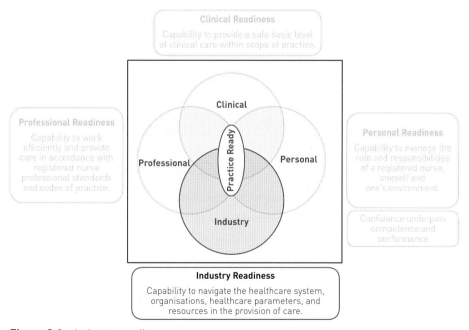

Figure 9.1 Industry readiness

Industry readiness broadly refers to a graduate nurse's capability to effectively navigate and understand the healthcare industry in which they work as a registered nurse (Harrison et al., 2020). New nurses need to know the healthcare system and organisations, and the resources available to them that are necessary for the provision of healthcare. This includes knowing and adhering to industry and organisational regulations (Harrison et al., 2020). Industry readiness is aligned with the concept of organisational acumen (Caballero et al., 2011; Walker et al., 2015). Early conceptualisations of work readiness led to the development of the Work Readiness Scale (WRS), a measure developed to assess work readiness in graduates from degree programs across different professions (Caballero et al., 2011) and, more recently, graduate nurses (Walker et al., 2015). The WRS identified organisational acumen as one of four measurable factors contributing to the work readiness of graduates. Organisational acumen incorporates aspects of professional readiness and refers to graduates' awareness of organisational systems, their professional work ethic, self-directedness and approach to lifelong learning, developmental feedback and professional development (Caballero et al., 2011; Walker et al., 2015). In particular, a graduate nurse's abilities to learn, implement feedback and identify with their health organisation have been identified as important factors in developing organisational acumen (Walker et al., 2015).

The importance of industry readiness

Industry readiness supports nurses to function responsibly, safely and effectively as a member of the healthcare workforce (Harrison et al., 2020). Nurses who are industry ready are more likely to practise safely. Several researchers have demonstrated the positive association between safe practice and patient outcomes (Aiken et al., 2012, 2017; Lake et al., 2016; Murray et al., 2018; Savitz et al., 2005). Knowing and understanding the industry and organisational rules (policies, procedures and guidelines) and boundaries of practice is an important aspect of safe practice, as is knowing your limitations in relation to practice and seeking assistance when needed. As discussed in Chapter 7, being able to acknowledge limitations and seek assistance when necessary requires new nurses to be self-aware, reflective, confident and resilient. The nursing environment and culture can influence a new nurse's confidence and resilience (Harrison et al.,

2020). Research indicates that many new nurses lack professional confidence when they commence practice (Ortiz, 2016); however, over time, with a nurturing environment and support, they can build this confidence. A qualitative systematic review of Australian research by Walker et al. (2017) found that supportive environments enhanced new nurses' perceived value and self-esteem, while a negative culture undermined confidence, leading to feelings of vulnerability and disillusionment with the nursing profession. When a new nurse's professional confidence is undermined or diminished, they are less likely to be proactive and take a role in seeking resources and support to guide their practice (Harrison et al., 2020; Ortiz, 2016).

Industry readiness is also important for the transition and integration of new nurses into the health workplace and for retaining them in the profession. Walker and colleagues (2020) conducted a time series study with 203 new Australian graduate nurses. The aim was to determine how four dimensions of pre-employment work readiness (organisational acumen, work competence, social intelligence, industry work characteristics) predicted three work outcomes of graduate nurses at the end of the first year of work (job satisfaction, work engagement, intention to remain in the profession). Organisational acumen (industry readiness) was found to be the strongest and most consistent predictor of all three work outcomes. This implies that new nurses who perceive they are industry ready at the commencement of their graduate nurse year feel more satisfied and engaged with their work by the end of their first year, and are also more likely to remain in the nursing profession long term. Patterson and colleagues (2017) investigated how different clinical placement models impacted new nurses' transition into the workplace and their perceptions of work readiness. Despite the small sample size of 28 graduate nurses, the authors found that the nurses who had participated in a collaborative university–organisation fellowship program rated themselves more highly on three of the four work readiness dimensions (organisational acumen, work competence, social intelligence). The authors concluded that these nurses were more familiar with and better understood how the health organisation functioned (i.e. were more industry ready), enabling a smoother transition into the workplace and better preparation for practice overall.

Portfolio Activity 9.1: Stop, reflect and think

What do you think about the concept of industry readiness? Had you given it much thought before reading this textbook? How much of the content in your nursing program is directly related to industry readiness? How much is indirectly related?

Capabilities associated with industry readiness

Some knowledge and skills related to industry readiness you will acquire as a nursing student, for instance, understanding the regulations that govern healthcare in Australia and New Zealand. Other aspects, however, can only be developed once you commence work within an organisation as a qualified nurse. For instance, while you need to have a solid understanding of your organisation's policies and processes and how these intersect in your practice, and understand the organisation's values and culture, you cannot know these aspects and consolidate your knowledge and skills in these areas, until you are working within the industry.

As a graduate nurse you will have attained a vast body of knowledge over the course of your studies, and developed competencies that are crucial to you being able to practise as a registered nurse. Entering the workforce, however, highlights that to be an effective registered nurse there is still much learning to be done. Often this will be outside the technical and clinical aspects of your role, as is the case with industry readiness. With this, the transition from learning in the educational environment as a student to learning in the workplace as a qualified nurse, requires a significant shift in a graduate's approach to learning and level of accountability (Fisher et al., 1990). Learning in the educational environment is highly structured, directed and supported by educators. In this context, nursing students adopt a dependent pedagogical learning approach, which is reliant on the educator identifying learning needs, establishing objectives, and creating plans, activities and assessments to develop and evaluate learning. In contrast, the

OXFORD UNIVERSITY PRESS

work context offers a much less structured and guided environment for learning. While organisations offer graduate nurses support from facilitators, clinical training staff, nurse unit managers, preceptors or mentors, the realities of the workplace and competing workplace demands can mean that these individuals may not be available as often as or when needed. This can result in graduates feeling stressed and less supported in their learning and practice (Newton & McKenna, 2007; Phillips et al., 2014).

Therefore, as a graduate nurse transitioning into the workplace, it is important you develop your ability to be self-directed and take responsibility for identifying and addressing your learning needs, rather than relying on your education and the organisation to provide you with this direction. As the nursing profession, contexts of practice and organisational systems advance and evolve over time, your development in industry readiness, like the other domains of readiness, will be cumulative and lifelong. Being a self-directed, lifelong learner will be invaluable to ensure you maintain the professional standard and quality of practice required by the industry. Knowing about these aspects of industry is both part of industry readiness and relevant to developing your industry readiness, given that much of the development and consolidation of this capability will take place in your graduate year. As there are a number of capabilities associated with industry readiness, for convenience, we will discuss these as industry readiness attitudes, attributes and abilities (Table 9.1).

Table 9.1   Capabilities associated with industry readiness

Industry readiness knowledge	Industry readiness attributes	Industry readiness abilities
• Healthcare systems and organisations • Industry and organisational regulations	• Adaptation to reality • Appropriate workplace behaviour	• Critical self-assessment • Self-development planning

Industry readiness knowledge

The first capability of industry readiness knowledge relates to understanding healthcare systems and organisations that operate within this healthcare system. As discussed in Chapter 2, the Australian and New Zealand healthcare systems and the health organisations in which nurses work are overseen by national and, in Australia, state and territory governments. There are several public and private healthcare providers across both countries delivering health services to the population via acute and/or community services. Australian and New Zealand governments legislate how health organisations should operate, to ensure they are accountable for the health services they deliver. However, the workplace environment and culture of each provider is unique and will depend on the context of specific communities and the nature of the people who work within each health service. To work effectively as a team member within a health organisational context, nurses need to not only understand the values and culture of their specific workplace, but also how their organisation functions and operates within a broader, multidisciplinary health system that runs 24/7. When new nurses are acquainted with the health organisation in which they work, and its processes, they are more likely to perceive themselves as industry ready (Patterson et al., 2017). New nurses in an unfamiliar environment need guidance and reassurance to ensure smooth transition into the health system, ongoing skill development and safe practice (Patterson et al., 2008). As discussed in Chapter 11, the provision of adequate orientation and ongoing support can assist new nurses with transition and integration into the health organisation context, especially during the first year of work (Walker et al., 2017).

New nurses also need to understand and comply with industry and organisational regulations that govern healthcare and safe clinical practice in Australia and New Zealand. Industry regulations include the various national, state and territory **employment awards** regularly negotiated by relevant nursing unions and communicated via employment agreements. These employment awards determine nurses' level of employment and remuneration, as well as the expectations and responsibilities for each level of the award. Such documents can also establish policy and procedures for health service delivery, such as nurse to patient ratios, and can be used to inform organisational regulations in relation to service provision, risk and safe practice. In addition to being aware of their health organisation's key performance indicators (KPIs), nurses also need to know, understand and work in accordance with their organisation's policies and practices and other important operational frameworks. These include standards, policies and procedures that guide clinical practice, eHealth systems and performance development. When new nurses are aware of a hospital's policies and procedures, have relevant ward knowledge including knowing where, how and from whom to access resources, information and assistance, they appear more confident and enjoy a smoother transition into the health workplace (Patterson et al., 2008; Walker et al., 2013).

Employment awards

Agreements between industry bodies and unions that determine employment levels and remuneration.

Case Study 9.2: Industry readiness knowledge

Janice is completing her graduate nursing year at a large hospital, currently undertaking a rotation in the geriatric acute ward. While she is enjoying how much she is learning on the job, she has found adjusting to the workload particularly challenging. She knew the shift work would take getting used to, but underestimated the workload and what she would be expected to achieve on an average shift. Janice considers herself a fast learner; however, it has been a steep learning curve and she still finds doing her job takes her longer than the more experienced nurses.

- What resources (tangible, informational or human) could Janice utilise to support her adaptation to the pace of the ward and improve her work efficiency?

Industry readiness attributes

In Chapter 6 we explored the capabilities associated with personal readiness for practice. The industry capabilities discussed in that chapter include commitment, resilience, confidence, relationship management, emotional intelligence and self-management. We also considered the concept of attributes, which are a person's inherent characteristics that determine how they approach and manage their day-to-day activities. The attributes associated with industry readiness are the abilities to adapt to practice in the work context and to align values and beliefs with those of the organisation.

As discussed in Chapter 4, many graduates experience transition shock when they commence work and are exposed to the realities that accompany the adaptation to reality. As part of nursing studies, students undertake clinical placements in acute, aged care and/or community settings. These placements are useful for consolidating your nursing knowledge and clinical skills and for introducing you to the health industry. However, it is not until you are working in an ongoing nursing position that you will get to experience the various nuances of the health industry and the organisation. For example, one of the things that adds great variety to nursing is the opportunity to undertake shift work. Often students get little, if any, experience working different shifts while on clinical placement. Adjusting to shift work can be a major job-related stressor that can impact the health and well-being of new graduate nurses (Walker et al., 2013). Other realities of the healthcare environment that new nurses need to be aware of involve understanding the pace and complexity of the work, including the intricacies of managing patients, clients, colleagues and other healthcare professionals. It is not uncommon for new nurses to feel unprepared for these realities of their professional role (Walker et al., 2017). Personal readiness attributes associated with a positive attitude and being flexible and resilient, augment industry readiness and your ability to adapt to reality. Coupled with your industry knowledge and the resources available in healthcare organisations, these attributes can help make your adaptation to the healthcare environment not only smoother but more enjoyable and rewarding.

 Portfolio Activity 9.2: Stop, reflect and think

Are you anticipating encountering any problems adapting to the reality of practice? What resources – personal, industry and professional – could you draw on to assist in smoothing your transition?

Professional workplace behaviour

The ability to consistently engage in professional workplace behaviour and manage the unprofessional behaviour of others.

The professional readiness capabilities discussed in Chapter 7 underpin appropriate workplace behaviour. This attribute of industry readiness incorporates the ability to consistently engage in **professional workplace behaviour** and have the capability to manage the unprofessional behaviour of others. It requires a professional work ethic that is aligned to the organisation's culture and values. It is well documented in the literature (Merga, 2016) that new nursing graduates are often exposed to bullying, horizontal violence and power games, as victims or as observers, and that this behaviour can impact successful transition into the workplace. Knowledge of your professional standards and codes of ethics and behaviour, and your organisational policies related to conduct and performance, will guide you to not only demonstrate appropriate workplace behaviour but learn how to manage unacceptable workplace behaviour. Personal readiness attributes and skills related to confidence, resilience, communication and relationship management will also support you to demonstrate professional workplace behaviour and respond appropriately to unprofessional behaviour.

As we will discuss in the following section, new nurses can also demonstrate industry ready capability by taking a continuous improvement approach to professional practice.

Case Study 9.3: Industry readiness knowledge and attributes

On one of her shifts, Janice is feeling particularly overwhelmed by looking after a high volume of patients and facing competing demands. There seem to be more ad hoc patient requests than usual, which are making it difficult to stay on top of her other tasks, including documentation and medication administration. Being constantly pulled in different directions, she is finding it difficult to manage her time effectively and is conscious that she has fallen behind on medication administration for two patients. On her way to administer the medication, a different patient of hers, Victor, calls out as she is passing his room. He requires assistance to move about, including transferring in and out of his wheelchair. He is frustrated, complaining that he has been calling out for help for some time and urgently needs the bathroom. Due to Victor's stature, normally two nursing staff are required to transfer and support him, or mechanical lifts are required.

Janice is conscious that her colleagues are busy with their patients and she has already asked for assistance on other matters. She is aware that the hospital has a policy for transferring and handling patients, but she feels under pressure and her other patients are waiting for medication. Given the short distance to the bathroom, Janice decides to transfer Victor on her own without the use of any mechanical devices. Janice assists Victor to the bathroom. Upon returning him to his bed, she lifts him from the wheelchair. Victor loses his balance and Janice loses her grip, resulting in Victor falling onto the bed. Janice's manager happens to be walking past and is able to assist Janice with transferring Victor safely into his bed.

Fortunately, Victor did not sustain any injuries; however, Janice is required to file a report and discuss the situation with her manager. Janice's nurse manager has also noticed that Janice has been late in administering some of her patients' medications.

- What is the main issue here for Janice?

- What industry readiness knowledge and attributes is Janice lacking in this scenario?

- What are the implications for Victor as the patient, as a result of Janice's actions?

- What are the implications for the manager and the organisation as a result of Janice's actions?

Industry readiness abilities

Perhaps more than any other domain of practice readiness, industry readiness is dependent on 'on the job' experience as a registered nurse. Adapting to a work context does not, however, occur automatically. It depends on your ability to apply your knowledge of healthcare organisations and regulations in the workplace. The knowledge and attributes associated with industry readiness must not only serve you as you navigate the healthcare system as a newly graduated registered nurse, they must also continue to support you as you progress throughout your career.

It is unlikely that you will spend your entire career in one facility. Even if you work in one place for a long period of time, organisational change means that industry readiness is not set; rather, it is dynamic and determined by context. In practice, this means that the industry readiness you possess today may not be sufficient tomorrow. You will need to constantly monitor your industry readiness, as you do all other domains of readiness. For this reason, it is important to use a structured approach to cultivating and maintaining industry readiness.

Your nursing education to this point has provided you with basic industry readiness knowledge, such as that discussed in the previous section. This information ensures that you know what to expect when you commence your role as a healthcare professional in an employing organisation. Your industry readiness with respect to nursing practice will, however, be influenced by your background and work experience to date, such as undertaking paid employment, as discussed in Chapter 5. All graduates will therefore possess different levels of industry readiness, and it is unlikely that any will have sufficient readiness for a specific place of employment at the time of graduation. As is discussed in Chapter 11, organisations provide support, such as orientation and training, to assist you in consolidating knowledge and skills aspects of industry readiness pertaining to that context. While this organisation-specific knowledge is important, it cannot address all the unique learning deficits in each individual graduate. For this reason, it is important that you take a proactive approach to identifying and addressing your individual industry readiness abilities, both as you embark on your new profession and throughout your career.

The first thing you will need to do to address your industry-related learning needs is to assess your current knowledge and attributes and identify your areas for development. Doing so requires you to have both insight and self-awareness. We discussed reflective practice as an important component of professional readiness in Chapter 7. A dynamic relationship exists between reflective practice and critical self-assessment. In order to self-assess, you require the ability to reflect effectively on your own practice. Conversely, to reflect effectively, you require the ability to accurately self-assess (Mann et al., 2009). Hence, to build industry readiness capability, it is important to build self-awareness of your learning needs and critically reflect to consolidate your learning. Self-awareness through assessment of your strengths and limitations in respect of industry readiness is the first important step in addressing any deficits.

 Portfolio Activity: Making the transition

Use the self-assessment checklists in Appendices 10–13 to assess your capabilities in respect of industry readiness knowledge and attributes. You will need to rate your current level of competence in each area of industry readiness. Upon completion of these self-assessment checklists, you should have a clearer idea about and be able to identify your industry readiness development needs.

Having identified your areas for industry readiness development, the next step is to develop a plan for addressing those needs. The first stage of self-development planning is the identification of specific goals. Goals are broad statements of intent that specify the intended outcomes of your plan. You may have several goals around developing industry readiness, depending on the outcome of your critical self-assessment. While goals generally describe where you are going, they also need to include specific objectives that describe the steps and actions you will take to achieve each goal (MacLeod, 2012). To be effective, your goals need to be SMART – that is, they are written in terms that are specific, measurable, achievable, relevant and time-bound. Likely you have learnt about **SMART goals** during your nursing program. Well-written objectives provide a foundation for evaluating your progress towards your goals.

SMART goals

Goals that are written in terms that are specific, measurable, achievable, relevant and time-bound.

Engaging in a structured critical reflection process, as discussed earlier in this chapter, can assist you to reflect on the successes and challenges of implementing your self-development plan and inform how things can be done differently in future. Critical reflection is a process that is typically carried out individually; however, it can also be used to debrief objectives or learning with a supervisor, mentor or trusted colleague. Involving others in the critical reflection process provides an opportunity to seek feedback, which is an important part of the learning and development process. Seeking feedback about your industry readiness development could feedback specific questions, such as those shown in Box 9.1.

Box 9.1 Feedback questions

- What's one thing I could improve in relation to ...?
- What do you think I could do differently?
- How could I be more helpful/supportive to you/my colleagues/my team?
- What improvements do you feel can be made to improve my current skills and knowledge?
- What are the most important goals in our area?

Case Study 9.4: Self-development planning

Janice has developed an industry readiness self-development plan (Table 9.2). Review this plan and consider whether there are any other elements you feel should be added or amended.

 ## Portfolio Activity: Making the transition

Use the framework in Table 9.2 to develop a plan to address one of the learning needs identified through your completion of the self-assessment checklists (Appendices 10–13).

Table 9.2 Self-development plan (adapted from Miller & Rollnick, 2012; Cooper, 2009)

Describe the goal What is the outcome you are hoping to achieve?	• *To ensure decisions and behaviours are informed and in line with organisational policies and procedures.*
Why is it important for you to achieve this goal? What are the benefits?	• *Important to ensure patient safety.* • *To improve my nursing practice and enable me to perform more competently and effectively.*
Current behaviour Is there behaviour that might interfere with attaining your goal? Describe relevant behaviours you may need to stop.	• *My tendency to be patient-centred, empathic and wanting to please others can sometimes be a barrier to me being more assertive and making decisions that seem harder but are in the patient's best interest. I need to be more conscious of this.*

Objectives: What are the specific steps and actions that need to be taken to achieve the goal? NB: Need to be **S**pecific, **M**easurable, **A**chievable, **R**elevant, **T**ime-bound
Read the policy for transferring and handling patients within 2 weeks.
Complete competency training in relation to transferring and handling patients within 3 weeks.
Obtain and read all organisational policies in relation to nursing work within 6 weeks.
Seek feedback from colleagues regarding performance and alignment with organisational policies and procedures over the next 3 months.

Support: Who can assist/support you in achieving your objectives?	• *My manager and colleagues can provide me with guidance on all relevant organisational policies.*
Resources: What resources can you access to assist you in achieving your objectives?	• *Access to organisational policies.* • *Access to competency training modules that are available to graduates regarding policies and procedures.*
Challenges: Identify any barriers that could interfere with your objectives and ways you will overcome them.	• *Sometimes find it difficult to be assertive and explain why decisions need to be made due to hospital policies.* • *I need to remember and be conscious of the importance of patient safety.*
Evaluation: How will you know you have been successful?	• *By achieving objectives above.* • *Completion of competency training.* • *Increased confidence in policy and procedural knowledge and skills.*
Feedback: Identify people who you can seek feedback from during and at the end of your objectives.	*Seek feedback from:* • *Manager* • *Colleagues* • *Other graduate nurses*

Conclusion

Industry readiness is perhaps the most overlooked domain of practice readiness, but by now you will have increased your understanding of why it is important. Industry readiness consists of generic health system and specific organisational knowledge, attributes that support agile and flexible adaptation to the professional role, and a structured approach to development within dynamic, complex contexts. While dependent on workplace experience in the professional role, industry readiness draws on a number of personal, professional and clinical capabilities. Similarly, new graduates will find it easier to make the transition to the role of registered nurse as they develop their industry readiness. Understanding the need for critical self-reflection to inform approaches to building and maintaining industry readiness is key to entering your first year of practice as a well-rounded graduate.

Key summary points

- Industry readiness is the capability of graduates to navigate the healthcare system, organisations, healthcare parameters and resources in the provision of care.

- The realities of the workplace and competing workplace demands can place enormous pressure on graduate nurses. It is important to take accountability and be self-directed in identifying and addressing your industry readiness learning needs.

- Capabilities for industry readiness include industry readiness knowledge, industry readiness attributes and industry readiness abilities.

- Graduate nurses need to possess industry readiness knowledge in respect of healthcare systems and organisations, and industry and organisational regulations.

- Attributes for industry readiness draw in capabilities from all other readiness domains to assist graduates to adapt to reality and demonstrate appropriate workplace behaviour.

- The ability to achieve and maintain industry readiness requires abilities in critical self-assessment and self-development planning to ensure appropriate use of industry ready knowledge and attributes.

OXFORD UNIVERSITY PRESS

Critical thinking questions

1. What would you consider are the important aspects of industry readiness, and why?

2. What is the difference between capabilities, attributes and abilities in respect of industry readiness? How do they relate in practice?

3. As a new nurse, describe how being industry ready will support you during your transition to practice as a registered nurse.

4. How important has industry readiness been in your clinical placement experiences? How might your learning have been enhanced with greater attention to industry readiness?

References

Aiken, L. H., Sermeus, W., Van den Heede, K., Sloane, D. M., Busse, R., McKee, M., Bruyneel, L., Rafferty, A. M., Griffiths, P., Moreno-Casbas, M. T., Tishelman, C., Scott, A., Brzostek, T., Kinnunen, J., Schwendimann, R., Heinen, M., Zikos, D., Sjetne, I. S., Smith, H. L., & Kutney-Lee, A. (2012). Patient safety, satisfaction, and quality of hospital care: Cross-sectional surveys of nurses and patients in 12 countries in Europe and the United States. *BMJ, 344*, Article e1717. https://doi.org/10.1136/bmj.e1717

Aiken, L. H., Sloane, D., Griffiths, P., Rafferty, A. M., Bruyneel, L., McHugh, M., ... RN4CAST Consortium. (2017). Nursing skill mix in European hospitals: Cross-sectional study of the association with mortality, patient ratings, and quality of care. *BMJ Quality & Safety, 26*(7), 559–568. https://10.1136/bmjqs-2016-00556

Caballero, C., Walker, A., & Fuller-Tyszkiewicz, M. (2011). The work readiness scale (WRS): Developing a measure to assess work readiness in college graduates. *Journal of Teaching and Learning for Graduate Employability, 2*(2), 41–54. https://doi.org/10.21153/jtlge2011vol2no1art552

Cooper, E. (2009). Creating a culture of professional development: A milestone pathway tool for registered nurses. *Journal of Continuing Education in Nursing, 40*(11), 501–508. https://doi.org/10.3928/00220124-20091023-07

Fisher, M., King, J., & Tague, G. (1990). Development of a self-directed learning readiness scale for nursing education. *Nurse Education Today, 21*(7), 516–525. https://doi.org/10.1054/nedt.2001.0589

Harrison, H., Birks, M., Franklin, R., & Mills, J. (2020). An assessment continuum: How healthcare professionals define and determine practice readiness of newly graduated registered nurses. *Collegian, 27*(2), 198–206. https://doi.org/10.1016/j.colegn.2019.07.003.

Lake, E. T., Germack, H. D., & Viscardi, M. K. (2016). Missed nursing care is linked to patient satisfaction: A cross-sectional study of US hospitals. *BMJ Quality & Safety, 25*(7), 535–543. https://10.1136/bmjqs-2015-003961

MacLeod, L. (2012). Making SMART goals smarter. *Physician Executive, 38*(2), 68–70, 72.

Mann, K., Gordon, K., & Macleod, A. (2009). Reflection and reflective practice in health professions education: A systematic review. *Advances in Health Science Education, 14*(4), 595–621. https://doi.org/10.1007/s10459-007-9090-2

Merga, M. (2016). Gaps in work readiness of graduate health professionals and impact on early practice: Possibilities for future interprofessional learning. *Focus on Health Professional Education: A Multi-Disciplinary Journal, 17*(3), 14–29. https://doi.org/ 10.11157/ fohpe.v17i3.174

Miller, W. R., & Rollnick, S. (2012). *Motivational interviewing* (3rd ed.). Guilford Press.

Murray, M., Sundin, D., & Cope, V. (2018). The nexus of nursing leadership and a culture of safer patient care. *Journal of Clinical Nursing, 27*(5–6), 1287–1293. https://doi.org/10.1111/ jocn.13980

Newton, J. M., & McKenna, L. (2007). The transitional journey through the graduate year: A focus group study. *International Journal of Nursing Studies, 44*(7), 1231–1237. https://doi. org/10.1016/j.ijnurstu.2006.05.017

Ortiz, J. (2016). New graduate nurses' experiences about lack of professional confidence. *Nurse Education Practice, 19*, 19–24. https://doi.org/10.1016/j.nepr.2016.04.001

Patterson, C., Curtis, J., & Reid, A. (2008). Skills, knowledge, and attitudes expected of a newly graduated mental health nurse in an inpatient setting. *International Journal of Mental Health Nursing, 17*(6), 410–418. https://doi.org/10.1111/j.1447-0349.2008.00572.x

Patterson, E. E., Boyd, L., & Mnatzaganian, G. (2017). The impact of undergraduate clinical teaching models on the perceptions of work-readiness among new graduate nurses: A cross sectional study. *Nurse Education Today, 55*, 101–106. https://doi.org/10.1016/j. nedt.2017.05.010

Phillips, C., Kenny, A., Esterman, A., & Smith, C. (2014). A secondary data analysis examining the needs of graduate nurses in their transition to a new role. *Nurse Education in Practice, 14*(2), 106–111. https://doi.org/10.1016/j.nepr.2013.07.007

Savitz, L. A., Jones, C. B., & Bernard, S. (2005). *Quality indicators sensitive to nurse staffing in acute care settings.* In K. Henriksen, J. B. Battles, E. S. Marks & D. I. Lewin (Eds.), *Advances in patient safety: From research to implementation. Vol. 4. Programs, tools, and products* (pp. 375–385). Agency for Healthcare Research and Quality.

Walker, A., & Campbell, K. (2013). Work readiness of graduate nurses and the impact on job satisfaction, work engagement and intention to remain. *Nurse Education Today, 33*(12), 1490–1495. https://doi.org/10.1016/j.nedt.2013.05.008

Walker, A., Yong, M., Pang, L. Fullarton, C., Costa, B., & Dunning, A. M. T. (2013). Work readiness of graduate health professionals. *Nurse Education Today, 33*(12), 116–122. https://doi.org/10.1016/j.nedt.2012.01.007

Walker, A., Storey, K., Costa, B. M., & Leung, R. K. (2015). Refinement and validation of the Work Readiness Scale for graduate nurses. *Nursing Outlook, 63*(6), 632–638. https://doi. org/10.1016/j.outlook.2015.06.001

Walker, A., Costa, B. M., Foster, A. M., & de Bruin, R. L. (2017). Transition and integration experiences of Australian graduate nurses: A qualitative systematic review. *Collegian, 24*(5), 505–512. https://doi.org/10.1016/j.colegn.2016.10.004

Walker, A., Smith, I., Dimitrovski, N., Caballero, C., & Hyder, S. (2020). *The impact of graduate nurses' pre-employment work readiness on work experiences and work outcomes during the first year of work.* [Manuscript under review.] School of Psychology, Deakin University.

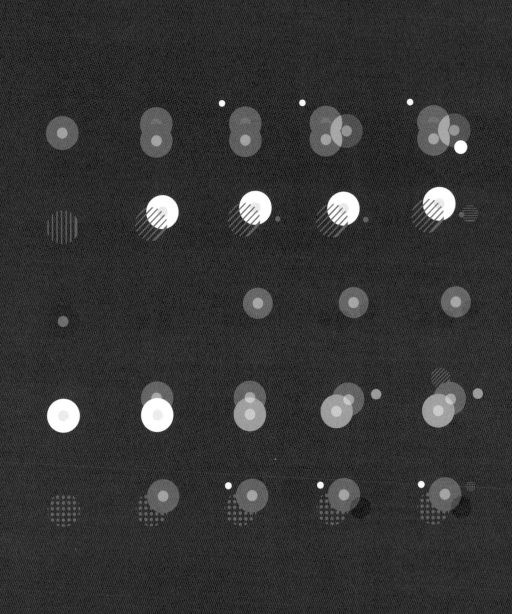

PART IV

JOINING THE
PROFESSION

Making the Transition

The first day of being a registered nurse is the most daunting,
I think. You suddenly realise the responsibility you have and
that you are accountable. You can no longer say 'I'm the
student nurse', because you are the nurse. You feel terrified but
enthusiastic at the same time.

Tara, Graduated 2019, New Zealand

Chapter 10

Becoming Practice Ready

Karen Missen and Naomi Byfieldt

Learning Outcomes

Following completion of this chapter, you will be able to:

1. Explain the importance of being ready for practice.

2. Analyse the contribution of clinical placements to practice readiness.

3. Describe the responsibilities of the undergraduate nurse in respect of clinical placements.

4. Evaluate external employment while studying as a means to enhance preparation for practice.

Key terms

Supernumerary   Tacit knowledge   Transferable skills

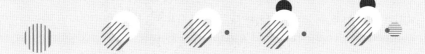

Introduction

Being ready for practice and able to demonstrate the capabilities described in previous chapters is important for both the new graduate nurses and the health service that employs them. Graduate nurses want to make a contribution to the healthcare team and are keen to consolidate their skills. The health service values and relies on the contribution these new nurses make. It is not unusual, however, for new graduate nurses to lack confidence and feel apprehensive in the early stages of their graduate year. While this is an exciting time, it is also a significant phase of learning and development. The more practice ready you are on commencing your first year of practice, the smoother your transition to the professional role. In this chapter we discuss the things you can do during your time as a nursing student to increase your practice readiness and optimise your preparation.

Case Study 10.1: Introducing Melinda

Melinda is a 24-year-old nursing student who is in her third year at university. She has been working in a local nursing home since she left school almost six years ago – she started out in food services and then decided to become an Assistant in Nursing. Melinda plans to work in aged care eventually. She wants to be well prepared for her new role and is thinking about the things she might do to make sure she is ready.

Opportunities to develop practice readiness

As explained in Chapter 5, the transition to become a registered nurse moves along a continuum that begins when a person commences their nursing education and continues through to the end of their first year of practice as a registered nurse (Harrison et al., 2020). During this time, new graduates demonstrate different levels of readiness as they move along the continuum to develop their competence, confidence and capabilities as safe registered nurses. In order to provide the best possible chance of a productive and successful first year as a registered nurse, nursing students need to take an active role in their learning and development from day one of their studies and continue this throughout their first year of practice. As discussed in Chapter 5, there are a number of strategies that contribute to your preparation for practice along this readiness continuum. We will discuss these under the headings of quality clinical placements and external work opportunities.

Quality clinical placements

Quality clinical experiences that provide authentic practice in the healthcare environment are essential for developing the capabilities necessary to work as a registered nurse. While in Chapter 5 we discussed the first year of practice as a registered nurse as being the critical final phase of the transition continuum, the most significant clinical experience is that obtained through undertaking placements as a nursing student. In this section, we will discuss the importance of clinical placements, particularly those in your final year, and consider how to make the most of these experiences to prepare yourself for your transition year.

In Australia and New Zealand, clinical placements begin in the nursing student's first academic year of study and continue throughout the three-year full-time program, with the number of clinical hours increasing at each year level. Clinical placements are a mandatory requirement and a formally assessed element of nursing degree programs. Students must complete all prescribed placement hours and assessment tasks and exhibit satisfactory levels of competence to achieve a passing grade in each clinical subject.

Clinical placements provide an opportunity for nursing students to learn experientially and to convert theoretical knowledge to a variety of mental, psychological and psychomotor skills that are significant in the delivery of holistic patient care (Jamshidi et al., 2016). Although you have already attended a number of clinical placements, it is essential to understand that enhancing practice readiness relies on the quality of the clinical placement and on how actively you, as a nursing student, engage in the learning process. The placements need to build on previous learning and experiences, and include clear learning goals and opportunities to apply knowledge through repetition in practice.

Models of clinical placement and supervision

Well-designed clinical placements during a nursing degree provide valuable learning experiences for nursing students to integrate their knowledge with practice and learn about the 'real work' of nursing while practising with experienced registered nurses. Nursing students are exposed to the **tacit knowledge** and capabilities of experienced registered nurses – those which are necessary for clinical practice, yet not readily articulated and learnt from a textbook in the university setting. These experiences provide a platform for on-the-job learning, helping students to develop their competence, build their confidence and enhance their understanding of their career choice (Ford et al., 2016). Through this process of experiential learning, nursing students begin to realise and develop a sense of their professional self, while learning to navigate the often complex nature of the healthcare environment while on placement (Ford et al., 2016). For these reasons, clinical placements are essential for developing practice readiness and preparing nursing students for the responsibilities of a registered nurse.

Tacit knowledge

Knowledge that is implicit and communicated through consistent and extensive relationships, contact or experiences with others.

There are a number of different modes used for allocating clinical placements to students, depending on how the education provider has designed their curriculum (Walker et al., 2013). As a nursing student you will have experienced one of these modes. The traditional mode is 'block' placement, where students are allocated clinical placements in weekly blocks, usually two to four week blocks at a time. A variant is the 'distributed' approach to placement, where the student spends two or three days a week on placement and the rest of the week on campus (Birks et al., 2017). Whichever placement mode is used, prior to attending placement nursing students need to possess theoretical knowledge and have sufficient practice in the clinical skills equivalent to their stage in their nursing program. This aligns learning in the classroom with the clinical setting, and consequently scaffolds and assists students to merge theoretical knowledge with what they are practising as nursing students in the healthcare environment.

Portfolio Activity 10.1: Stop, reflect and think

Which model(s) of placement have you experienced in your nursing program? What aspects of these models did you find most conducive to learning? Why?

OXFORD UNIVERSITY PRESS

Nursing students begin to identify and practise the roles, functions and skills involved in caring for patients, managing workloads and making independent decisions while on clinical placements. Accreditation standards require that nursing students are under the supervision of an appropriately qualified and experienced registered nurse (Nursing Council of New Zealand [NCNZ], 2020; Australian Nursing & Midwifery Accreditation Council [ANMAC], 2019), and for the duration of the placement the student is **supernumerary**. Being supernumerary and not responsible for a patient workload throughout their undergraduate program allows nursing students to be free to pursue learning opportunities as they arise in the clinical unit.

Supernumerary

When a person is not included in the rostered numbers to cover the clinical area but makes an active contribution to care delivery.

Case Study 10.2: Supervision on placement

Melinda is undertaking her third-year placement in an extended care facility. She mentions to her preceptor, Peta, that she works as an AIN on the weekends. Peta has a full patient load during that shift so allocates two patients to Melinda to manage unsupervised. Melinda is not comfortable working without supervision.

- What should Melinda do in this case?

- Is there a degree of autonomy that Melinda can exercise as a third-year nursing student?

- What relevance does her AIN experience have to the current situation?

There are a number of models of clinical supervision used in healthcare organisations. The usual model is where registered nurses assume the role of a preceptor and predominantly supervise nursing students in practice, one on one, with a clinical educator and/or facilitator, who is from either the education provider or the health organisation, overseeing all of the students on placement (Health Workforce Australia [HWA], 2014a; Levett-Jones et al., 2018). The clinical educator or facilitator is also a registered nurse who works closely with both the preceptors and students to make sure they have a quality clinical learning experience. Together, the preceptor, clinical educator and/or facilitator teach and provide guidance and support for nursing students through education, role modelling and socialisation (Levett-Jones et al., 2018). They ensure assessments are completed, support achievement of learning outcomes, work with students who are not performing to standard, remove students from placement if they are deemed unsafe, give feedback to the education provider on student preparation, undertake regular debriefing, and deliver tutorial sessions to students as needed (HWA, 2014a; Levett-Jones et al., 2018).

Even though the nursing student is supervised by a preceptor, all health professionals on the team play an important role in the student's acquisition of non-technical skills by coaching them in the attitudes and behaviours expected within the clinical environment (Fukuta & Iitsuka, 2018). Nursing students need to develop and learn the importance of professional attributes such as effective communication, situational awareness, teamwork, decision-making and leadership (Fukuta & Iitsuka, 2018; Murray et al., 2016) and continually demonstrate these in their practice to enhance patient safety. Everyone on the healthcare team is a role model who can support new nurses to know and understand a raft of personal, professional, clinical and industry readiness capabilities for practice.

Maximising learning on placement

Learning is the aim and main priority for nursing students undertaking clinical placements. Every interaction within the clinical setting is an opportunity to engage in activities to become practice ready. It is important for nursing students to take the lead, be resourceful and actively engage in healthcare placements to make the most of the opportunities presented (Mellor & Gregoric, 2016). An important element of a student's clinical placements is the prospect of developing professional relationships and networks with potential post-graduation employers and co-workers. The clinical placement environment provides students with the opportunity to foster relationships with nurses who may be potential referees for graduate year applications.

Clinical placements need to be designed with elements that reflect the work of a registered nurse, to maximise the benefits. Exposure to various clinical areas and locations, and engaging in all shift times and days, including weekends, help to ensure that nursing students are suitably prepared on graduation. Clinical placement areas can be geographically dispersed and in tertiary, secondary and primary care. Exposing nursing students to a variety of clinical settings and situations enables them to apply their knowledge and skills in different situations (Benner et al., 2010). The variety will also engender flexible critical thinking and fosters the ability to adapt to and manage change. Working various shifts provides an excellent opportunity for nursing students to gain a good understanding of what it is like to work unsociable hours, and the effect it can have on their physical well-being (Missen et al., 2018). In doing so, nursing students become more prepared for the experience and plan more effectively for this when they commence practice.

 ## Portfolio Activity: Making the transition

Reflect on the variety of placements you have undertaken in your nursing program. Do you feel you have experienced sufficient variety in terms of clinical setting, geographical diversity and shift work?

Preparing for clinical placements

Being exposed to real patients, performing skills under scrutiny and in unfamiliar situations, can make clinical placements both intimidating and stressful for nursing students. This can compromise learning (Miller, 2014). Thorough preparation, using the clinical placement guidelines provided by your education provider and industry partners, assists in reducing anxiety and enhancing the learning experience. In actual fact, when you prepare and know what is required, you shift your focus from trying to recall these requirements, to achieving them and seeking additional learning experiences above the requirements.

Regardless of how many placements you have already completed, the increasing duration and significance of placements as you progress through your program makes adequate preparation even more important. In particular, students tell us that the consolidation placements in their final year are the most exciting and rewarding time of their studies. In Box 10.1, we have summarised specific points that you need to focus on so that you are adequately prepared and ready for your clinical placements and can maximise and enhance your learning during these experiences. They will be specifically important to your final extended clinical placement.

Box 10.1   Preparation for placement

- **Healthcare setting preparation:** Develop an understanding of the healthcare setting and clinical area you are allocated. Review the placement profile to find out about the facility, patient profile, clinical areas, health conditions, treatments and investigations.
- **Financial preparation:** Be aware that costs may include accommodation, parking and fuel, childcare and lost earning capacity while on clinical placements, particularly in your final year where placements are longer.
- **Knowledge preparation:** Revise notes and clinical course objectives. Read up on common diagnoses, medications and terminologies.
- **Learning preparation:** Make a list of what you need and what you want to learn during the placement. Then create achievable learning objectives and goals specific to the clinical area of practice. Align these to what you have been studying in classes and adhere to your scope of practice. These learning objectives and goals can build upon previous experience and be refined with your preceptor on the first day of your clinical placements.
- **Professional preparation:** Review the registered nurse standards for practice, code of conduct and code of ethics. Understand the scope of practice that is commensurate to the year level of your nursing program.
- **Orientation:** Read your induction material prior to the clinical placement. Attend the clinical briefing and, if available, the orientation provided by the healthcare organisation. Know your initial meeting place for placement and be on time. Know the location, transport, access and security arrangements if working shift work. If needed, explore this ahead of time.
- **Documentation:** Prior to attending placement, review what is involved in completing the clinical appraisal and assessment documentation, both interim and final, for assessing your competence on clinical placement.

Engaging in clinical placements

It is important that you work to make the most of clinical placement opportunities in order to be adequately prepared for your graduate year. By the final year, you will be ready to take responsibility and prioritise your learning opportunities while on placement. Remember that you are less likely to get the most out of these experiences if you simply stand back and observe; make an effort to be proactive and demonstrate willingness to be actively involved in patient care in respect of both clinical and non-clinical tasks. Finishing a placement with unfulfilled goals or a poor performance report can be demoralising and impact on study progression. Regularly review your performance and engage in activities to remediate gaps in your performance, to be the best you can be during this time.

During clinical placements, it is important to ensure you are given some responsibility and accountability for patient care, especially in your final year of study. Again, this facilitates learning in all domains of practice readiness but specifically professional and clinical readiness capabilities associated with critical thinking, time management, and clinical capabilities in assessment, planning and evaluating care (Missen et al., 2016). Table 10.1 provides guidelines for the expected performance level of nursing students relative to their year of study.

Table 10.1   Level of performance relative to year of study

Year level	Performance level
Year 1	Preceptor closely directs and/or observes and the student observes, participates and assists in care. *We teach you the rules and hold your hand as you cross the road.*
Year 2	Preceptor provides some supervision and/or guidance. The student actively participates, planning most activities and leading on some. *We remind you of the rules and walk beside you as you cross the road.*
Year 3	Preceptor provides minimal to indirect supervision. The student actively participates, planning all activities and leading most. *We remind you of the rules and watch as you cross the road. As a graduate nurse, you are expected to know the rules (or know where to find them) and cross the road on your own.*

Final clinical placement

One of the most exciting things about the final stages of nursing study is that you will get the opportunity to be more actively and independently involved in patients' care. Relying less on shadowing your preceptors gives you the opportunity to reinforce your learning and build confidence in your nursing skills. The consolidated time and continuity of your final clinical placement is crucial for cultivating higher levels of practice readiness. Your familiarity with the healthcare team and environment increases, which helps you to adapt and prepare to manage your responsibilities as a new graduate nurse. Kaihlanen et al. (2018) explored the impact of the final clinical placement and found that it provides a particular opportunity to develop confidence and competence with many aspects of the registered nurse role.

Gaining employment as newly graduated registered nurse can be very competitive, so the more you seek out and remain open to available opportunities during your final placement, the better placed you will be to secure a position as a new graduate. This can be particularly important if the organisation in which you are seeking employment as a new graduate, is where you are undertaking your final clinical practicum (Harrison et al., 2020). As part of your learning goals, ask your preceptors to provide you with opportunities to observe and to demonstrate your capabilities in areas that align with the registered nurse standards of practice. Importantly, nursing students in their final year placement need to practise initiating patient care and, if possible, managing a full patient load. Your preceptor needs to supervise you, but you will have the chance to demonstrate your ability to prioritise care and take on more responsibility.

Box 10.2 outlines the behaviours that healthcare organisations are looking for in healthcare professionals, and specifically in new graduate registered nurses who are considered practice ready. As you will learn in Chapter 12, nursing students, particularly those in their final year, are continually assessed as to their readiness for practice, and therefore as potential future employees in new graduate programs. Make each moment in the healthcare setting count. While you may have attended many clinical placements and know what these involve, we encourage you to review the list carefully to ensure you engage in these behaviours during your clinical placements.

Box 10.2   Engaging in clinical placement

- **Demonstrate professionalism and maintain safety:** Dress according to the specified uniform. Be punctual – arrive early on the first day and at least 15 minutes prior to the commencement of all shifts. This allows time to introduce yourself to staff, find handover and review your learning goals for the day. Notify appropriate staff (healthcare and education provider) in a timely manner when unable to attend a shift or placement, and report injuries and near misses immediately.
- **Adhere to standards and scope of practice:** Follow appropriate clinical procedures and protocols under the supervision of a registered nurse and work only to the level of practice commensurate with your nursing program.
- **Be self-directed:** Meet with your preceptor on your first day of placement and go through your learning objectives. Identify your strengths and limitations and set goals each week to work on both enhancing and developing your capabilities.
- **Acknowledge limitations:** Intellectual honesty is critical to safe practice. Acknowledge when you do not know something – be honest with yourself and others. Ask questions, seek help and support. This is an important habit for practice readiness and something healthcare staff will expect you to do.
- **Seek regular feedback:** Feedback is an essential component of learning. Actively request feedback from staff you are working with. Be aware that feedback can be formal or informal, so be sure to monitor verbal and nonverbal communications.
- **Access resources:** Read local policies, procedures and guidelines. These might include infection prevention and control, dress code, manual handling, equality and diversity, electronic devices and the use of social media. Organise resources specifically designed for quick access to medication information, calculation formulas and other essential reference material pertinent to your learning.
- **Engage proactively in learning and developing:** Seek and engage in a diverse range of experiences aimed at meeting your learning goals and developing your capability as a registered nurse.
- *Learn about diagnoses and procedures pertinent to your patients.*
- *Practise procedures even if you have done them before. If you need more practice on a specific procedure – ask for more.*
- *Reflect on what you have learnt at the end of each shift to reinforce learning. Keep a de-identified record of these reflections for your portfolio.*

One last important point regarding clinical placement – ensure all your clinical appraisal and assessment documentation is finalised on completion. This is your responsibility, not your preceptor's. Ensure your timesheet or attendance record is signed off by your preceptor each shift. As the final activity of any placement, update your professional portfolio. Keep a record of your assessments, learning plan and reflective pieces. These artefacts will support your application for a new graduate position when you complete your nursing program.

Challenges with clinical placements

Sometimes the quality of nursing students' clinical learning experiences can be affected by matters outside their control. The clinical environment can be a difficult and, occasionally, a hostile place for nursing students that can affect their ability to learn. A study by Budden et al. (2017) revealed that 50% of nursing student respondents experienced bullying and harassment behaviours while undertaking clinical placements, and that the main perpetrators were registered nurses. Bullying and harassment of any health professional, including nursing students, is unacceptable and has zero tolerance within the profession (Birks et al., 2018). The repercussions of bullying and harassment of nursing students are profound. Nursing students who have been bullied reported the loss of learning opportunities and being unable to meet learning objectives, loss of motivation and wanting to leave their nursing program (Minton & Birks, 2019). Not only does bullying impact on the well-being of students, it can contribute to workplace errors and concerns for patient safety (Birks et al., 2018). If a nursing student is subjected to bullying or harassment, they need to report this behaviour to their clinical educator or facilitator at the healthcare organisation immediately. If students feel uncomfortable with speaking to someone at the healthcare organisation, they need to contact and speak to the clinical coordinator or equivalent staff member at their educational institution.

Another challenge that has been highlighted in the literature, and one that students need to prepare for, is the witnessing of poor nursing practices on clinical placements (Bickoff et al., 2017). These practices include physical or emotional abuse of patients, breaches of patient safety, privacy and dignity, the provision of substandard or outdated care, and clinical errors (Bickoff et al., 2017). Research on nursing students who have witnessed poor practice during clinical placements found it resulted in negative feelings about themselves and the nursing profession, with some students questioning whether they should continue with their studies (Bickoff et al. 2017). Nursing students have reported that if they speak up about poor practices, it could result in a range of ramifications such as being ostracised and potentially experiencing horizontal violence from the nurses in that unit (Bickoff et al. 2016). Another consequence of speaking up is that nursing students thought it would affect their clinical placement assessment and ultimately their chances of working at the healthcare organisation post-graduation. As a result, students would stay silent to avoid confrontation (Bickoff et al. 2017).

Bickoff et al.'s (2016) study found that students' degree of morality increased as they progressed through their nursing program, with each new clinical placement experience and semester studies giving them more confidence to speak up if they were confronted with poor nursing practice. For the nursing profession to maintain high standards of practice, it is important that poor practice is challenged, not condoned. Clinical facilitators were noted as being trusted authority figures that students could turn to for encouragement as well as practical advice on how to communicate effectively with other nurses and debriefing if the need arose (Bickoff et al. 2016).

Case Study 10.3: Witnessing poor practice

Melinda is working night shift with her preceptor Peta. Peta asks Melinda to check a narcotic drug order for a terminally ill patient, Mrs Mitchell. Peta has been caring for Mrs Mitchell for a number of months and has become close to her. She is distressed to see her in pain. The drug order calls for ¾ of the vial to be administered to the patient, with the rest discarded according to protocol. Peta informs Melinda that she is giving Mrs Mitchell the full dose as she doesn't believe the prescribed amount is adequate. Peta hands Melinda the pen to sign the drug register.

- What should Melinda do in this situation?

- What are the potential consequences if Melinda refuses to sign?

- What are the consequences if she complies with Peta's request?

- If Peta believes the prescribed medication is inadequate, what should she do?

OXFORD UNIVERSITY PRESS

External work opportunities

Throughout this chapter, we discuss how seeking opportunities to develop the capabilities outlined in Chapter 5, and detailed further in Chapters 6, 7, 8 and 9, will help you become well prepared for your new role so that you can perform with a measure of competence and safety when you commence practice. Taking the initiative to be exposed to and practise the capabilities required of a registered nurse during a nursing program increases the ability of new graduate nurses to function independently (Missen et al., 2016). In addition to clinical placements, nursing students can enhance their readiness for practice through paid employment in both the healthcare facilities and in other settings, and through volunteering.

Paid employment in the healthcare setting

One of the most effective ways a nursing student can gain authentic experience to enhance their learning and practice readiness is through paid employment in a healthcare role. Many nursing students work in paid employment in a healthcare role during their nursing program. Paid employment provides first-hand experience of the realities of the workplace as an accountable professional.

While the pre-registration clinical placements garnered through university are necessary, these are structured, supervised and specifically tailored for learning. Working in the healthcare environment provides a lived experience as a healthcare professional that enhances learning in different ways. As an employee, the focus is on 'working' and meeting workplace responsibilities. In doing so, the nursing student becomes a respected, responsible member of the healthcare team, accountable for their nursing practice. Working in this role, they are exposed to the reality of practice and therefore have the opportunity to develop the capabilities necessary for their practice as a registered nurse, such as time management, communication and teamwork (Salamonson et al., 2020).

In Australia and New Zealand, there are various options for paid employment as a healthcare worker that nursing students can consider (Mitchell, 2020). Clinical experience gained through student in nursing (SIN), assistant in nursing (AIN) or enrolled nurse (EN) positions are thought to be some of the best options (Phillips et al., 2016; Salamonson et al., 2020). A SIN is a paid role in a healthcare facility that is aimed at complementing a nursing student's formal education programs and providing increased exposure to the clinical environment. You may be familiar with this role, through past or current work as a SIN. The role is independent from and not a requirement of a student's clinical placement experiences. A SIN works to a defined level of practice, depending on their stage of study in their nursing program and according to the health facility's policy, and they must be registered with AHPRA (Australian Nursing & Midwifery Federation [ANMF], 2017).

 ## Portfolio Activity: Making the transition

Are you currently working in a paid position in the healthcare setting? How has this contributed to your preparedness for your professional role? What specific skills relevant to your studies have you developed through this work?

AINs, also referred to as personal care assistants (PCAs), aged care workers (ACWs), disability support workers or care support workers, are paid employment healthcare roles but those positions are not professional nursing positions. It is important to note that there is no formal regulatory oversight of AINs, no standard educational requirement and no national practice standards (Schwartz, 2019). These are predominantly carer roles that assist people with activities of daily living (ADLs) such as feeding, toileting, showering, dressing and mobility. The responsibilities are defined by a specific role or job description and AINs work under the supervision of regulated nurses, such as enrolled and registered nurses (Schwartz, 2019). Most often AINs are employed in aged care facilities, primary healthcare clinics and hospitals.

Before entering a Bachelor of Nursing degree to become a registered nurse (RN), some students commence their nursing career as an enrolled nurse (EN). Nursing students who have qualified as an EN can continue to work as an EN while completing their nursing program. As outlined in Chapter 1, this is the first tier of nursing in both Australia and New Zealand. For an individual to become an EN, they must complete a Diploma of Nursing via a registered training organisation such as a Technical and Further Education (TAFE) institute in Australia or a Polytechnic in New Zealand. These courses of study can take up to two years, depending on the training organisation (Schwartz, 2019). EN training requires competency in a number of areas before students can complete the course and, while ENs can independently perform many tasks, they are required to work under the direct or indirect supervision of registered nurses (Schwartz, 2019).

 Portfolio Activity 10.2: Stop, reflect and think

What is your understanding of the distinction between enrolled and registered nursing roles? How does the scope of practice vary? How much does the specific workplace context determine how each role functions?

Working in one of these roles in a healthcare setting provides an opportunity to consolidate some nursing knowledge and skills in practice. There are, however, differences in scope of practice and therefore permission to perform certain tasks needs to be secured even if competency has been achieved as a nursing student. Such opportunities can help strengthen new graduate nurses' ability to work independently and competently; an area that has been identified as one that nursing graduates need to improve (Missen et al., 2016; Stuhlmiller & Tolchard, 2015; Woods et al., 2015). Further, these roles offer nursing students the chance to work with and observe registered nurses performing in their role. Nursing students can therefore gain tacit nursing knowledge, referred to previously, which can only be communicated through experience and is difficult to obtain in a coded, tangible form.

In addition to SIN, AIN and EN roles, there are a number of other roles within healthcare settings which can benefit nursing students. Working within a healthcare organisation can provide nursing students with valuable experience, particularly in relation to gaining exposure to the workings of the healthcare environment and healthcare professionals. A healthcare organisation may not necessarily be a hospital or aged care facility. Pharmacies, primary care clinics, community health centres, blood donor centres and private medical clinics are also useful places to learn and consolidate the skills required for nursing.

A hospital orderly (also known as a patient transport assistant, patient services assistant or wards person), for example, performs a number of tasks including assisting with transporting, lifting or turning patients; maintaining the cleanliness of the clinical environment; restocking equipment; bed making; and meal delivery. Options also exist for nursing students to work as phlebotomists or pathology collectors. Pathology collection requires the ability to strictly follow procedures and comply with hygiene regulations, both of which are essential components of nursing. Additionally, this position requires regular contact with patients, and good communication skills are required to ensure procedures and instructions are explained clearly to those being cared for (TAFE Courses Australia, 2018). Roles such as orderly and phlebotomist require completion of a certificate from a registered training organisation (RTO), and you may be able to secure advanced standing for studies completed in your nursing program.

Clerical workers or ward clerks are vital to healthcare facilities. Sometimes these positions may be referred to as admissions clerk, administration officer or medical receptionist. While the title may vary, the position is essentially a combination of customer service and administration skills, requiring interaction with patients and visitors. The role includes arranging and recording appointment information, managing enquiries, complaints, correspondence and sometimes medical record information. To undertake this role, some organisations require the completion of a certificate from a registered training organisation. These positions require time management, communication skills and the ability to work independently under supervision, all of which are essential capabilities for your role as a beginning registered nurse.

Paid employment in other roles

Transferable skills

Skills and abilities that are relevant and able to be applied across different areas. They are sometimes referred to as portable skills.

While it would be ideal for all students to have extended exposure to healthcare settings in healthcare roles, the reality is that this is not always possible. When contemplating paid employment that is not in a healthcare role or is outside a healthcare setting, it is important to consider positions that support the development of skills that are **transferable** and can be applied to nursing roles.

Areas of employment that augment preparation for practice include those that enhance personal and professional readiness capabilities such as communication, critical thinking and problem solving, working independently and delegation, customer service, time management, task prioritisation and conflict management (Mellor & Gregoric, 2016; Missen et al., 2016; Woods et al., 2015). Any type of leadership, management and teamwork role, whether in healthcare, retail or another area, will aid to prepare nursing students with skills required for their nursing role. Nurses take on leadership roles and work in teams throughout their career, and it is these qualities that contribute to ensuring patient safety and high-quality care (Ellis, 2018). Phillips et al. (2016) identified a number of positive factors that support engaging in paid employment while studying a nursing degree, whether in health or a non-clinical role. Working in hospitality or retail has benefits for nursing students by improving confidence, communication, teamwork and time management. For those in healthcare employment, there is the additional benefit of consolidation of nursing skills.

Working in a retail store provides the opportunity to develop customer service skills and therefore communication, problem solving and conflict resolution. Working in hospitality will develop essential communication, multi-tasking, teamwork and customer service skills, as well as conflict resolution and potentially heightened cultural awareness. Working in the hospitality industry also enables the development of a strong work ethic and excellent time management skills, with multi-tasking and customer service being at the forefront of good service. This type of work provides exposure to shift work and how to manage it in relation to other lifestyle commitments. These skills have been identified as ones in which nursing students often have reduced confidence or proficiency (Missen et al., 2016).

Volunteering

Volunteering is an avenue through which students can gain exposure to the healthcare environment. Through volunteering, nursing students can improve their psychosocial skills, including communication and social interaction skills, while helping others. Non-profit organisations, aged care facilities and hospitals are great places to apply for a volunteer role; however, it is important to remember that this work will be within the scope of the volunteering role, not a nursing position. Education providers sometimes have opportunities for volunteering placements and will send out announcements to nursing students when they are available. Often these opportunities are limited and competitive, and an application process is used to select volunteers (Baumann et al., 2018). Nursing students can use this as an opportunity to practise applying for jobs and interviews, regardless of the outcome.

 Portfolio Activity: Making the transition

After reading and reflecting on the opportunities available for you, think about where you are at now and the time remaining in your nursing program. Consider whether there is more you could be doing to access and engage in relevant opportunities to further enhance your practice readiness capabilities.

Working while studying

Christiansen et al. (2019) maintain that there is a fine balance between work, study and home life, which not all students can manage. Working in a healthcare setting during nursing studies ties together theoretical knowledge and practice and can assist some students with prioritisation and time management skills; however, working while studying requires resilience and tenacity to succeed (Christiansen et al., 2019). Maximising the benefits requires solid time management and the ability to recognise when your employment is affecting your ability to study, or vice versa. Some nursing students can struggle to get real value from clinical placements because they are exhausted from their extracurricular workload (Christiansen et al., 2019). Therefore, it is essential that, if you do choose to work during your nursing studies, you monitor your progress and adjust your work or study to ensure that neither detrimentally affects the other. In particular, it may be necessary to suspend your usual employment while undertaking placement.

It is advisable that nursing students who are employed in a healthcare setting do not undertake clinical placements at their place of employment. When this happens, there is a risk that the nursing student will end up working within the scope of their employment rather than the scope of a nursing student role. This can compromise the learning experience and leave the student frustrated at the expected level of knowledge from their peers (Brown et al., 2015). Further, most education providers recommend that nursing students not undertake paid work while on clinical placements. Completing a 40-hour week of shift work while also attempting to work can lead to extreme tiredness and affect a student's well-being. This can have detrimental effects on clinical reasoning and patient safety (Christiansen et al., 2019). These are important factors for nursing students to consider when working and studying. Clinical placements are a significant component of a nursing student's development as a registered nurse. It is essential that, as key learning experiences, they are not compromised. Balancing work and study and being well prepared for the physical and mental demands of professional experience is vital.

Case Study 10.4: Working while studying

Melinda's car insurance payment is due and she is struggling to get the money together. She decides to take some extra shifts at the aged care facility. She is presenting at work for an early shift straight from her overnight placement.

- What are the potential risks in this situation?
- What codes and standards of practice is Melinda breaching?
- If you were a colleague of Melinda's, what would your responsibilities be in this case?

Conclusion

Throughout this text we have emphasised the importance of practice readiness and its impact on your transition to the professional role, patient safety and workforce retention. New nurses need to be prepared with the capability to provide safe professional practice within a demanding and evolving healthcare system (Harrison et al., 2020). Through quality learning experiences in the clinical environment, students are provided with the opportunity to combine theory and practice, consolidating their foundational knowledge and skills, and become lifelong learners. Work experiences in more diverse settings can contribute to practice readiness in indirect ways, further helping to smooth the transition to the professional role.

Key summary points

- New graduate nurses must be well prepared, self-directed and as ready as possible to manage the responsibilities of their new role.

- There are a number of strategies that contribute to a graduate's preparation for practice along the readiness continuum, including quality clinical placement experiences and external work opportunities.

- Quality clinical experiences that provide authentic practice in the healthcare environment are essential for developing the capabilities necessary to work as a registered nurse.

- Thorough preparation for clinical placements will assist in reducing anxiety and enhancing the learning experience.

- Nursing students will be more adequately prepared for practice if they take responsibility and prioritise learning opportunities while on placement.

- Nursing students need to take the opportunity to be actively involved in patients' care rather than simply observing and shadowing their preceptors, particularly during their final clinical practicum.

- At times, the clinical environment can raise challenges for nursing students and affect their ability to learn; students should be comfortable seeking support when this occurs.

- In addition to clinical placements, nursing students can enhance their readiness for practice through paid employment and/or volunteering.

- Nursing students must be careful to ensure a balance between work and study, particularly while on placement, and should avoid undertaking placement at their place of employment.

Critical thinking questions

1. What strategies have you used to maximise your learning opportunities when on clinical placements?

2. Analyse and evaluate the advantages and disadvantages of working while studying.

3. What strategies can nursing students utilise to enhance their practice readiness while working in a paid employment position?

OXFORD UNIVERSITY PRESS

4. In this chapter we discuss the need for nursing students to avoid undertaking placements at their place of employment. Do you agree with this position? Provide a rationale for your answer.

References

Aiken, L., Cerón, C., Simonetti, M., Lake, E. T., Galiano, A., Garbarini, A., Soto, P., Bravo, D., & Smith, H. L. (2018). Hospital nurse staffing and patient outcomes. *Revista Médica Clínica Las Condes, 29*(3), 322–327. https://doi.org/10.1016/j.rmclc.2018.04.011

Australian Nursing & Midwifery Accreditation Council. (2019). *Registered nurse accreditation standards 2019.* https://www.anmac.org.au/search/publication

Australian Nursing & Midwifery Federation. (2017). *ANMF position statement: Employment of undergraduate students of nursing and midwifery.* http://anmf.org.au/documents/policies/PS_Employment_UG_students_nursing_midwifery.pdf

Baumann, S. L., Sharoff, L., & Penalo, L. (2018). Using simulation to enhance global nursing. *Nursing Science Quarterly, 31*(4), 374–378. https://doi.org/10.1177/0894318418792877

Benner, P. E., Sutphen, M., Leonard, V., & Day, L. (2010). *Educating nurses: A call for radical transformation.* Jossey-Bass.

Bickoff, L., Levett-Jones, T., & Sinclair, P. M. (2016). Rocking the boat – Nursing students' stories of moral courage. A qualitative descriptive study. *Nurse Education Today, 42,* 35–40. https://doi.org/10.1016/j.nedt.2016.03.030

Bickoff, L., Sinclair, P. M. & Levett-Jones, T. (2017). Moral courage in undergraduate nursing students: A literature review. *Collegian, 24*(1), 71–83. https://doi.org/10.1016/j.colegn.2015.08.002

Birks, M., Bagley, T., Park, T. L., Burkot, C., & Mills, J. (2017). The impact of clinical placement model on learning in nursing: A descriptive exploratory study. *Australian Journal of Advanced Nursing, 34*(3), 16–23.

Birks, M., Budden, L. M., Biedermann, N., Park, T., & Chapman, Y. (2018). A 'rite of passage?' Bullying experiences of nursing students in Australia. *Collegian, 25*(1), 45–50. https://doi.org/10.1016/j.colegn.2017.03.005

Brown, C., Baker, M., Jessup, M., & Marshall, A. P. (2015). EN2RN: Transitioning to a new scope of practice. *Contemporary Nurse, 50*(2–3), 196–205. https://doi.org/10.1080/10376178.2015.1111766

Budden, L. M., Birks, M., Cant, R., Bagley, T., & Park, T. (2017). Australian nursing students' experience of bullying and/or harassment during clinical placement. *Collegian, 24*(2), 125–133. https://doi.org/10.1016/j.colegn.2015.11.004

Christiansen, A., Salamonson, Y., Crawford, R., McGrath, B., Roach, D., Wall, P., Kelly, M., & Ramjan, L. M. (2019). 'Juggling many balls': Working and studying among first-year nursing students. *Journal of Clinical Nursing, 28*(21–22), 4035–4043. https://doi.org/10.1111/jocn.14999

Doughty, L., McKillop, A., Dixon, R., & Sinnema, C. (2018). Educating new graduate nurses in their first year of practice: The perspective and experiences of the new graduate nurses and the director of nursing. *Nurse Education in Practice, 30,* 101–105. https://doi.org/10.1016/j.nepr.2018.03.006

Duchscher, J. E. B. (2008). A process of becoming: The stages of new nursing graduate professional role transition. *Journal of Continuing Nursing Education, 39*(10), 441–450. https://doi.org/10.3928/00220124-20081001-03

Duchscher, J. E. B. (2009). Transition shock: The initial stage of role adaptation for newly-graduated registered nurses. *Journal of Advanced Nursing, 65*(5), 1103–1113. https://doi.org/10.1111/j.1365-2648.2008.04898.x

El Haddad, M., Moxham, L., & Broadbent, M. (2013). Graduate registered nurse practice readiness in the Australian context: An issue worthy of discussion. *Collegian, 20*(4), 233–238. http://dx.doi.org/10.1016/j.colegn.2012.09.003

Ellis, P. (2018). *Leadership, management and team working in nursing*. Learning Matters.

Ford, K., Courtney-Pratt, H., Marlow, A., Cooper, J., Williams, D., & Mason, R. (2016). Quality clinical placements: The perspectives of undergraduate nursing students and their supervising nurses. *Nurse Education Today, 37*, 97–102. https://doi.org/10.1016/j.nedt.2015.11.013

Fukuta, D., & Iitsuka, M. (2018). Nontechnical skills training and patient safety in undergraduate nursing education: A systematic review. *Teaching and Learning in Nursing, 13*(4), 233–239. https://doi.org/10.1016/j.teln.2018.06.004

Harrison, H., Birks, M., Franklin, R., & Mills, J. (2020). Fostering graduate nurse practice readiness in context. *Collegian, 27*(1), 115–124. https://doi.org/10.1016/j.colegn.2019.07.006

Health Workforce Australia. (2014a). *Clinical training profile: Nursing March 2014*. Retrieved October 13, 2020 from https://www1.health.gov.au/internet/main/publishing.nsf/Content/hwa-archived-publications

Health Workforce Australia. (2014b). *Australia's future health workforce: Nurses overview report August 2014*. Retrieved October 13, 2020 from https://www1.health.gov.au/internet/main/publishing.nsf/Content/hwa-archived-publications

Jamshidi, N., Molazem, Z., Sharif, F., Torabizadeh, C., & Najafi Kalyani, M. (2016). The challenges of nursing students in the clinical learning environment: A qualitative study. *The Scientific World Journal, 2016*, Article 1846178. https://doi.org/10.1155/2016/1846178

Kaihlanen, A.-M., Salminen, L., Flinkman, M., & Haavisto, E. (2018). Newly graduated nurses' perceptions of a final clinical practicum facilitating transition: A qualitative descriptive study. *Collegian, 26*(1), 55–61. https://doi.org/10.1016/j.colegn.2018.03.003

Levett-Jones, T., Reid-Searl, K., & Bourgeois, S. (2018). *The clinical placement: An essential guide for nursing students* (4th. ed.). Elsevier.

Mellor, P., & Gregoric, C. (2016). Ways of being: Preparing nursing students for transition to professional practice. *Journal of Continuing Education in Nursing, 47*(7), 330–340. https://doi.org/10.3928/00220124-20160616-10

Miller, S. L. (2014). Assisting students to prepare for a clinical practice placement. *Nursing Standard, 29*(15), 51–59. https://doi.org/10.7748/ns.29.15.51.e9274

Milton-Wildey, K., Kenny, P., Parmenter, G., & Hall, J. (2014). Educational preparation for clinical nursing: The satisfaction of students and new graduates from two Australian universities. *Nurse Education Today, 34*(4), 648–654. https://doi.org/10.1016/j.nedt.2013.07.004

Minton, C., & Birks, M. (2019). 'You can't escape it': Bullying experiences of New Zealand nursing students on clinical placement. *Nurse Education Today, 77*, 12–17. https://doi.org/10.1016/j.nedt.2019.03.002

Missen, K., McKenna, L., & Beauchamp, A. (2014). Graduate nurse program coordinators' perceptions of role adaptation experienced by new nursing graduates: A descriptive qualitative approach. *Journal of Nursing Education and Practice, 4*(12), 134–141. https://doi.org/10.5430/jnep.v4n12p134

Missen, K., McKenna, L., & Beauchamp, A. (2015). Work readiness of nursing graduates: Current perspectives of graduate nurse program coordinators. *Contemporary Nurse, 51*(1), 27–38. https://doi.org/10.1080/10376178.2015.1095054

Missen, K., McKenna, L., & Beauchamp, A. (2018). Are we there yet? Graduate readiness for practice, assessment and final examinations. *Collegian, 25*(2), 227–230. https://doi.org/10.1016/j.colegn.2017.06.006

Missen, K., McKenna, L., Beauchamp, A., & Larkins, J.-A. (2016). Qualified nurses rate new nursing graduates as lacking skills in key clinical areas. *Journal of Clinical Nursing, 25*(15–16), 2134–2143. https://doi.org/10.1111/jocn.13316

Mitchell, J. (2020). Juggling employment and studies: Nursing students' perceptions of the influence of paid employment on their success. *Nurse Education Today, 92*, 104429. https://doi.org/10.1016/j.nedt.2020.104429

Murray, K., McKenzie, K., & Kelleher, M. (2016). The evaluation of a framework for measuring the non-technical ward round skills of final year nursing students: An observational study. *Nurse Education Today, 45*, 87–90. https://doi.org/10.1016/j.nedt.2016.06.024

Nursing Council of New Zealand. (2020). *Education: Educating and preparing competent nurses.* https://www.nursingcouncil.org.nz/Public/Education/NCNZ/Education.aspx?hkey=ad8e6aed-3834-4aef-bbd2-eaa223a5c113

Olds, D. M., Aiken, L. H., Cimiotti, J. P., & Lake, E. T. (2017). Association of nurse work environment and safety climate on patient mortality: A cross-sectional study. *International Journal of Nursing Studies, 74*, 155–161. https://doi.org/10.1016/j.ijnurstu.2017.06.004

Parker, V., Giles, M., Lantry, G., & McMillan, M. (2014). New graduate nurses' experiences in their first year of practice. *Nurse Education Today, 34*(1), 150–156. https://doi.org/10.1016/j.nedt.2012.07.003

Phillips, C., Kenny, A., & Esterman, A. (2016). Pre-registration paid employment practices of undergraduate nursing students: A scoping review. *Collegian, 23*(1), 115–127. https://doi.org/10.1016/j.colegn.2014.09.012

Salamonson, Y., Roach, D., Crawford, R., McGrath, B., Christiansen, A., Wall, P., Kelly, M., & Ramjan, L. M. (2020). The type and amount of paid work while studying influence academic performance of first year nursing students: An inception cohort study. *Nurse Education Today, 84*, 104213. https://doi.org/10.1016/j.nedt.2019.104213

Schwartz, S. (2019). *Educating the nurse of the future: Report of the Independent Review into Nursing Education.* Australian Government Department of Health. https://www.health.gov.au/resources/publications/educating-the-nurse-of-the-future

Stuhlmiller, C., & Tolchard, B. (2015). Developing a student-led health and wellbeing clinic in an underserved community: Collaborative learning, health outcomes and cost savings. *BMC Nursing, 14*(1), 1–8. https://doi.org/10.1186/s12912-015-0083-9

TAFE Courses Australia. (2018). *Compare courses from Australia's leading TAFEs and Colleges.* https://www.tafecourses.com.au/

Walker, A., & Campbell, K. (2013). Work readiness of graduate nurses and the impact on job satisfaction, work engagement and intention to remain. *Nurse Education Today, 33*(12), 1490–1495. https://doi.org/10.1016/j.nedt.2013.05.008

Walker, S., Dwyer, T., Moxham, L., Broadbent, M., & Sander, T. (2013). Facilitator versus preceptor: Which offers the best support to undergraduate nursing students? *Nurse Education Today, 33*(5), 530–535. https://doi.org/10.1016/j.nedt.2011.12.005

Wareing, M., Taylor, R., Wilson, A., & Sharples, A. (2017). The influence of placements on adult nursing graduates' choice of first post. *British Journal of Nursing, 26*(4), 228–233. https://doi.org/10.12968/bjon.2017.26.4.228

Woods, C., West, C., Mills, J., Park, T., Southern, J., & Usher, K. (2015). Undergraduate student nurses' self-reported preparedness for practice. *Collegian, 22*(4), 359–368. https://doi.org/10.1016/j.colegn.2014.05.003

Chapter 11

The Right Environment to Flourish

Caroline Rosenberg, Michael Leiter and Helena Harrison

Learning Outcomes

Upon completion of this chapter, you will be able to:

1. Describe the factors that cultivate environments in which new graduate nurses can flourish.
2. Recognise incivility and signs of burnout in yourself and others.
3. Evaluate the causes and impacts of burnout in the context of healthcare environments.
4. Formulate strategies that prevent, mitigate and manage negative workplace interactions.

Key terms

Attachment style
Burnout
Cognitive bias
Complex system
Confidence
Culture

Healthy workplace
environment
Incivility
Job Demands-Resources
(JD-R) model
Leadership

Psychological safety
Resilience
Self-determination
Self-efficacy
Tacit knowledge

Introduction

In this chapter, we bring the focus back to the healthcare environment and examine the key factors that can be both helpful and contrary to your development as a registered nurse. As a result, you will be able to identify the environments, individuals and resources that best support and facilitate your professional development. The right environment for new graduate nurses to flourish is a positive healthy one, where new graduate nurses feel safe and supported to grow and develop. We begin the chapter by exploring the key factors that drive a positive workplace environment. In the second part of the chapter we examine aspects of healthcare environments that can be challenging for new graduate nurses, with a focus on causes and impacts of negative workplace interactions. Leveraging on the readiness capabilities discussed in previous chapters, you will learn skills that will help you to navigate these situations as a new graduate nurse.

> ## Case Study 11.1: Introducing Felipe
>
> Felipe is a 22-year-old international student from Chile. He is enjoying his final year of study for his nursing degree but is nervous about making the transition to a registered nurse. He plans to seek permanent residency following his graduate year. Felipe is academically strong and has a solid command of English although he speaks with an accent. He believes he is practice ready.

What is the right workplace environment?

As a new nursing graduate celebrating the completion of your degree and feeling accomplished and ready to enter the workforce with enthusiasm and commitment, the reality of working life, as discussed in Chapter 4, can be a shock to the system. Your first year of practice will be your first engagement with the workplace as a registered professional, without the structure and supported conditions experienced in your nursing program. At this time, points of reference for support, and a workplace environment that enables you to learn and grow as a registered nurse, are yet to be established. Prior knowledge of the factors in the workplace that will support and facilitate your progress, and how to recognise these, can help support a successful transition period.

The right environment

For new graduate nurses, the right environment is one where factors present in the workplace interact to create a place where new graduates feel respected, safe and supported and can demonstrate, learn and develop their capability as a registered nurse. These environments reflect those described as healthy workplace environments. Research indicates that positive workplace environments are critical to a new graduate's transition to practice (Kramer et al., 2013a; Laschinger et al., 2016; Phillips et al., 2015; Walker et al., 2017). Definitions of a **healthy workplace environment** vary, with the term often referring to similar concepts but focusing on different aspects. For example, the term 'good work environment' includes aspects of the physical, psychosocial and organisational conditions (Lindberg & Vingård, 2012) and the term 'healthy work organisation' includes a healthy workforce as well as the financial success of the organisation (Lindberg & Vingård, 2012; Sainfort et al., 2001). Alternatively, the World Health Organization (WHO) defines a healthy workplace as one where managers and employees collaborate to continually improve, promote and protect the health, safety and well-being of all employees and the business of the workplace by focusing on the individual, environmental and organisational factors affecting an employee's well-being (Burton, 2010, p. 15).

Relative to new graduate nurses, Kramer et al. (2013a) defined a healthy workplace environment as an interrelated system of people, structures and practices that enable nurses to engage positively in work processes and relationships. This definition highlights the fixed fundamental elements of the workplace as a system, as well as the interrelated fluidity of elements that interact to create a workplace environment. Translating that into the characteristics of the 'right' workplace environment indicates two overarching categories. One is to meet the common core needs required by everyone who works and operates

Healthy workplace environment

The outcome of a collaborative, interrelated system of people, structure and practices that enables others to engage effectively in work processes and relationships to meet the core and subjective needs of all employees.

in the environment; and the other is to be adaptive to the subjective, individual needs that vary from person to person, which is particularly important to new graduate nurses commencing work for the first time.

Key elements of the right environment

While the right environment for anyone is subjectively determined and varies according to an individual's needs, there are key factors that are particularly important for new graduate nurses during their transition year. Workplace environments that are stable, predictable, familiar and consistent support successful transition processes (Duchscher, 2012). These elements help new graduate nurses gain a sense of stability, control and support while adapting to their new role and responsibilities (Duchscher, 2012). Creating an environment that cultivates these qualities takes time and is reliant on the interaction of certain elements present in the workplace. These include positive leadership, collegial teams, a positive workplace culture and structured support. The presence of these elements is a strong predictor of a healthy workplace environment, one that enables new nurses to thrive and evolve (Harrison et al., 2020).

 Portfolio Activity 11.1: Stop, reflect and think

Reflect on your clinical placements. Can you think of an experience that you really enjoyed and from which you learnt a lot? Can you recall why you found the experience so enjoyable? Was it the people, the type of nursing or patients? Was it the leadership and respect you felt while you worked with the team?

Leadership

The ability to influence and guide others toward achieving a common goal in a way that leaves them feeling motivated and accomplished.

Positive leadership

Leadership is an essential element for achieving key organisational outcomes, including staff motivation and engagement (Smith et al., 2013). In the healthcare context, leadership for new graduate nurses stems from many sources, including hospital executives, nursing unit managers and educators, senior staff and clinical nurses. The collective leadership from these individuals influences the experiences of graduate nurses both directly and indirectly.

There is a wealth of literature related to leadership and leadership styles and associated qualities. Each leader has their own leadership style, based on their personalities, preferences, past experiences and the needs of their current role. Traditionally, style categories are based on levels of control, ranging from highly controlled autocratic leadership, to moderately controlled democratic leadership, to low controlled laissez-faire leadership. In recent years, leadership researchers and professionals have invested more focus on styles that are based on particular functions. For example, transformational leadership focuses on change through inspiration and transactional leadership focuses on motivating through reward and correction. Other leadership styles, such as ethical leadership, servant leadership and authentic leadership, also emphasise one aspect of leadership functions that are needed in particular workplace environments.

Despite the popularity of some leadership styles, effective leadership is dependent on the workplace context and the preferences of the people in the workplace. According to the Leader-Member Exchange (LMX) framework, the quality of the relationships between leaders and followers is determined by the characteristics of the leader and the follower, as well as their perceived similarity and affect towards each other (Dulebohn et al., 2012). Effective leaders may naturally have different qualities and styles, but adapt these to the situational needs and preferences of their teams.

Leaders who cultivate positive healthy workplace conditions for new graduate nurses are themselves positive, approachable and encouraging, aim for equitable fair workplaces and prioritise staff and patients in how they manage resources (Harrison et al., 2020). These leaders are well connected to their staff and known to foster high-functioning teams that are respectful to each other and to newcomers (Kaiser, 2017). They are situationally aware; that is, they know what is going on in the environment, and aim to ensure that all staff are supported. As leaders, they collaborate with staff, provide resources that facilitate quality patient care and promote professional development (Kramer et al., 2013a). A supportive, welcoming and encouraging environment where staff facilitate learning and socialisation cultivates a sense of safety, belonging, autonomy and respect (D'Ambra & Andrews, 2014; Phillips et al., 2015; Walker et al., 2017). Belongingness or relatedness, autonomy or agency, and competence are core needs fundamental to human experience (Leiter & Maslach, 2017) and instil a motivation for work (Deci & Ryan, 1985). The right workplace environment is one where factors are present that help individuals meet these core needs.

Belongingness describes nurses' relationships with a particular group and people within that group. The need to belong by forming social attachments is a fundamental human motivation regardless of context (Baumeister & Leary, 1995). Given that working adults spend a significant portion of their waking hours at work, belongingness in the workplace is increasingly important. From a skill or competency perspective, in a healthcare context, other nurses are the most relatable team members for a new graduate nurse as they share similar work tasks and understand common work challenges. A new graduate nurse's belongingness and relatedness are fostered through working as part of a professional team with people, such as other nurses, who appreciate and respect their competency and autonomy. The sense of belongingness is also experienced through positive social interactions at work that may not be directly related to professional skills. For example, being included in social functions, especially with people who are perceived to be in the same workgroup, being treated fairly in workload allocation, or receiving recognition that indicates team membership.

The need for autonomy and competence motivate self-initiated behaviours as part of self-selected goals (Deci & Ryan, 1985). Workplace structures that provide opportunities for employees to make independent decisions and utilise their purposively acquired skills to make an impact, will fulfil the need for autonomy and competence. This cultivates essential capabilities that new graduate nurses need to develop in their first year – independent and autonomous practice. A sense of belongingness, autonomy and competence need to be nurtured and strengthened throughout the graduate year and the early career stages of newly registered nurses. These core needs are fundamental to human experience and essential for new graduate nurses to flourish.

Self-determination

The concept that people are motivated to participate and engage in activities because of their inherent human needs and intrinsic motives.

For new graduate nurses, working as a registered nurse gives meaning to the three years of full-time tertiary education. It provides a licence to be an autonomous agent in the health profession, and validates their professional competence. It also helps to solidify their identity and belongingness as a skilled member of a profession. From a perspective of **self-determination** theory, people are motivated to participate and engage in workplace activities because of the interplay between the extrinsic forces acting on them and the intrinsic motives and needs inherent in human nature (Deci & Ryan, 1985; Ryan & Deci, 2000). These circumstances engender positive transition experiences for new graduates that foster autonomy, competence, confidence and job satisfaction (Dawson et al., 2014; Kramer et al., 2012; Laschinger et al., 2012).

Positive, firm, approachable leaders are necessary for establishing relationships that encourage nurses to voice concerns and ask for help (Paterson et al., 2015). This is critical to developing safe practice and is particularly important when faced with difficult or conflicting situations, related staff interactions, or patient care that can compromise patient or staff safety. As discussed in Chapter 8, new nurses need to feel safe to speak up, identify and escalate concerns without fear of recuse. When leaders are approachable and encouraging, and can be relied upon for support, it is easier to speak with them and seek their advice and support.

Bowlby's (1969) attachment theory gives us some insight into why this type of leadership is so influential and important. Bowlby (1969) studied the nature and development of the bond between infants and their caregivers. His findings indicated that infants, driven by the core human need of belonging, are innately motivated to seek comfort and safety from an attachment figure in times of need (Baumeister & Leary, 1995; Bowlby, 1969, 1979). Bowlby (1969) defined this bond as attachment, and described three **attachment styles** to indicate the different patterns of behaviours in times of stress. These attachment styles are thought to influence an individual's relationship development into adulthood (Ainsworth, 1979; Bowlby, 1969). The attachment patterns are (Bowlby, 1969):

1. Secure: the result of consistent experiences of supportive care
2. Anxious: the result of inconsistent availability of supportive care
3. Avoidant: the result of consistently unavailable supportive care.

The attachment theory has been extended to organisational life and relationships at work. Advances have been made in understanding leadership dynamics, employee proactivity (Wu & Parker, 2012, 2017) and burnout (Leiter et al., 2015). In the workplace, leaders and managers are often perceived as attachment figures for employees, including new graduate nurses. Securely attached individuals experience more satisfaction at work, not only feeling competent with their own skills, but also having positive views about colleagues and the job. Conversely, individuals who are anxious or ambivalent tend to worry about acceptance or approval from others, while avoidant individuals

Attachment style

The pattern of behaviour an infant develops in response to stress, which is determined by the emotional bond and the consistency of supportive care provided by the caregiver.

tend to work alone and distance themselves from emotional connections with others (Wu & Parker, 2012, 2017). Because of the different attachment styles, professional relationships with colleagues and managers will vary.

Individuals who have an anxious or ambivalent attachment style are likely to have a more critical view about themselves and seek closer relationships from others (Mikulincer & Florian, 1995). Regular feedback and frequent reassurance from the attachment figure are needed to maintain performance. Individuals who have avoidant attachment style are likely to be critical of others, and do not seek to establish relationships. Therefore it is challenging to establish trust with colleagues and supervisors under stress (Collins & Read, 1990; Hazan & Shaver, 1990). Leaders need to appropriately challenge the existing beliefs of avoidant individuals, as trust is an essential element in teamwork, especially in healthcare professions.

Leaders who are firm and fair, prioritise staff and patients and value collaboration are more likely to take an interest in and address issues to preserve the workplace culture. Where a leader is responsive, adaptive and collaborative with staff, individuals will be more likely to have their individual core needs met. They are more likely to feel secure, competent and satisfied, and engender positive responses to work and the organisation. This influences the nature of the teams in the workplace.

 ## Portfolio Activity 11.2: Stop, reflect and think

Think about your clinical placements. Have you met leaders who reflect some or all of what is described here? Are they nurse managers or clinical nurses working alongside you, providing care? Can you describe their verbal and non-verbal interactions? Reflect on how these individuals make you feel and behave.

Collegial teams

The leadership of the workplace environment plays an indirect, but crucial, role in creating how teams relate and the workplace culture. As you recall from Chapter 2, healthcare teams are interprofessional; they can extend beyond nurses to medical and allied health professionals, technicians and other specialists. The multidisciplinary nature of the team introduces complexity to team relationships and tasks. Positive leadership can generate a positive healthy workplace; however, it can only be sustained by the collective of individuals in the team.

Positive engaged leadership and collaboration is associated with high-performing cohesive teams (Vaughn et al., 2018). Leaders who provide consistent support to the team, role modelling positive, equitable and collaborative interactions, will create healthcare teams that are collegial and supportive. Importantly, the leader's interactions with and attitude towards a new graduate nurse influences the attitude of staff and how they welcome and support that person. If leaders are positive about supporting new nurses, they will be embraced by the team and given opportunities to develop their nursing practice (Harrison et al., 2020).

Positive interactions dominate the relationships within a collegial healthcare team. These teams demonstrate mutual respect, open communication and shared expectations. Team members are supportive, respectful and helpful to each other and welcoming, inclusive and encouraging of new graduate nurses. All team members look for opportunities for new graduates to learn, and contribute to their growth and socialisation. As such, new graduate nurses are assimilated in the workplace and eased into the team – they have their core needs met. Consistent support and constructive feedback are given by the team members. Again, this is critical for new graduate nurses to cultivate a sense of autonomy, belonging and competence. Competence in your professional domain instils confidence in other healthcare professionals on the team. The collaboration and cohesiveness of the healthcare team in turn instils trust and confidence in the patients, who are often apprehensive about their health situation.

As a new graduate nurse entering a new social environment at work, positive healthy environments also offer the opportunity to develop positive working models of both yourself and others, and to feel secure when exploring the new work environment and building new social relationships at work (Leiter et al., 2015; Mikulincer & Florian, 1995). Developing relationships with positive professional role models can also lead to reciprocal role modelling, whereby those within the relationship become cognisant and accepting of each other's knowledge and skills, learn and adopt them to become better practitioners (Hoare, 2016). These experiences strengthen the relationship and enable the transfer of the necessary tacit knowledge that is held by experienced nurses and needed by new graduates for their professional development as a registered nurse. Observing how senior staff manage challenging situations will also help new nurses build up a repertoire of strategies for managing their own practice in similar situations. Given that the quality of leadership influences people's attitudes, goals and relationships in the workplace, leaders therefore have a significant influence on the workplace culture (Boamah et al., 2016).

 Portfolio Activity 11.3: Stop, reflect and think

Consider your clinical placements and the culture of the workplaces you have experienced. Is there one that stood out for making you feel positive and embraced as part of the team? Did you feel a sense of belonging in this team? Can you recall how the team interacted to support you? How did this make you feel and behave?

Positive workplace culture

Culture

Shared attitudes, social conventions, values, goals and practices that characterise a group or situation.

Culture represents the shared attitudes, social conventions, values, goals and practices that characterise a workplace. These are communicated through the interactions between those working in the environment. When positive leadership and collegial teams are present, a supportive workplace culture that promotes psychological safety develops. The concept of psychological safety has been recognised as an enabling condition for better workplace collaboration – which is a critical factor in understanding teamwork, team learning and other organisational outcomes (Edmondson & Lei, 2014).

Psychological safety

The experience of feeling safe to express yourself without fear of being negatively judged or ridiculed.

Psychological safety is experienced when individuals feel safe to express themselves without fear of being negatively judged or ridiculed (Kahn, 1990). When this experience is shared by everyone in a team or workplace, it depicts a workplace culture that is safe for interpersonal risk-taking (Edmondson, 1999). In the new graduate nurse context, psychological safety is essential for building your confidence and learning to be a registered nurse. A psychologically safe workplace culture prioritises an individual's needs and engenders trust. This means that a new graduate nurse can feel secure enough to apply learning to practice, seek help and demonstrate competence and autonomy without feeling the risk of negative consequences from either a relationship or the tasks. Consequently, new nurses build confidence to navigate the workplace safely and efficiently.

This is particularly important in healthcare, because the fear of negative consequences may cause less experienced nurses to be reluctant to speak up and ask for help. More concerningly, they may try to cover up incidents and thus miss the opportunity to recover and learn from such situations. A psychologically safe workplace culture helps graduate nurses to openly discuss their challenges and learnings with their peers or supervisors on a regular basis. The most effective way for nursing graduates to build competence and autonomy is through on-the-job learning. While trial-and-error is a reasonable approach in other work contexts, it carries higher risk and cost in healthcare contexts. Open communication from graduate nurses is crucial in proactively managing situations that could escalate, and potentially lead to patient harm. It is essential that new graduate nurses have an environment where they feel psychologically safe to openly communicate, ask questions and escalate concerns.

Case Study 11.2: A sense of belonging

Felipe is on his final clinical placement and is really enjoying it, even though it is a medical unit and he is more interested in ICU. The team is very respectful of his knowledge and is always looking for opportunities for him to practise his clinical skills. He is actually thinking he would like to work in this organisation as a graduate because they treat him like he is one of the team.

- Considering what you now know about positive healthy workplaces, why do you think Felipe is enjoying this placement and wants to work in this area?

- What do you think the manager of this unit is like?

Structured support

As we have discussed, the first year of practice for a new graduate nurse is a significant period of transition. New graduates need structure, stability and support to help them manage this transition effectively. Internationally, Graduate Nurse Transition Programs (GNTP) are used in organisations as the means by which support is provided (Adams & Gillman, 2016; Africa, 2017; Bakon et al., 2018, Missen et al., 2014; Rush et al., 2019). Programs vary in name and content, but demonstrate similar factors that are known to support and promote a successful transition. Well-structured, evidence-based programs with organisational commitment have been found to achieve the most successful outcomes for new graduate nurses (Bull et al., 2015; Spector et al., 2015; Tyndall et al., 2018). These are usually 12-month programs that are structured to align with the stages of transition and development that new graduates are known to experience on entry to practice (Bakon et al., 2018; Cochran, 2017). We discussed these in Chapters 4 and 5. When programs are structured in this manner, a new graduate nurse can be offered the right support at the right time, and is supported to progressively build their capability (Figure 11.1).

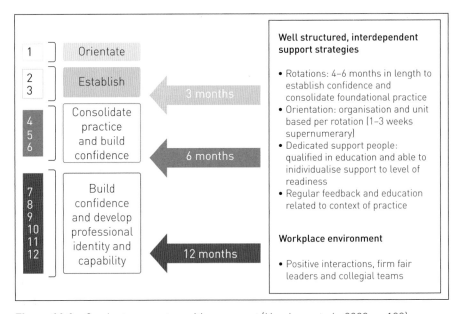

Figure 11.1   Graduate nurse transition support (Harrison et al., 2020, p. 122)

When seeking out a GNTP, there are certain elements to look for. These elements will help ease you into the workplace and create a level of stability and protection as you learn and develop. First, the program should have clear aims or objectives. These establish the expectations and shared goals for the program and the new graduate's performance. In Table 11.1 we have provided examples of what these might look like. Second, programs that offer organisational and unit-based orientation are more supportive, as they help to cultivate both industry and professional readiness (Harrison et al., 2020). As you recall, key aspects of practice readiness are knowing the organisation and system in which you are working, and being able to adhere to both professional and organisation standards. Orientation will familiarise you with the organisation and unit where you are working, including specific policies and procedures, and the layout of the organisation. It will also introduce you to key individuals who can be sources of information and support. If you are offered supernumerary time – take the opportunity. It will help you in the early stages to familiarise yourself with the team, workplace and overall functionality of the unit.

Third, look for programs with four- to six-month rotations. A critical point in establishing your confidence in clinical practice occurs at around three to four months of your first year (Duchscher, 2008, 2009; Harrison et al., 2020). Therefore, transition programs that offer four- to six-month clinical rotations will help you steadily build your confidence. Rotating prior to this point can undermine your confidence and development. A stable environment helps consolidate your practice and confidence and gives you a sense of control in dynamic environments (Duchscher, 2012). Constant change associated with frequent rotations can induce additional stress that could destabilise your confidence, learning and socialisation (Walker et al., 2017). Multiple rotations can reinforce your beginning status, as you constantly have to relearn how to work in unfamiliar environments. This can also disrupt your sense of belonging and autonomy in the healthcare team – as discussed, these are core needs that, when met, cultivate a smoother and more effective transition process.

Fourth, in addition to the length of the program, it is also important to consider the sequence of rotations. If possible, aim for a rotation in a generalist area prior to one in a specialty area unless there is additional support provided in the specialty area. Consider a specialty area on your second or third rotation. Commencing practice in a generalist area before moving to advanced areas of specialised practice is necessary to scaffold your learning and development (Harrison et al., 2020). The sequence also gives you time to develop confidence and establish the foundational capability needed for specialty or advanced practice (Benner, 1984). Your nursing program is not aimed at preparing you for practice in a specialty area, and working in these areas can add additional stress (Walker et al., 2017). Specialty area practice requires specific capabilities to work in the area and healthcare professionals find that new nurses perform better in specialty areas after having established their confidence and consolidated their foundational practice in a more generalist area (Harrison et al., 2020; Phillips et al., 2014).

Often, however, given the breadth and availability of positions, not all new nurses can initially be employed in a generalist area and some new nurses just want to work in specialty areas. If you do start in a specialty area, check that there is specific support designed to help you, as this will ensure you have the resources you need and you are more likely to be successful (Bortolotto, 2015; Aggar et al., 2017).

Fifth, effective support is support that is tailored to your needs. This relies on the availability of dedicated support people. These can be well-prepared, approachable nurse educators, clinical coaches and preceptors with the educational capability to establish positive relationships and facilitate meaningful learning (Edward et al., 2017; Fowler et al., 2018). These types of support people can enhance a new nurse's confidence, socialisation and independence (Edward et al., 2017; Fowler et al., 2018; Phillips et al., 2015), which helps them understand their responsibilities and adapt to their new role (Ankers et al., 2018; Edward et al., 2017). Because of their educational capability, support people are able to individualise their education strategies to each nurse's needs. As such, they are instrumental in facilitating meaningful learning, the type of learning that enables new nurses to translate learning into practice and promotes a sense of accomplishment and confidence. This level of learning leads to significant performance development (Sweet & Broadbent, 2017). The use of dedicated, skilled support people can help minimise unintended impacts on staff workloads and provide opportunities for moral support to discuss conflict, feel safe and practise skills.

A final element necessary for an effective GNTP program is the provision of regular educational opportunities that include simulation and hands-on practice to potentiate a new graduate nurse's clinical development (Rush et al., 2019; Walker et al., 2017). Dedicated study days aimed at developing specific skills including critical thinking and leadership, quality and safety, and consolidating old and introducing new capabilities can increase a new graduate registered nurse's confidence and capability for independent practice and provide an opportunity for confidential debriefing (Henderson et al., 2015; Murray et al., 2020). New nurses can benefit from having the additional time to deal with conflict, particularly that stemming from uncivil workplace behaviours. In the next section, we will examine why dedicated support people are paramount for new graduate nurses in times of conflict and stress.

Table 11.1 Structured support: Example of graduate nurse transition program

Aims or objectives
- Support new graduate nurses to apply learning to practice, build confidence and capability to work safely and efficiently in the environment.
- Foster gradual development for progressive development of capability: (novice – beginner – competent)

Structural elements	Details
Timeframe	• Minimum 8 to maximum 12 months
Orientation	• Organisational orientation • Rotation-based orientation – each rotation
Rotations	• 4–6-month duration
Sequence	• General to specialty
Shifts	• Mixed: night duty after initial six-week settling-in period
Education	• Dedicated support positions: available, approachable individuals with education expertise linked to GNTP • Available committed mentors and preceptors to guide and model • Facility relevant education to consolidate and extend development
Leadership	• Management: visible, supportive, collaborative and involved • Program managers: key person with oversight for the program • Passionate, knowledgeable and committed
New graduate nurse	• Positive, committed and seeks opportunities to learn • Asks questions – acknowledges limitations • Seeks support and is solution-focused – takes initiative
Key milestones	• 1–3 months: consolidate learning and establish confidence • 3–6 months: establish RN role and cultivate nursing practice • 6–8 months: acquire and extend nursing practice; gain experience • 8–12 months: consolidate RN role and nursing practice

Portfolio Activity: Making the transition

Early in your final year of your nursing program is the time to think about where you would like to work, and to plan your graduate transition year. Begin to explore the graduate transition programs available to you and the structural elements within those programs. While on your final placement, consider the factors we have outlined about positive workplaces and what you might look for as your first place of work.

Unhealthy workplace environments

While it is important for you as a new graduate nurse to recognise the characteristics of the right workplace environment, it is equally important to be prepared for the negative aspects of the workplace. As a new nurse, you may not have the option of being selective in your first professional position, and rotations to different teams or specialty areas can be destabilising. The cultures in work teams can be very different; some will not be aligned with your preferences or expectations and some workplaces will vary in the key elements necessary for a healthy workplace environment. Even if you completed student placements at the same workplace, the relationship dynamics can be very different when you are a registered nurse. Understanding negative workplace phenomena and how to manage them effectively is vital to ensuring a successful transition and a positive start to your nursing career.

Negative workplace experiences

In Chapter 2, the complex and dynamic nature of healthcare environments was discussed. Healthcare environments are constantly adapting to change and, as a result, healthcare professionals frequently work in environments that are constantly challenging and demanding. The consequences of long-term struggle and frustration in such conditions vary for each person depending on their individual characteristics and coping strategies; however, they generally include workplace burnout and incivility.

Burnout

Burnout is conceptualised as a response syndrome to problematic relationships between an employee and their work, resulting from chronic workplace stresses that are not successfully managed (Leiter & Maslach, 2014). It reflects an occupational phenomenon that is characterised by overwhelming exhaustion, feeling of mental distance or cynicism from your job, and the reduction of self or professional efficacy over time (Maslach et al., 2001; WHO, 2019).

Dimensions of burnout. The everyday use of the term 'burnout' often refers to the first dimension only: emotional exhaustion, the stress or depletion of energy from over-extended workload or interpersonal conflicts (Leiter, 2017). However, while it is the central dimension of burnout, emotional exhaustion alone cannot capture the complexity of burnout. Individuals react differently to stress, and have different levels of ability to recover from adversity; that is, psychological resilience (Fletcher & Sarkar, 2013), which is developed through past experiences in managing adversity. The second dimension of burnout, cynicism, is a negative response to the interpersonal context dimension of burnout (Maslach et al., 2001). Similar to avoidant attachment style, cynicism captures the feeling of distrust, distancing to protect yourself (Leiter et al., 2015). Individuals experiencing cynicism attribute their emotional exhaustion to extrinsic factors, such as difficult colleagues or unfair systems. The third dimension, reduced self or professional efficacy, represents the self-evaluation dimension of burnout (Maslach et al., 2001). Similar to anxious/ambivalent attachment style, individuals may intrinsically attribute the reason for their lack of accomplishment over time, despite continued effort, to their inability to control the environmental stressors or cope with the emotional exhaustion, resulting in reduced self or professional efficacy (Leiter et al., 2015).

The relationships among the three dimensions have been theorised and investigated through different developmental models (Lee & Ashforth, 1996; Leiter, 2017; Maslach et al., 2001). It is important for new graduate nurses to recognise that burnout does not occur spontaneously – time is an important dimension (Leiter, 2017). Stressors that persist over time are more likely to be systematic than incidental, and efforts by the individual to change the system are impossible. It is also helpful for new graduate nurses to understand the human tendency to see people as the inherent cause of the stressors. Personal

Burnout

A state of physical, mental and emotional exhaustion that stems from chronic workplace stress that is not successfully managed.

attributes and styles play a part in burnout, but evidence shows that burnout is best understood in terms of job-related situational sources (Maslach, 2003). Chapters 1 and 2 discussed the systematic challenges associated with the professional nursing role as well as the healthcare environment. These are some of the situational sources of stress.

Consequences of burnout. The consequences of burnout in healthcare professions are serious, and it can negatively impact personal, social and organisational outcomes. Burnout can lead to poor physical and mental health and increase the risk of depression; it can be a source of incivility causing interpersonal conflicts; individuals may choose substance abuse to cope, which in turn exacerbates problems; and individuals may have a stronger intention to leave the organisation or the profession. Most importantly, the impact on the quality of patient care provided by burnt out workers will increase the risk of patient mortality (Maslach & Leiter, 2017).

Recognising the signs of burnout in yourself and others is vital for new graduate nurses so that you can objectively assess and manage relationship issues at work. The warning signs of burnout may present differently in different people. Table 11.2 summarises the categories of signs into cognitive, affective, physical, behavioural and motivational aspects (Snarr et al., 2017). While the behavioural signs are more salient for observation, they are more likely to result from cynicism or inefficacy instead of the precursor dimension of emotional exhaustion (Leiter, 2017). Emotional exhaustion does not always lead to cynicism or inefficacy, depending on an individual's coping strategies and the stressors in the environment; however, elevation in one of the three burnout dimensions can be an early sign of burnout (Maslach & Leiter, 2008).

The time dimension of burnout is the other important aspect about which new graduate nurses need to be mindful. An individual's length of service or work experience does not necessarily combat or exacerbate burnout. Senior nurses or managers can develop skills to manage stressful events more effectively, and develop **resilience** through these experiences. It is also possible that they are struggling to manage or develop adequate coping strategies. Without appropriate intervention, the longer they hold their positions in the same condition, the more burnout behaviours they will present at work. When they are in a leadership position, these behaviours may have a negative impact on

Resilience

The ability to respond and adapt to changing and challenging situations.

Table 11.2 Signs of burnout (Snarr et al., 2017)

Category	Signs of burnout
Cognitive	• Abnormal thought processes (weakened memory, cynical attitude, trouble concentrating) • Dehumanising perceptions of traditional job tasks
Affective	• Emotional exhaustion • Abnormal emotional states (insecure, anxious, depressed, hostile)
Physical	• Chronic skeletal muscle pain • Decreases in strength • Loss of appetite • Sleep disturbances • Migraines • Recurring illnesses
Behavioural	• Absenteeism • Substance abuse • Increased conflicts in relationships • Impaired work performance
Motivational	• Lack of enthusiasm • Reduction in work ethic • Low motivation

the personal and professional development of graduate nurses. It is critical for you to understand that as a graduate nurse your leaders, supervisors and senior colleagues can also experience burnout. Such understanding will ensure that you respond appropriately or seek assistance if you find yourself the recipient of poor behaviour from these individuals.

Incivility

As the previous discussion has indicated, one of the outcomes of burnout is workplace incivility. **Incivility** is low-intensity deviance behaviour with ambiguous intent to cause harm (Pearson et al., 2000). It describes behaviours that are rude or disrespectful, and implies conflicts among members of a group with shared behavioural standards. Incivility is not limited to verbal interactions. It can be body language; for example, ignoring others. When individuals experience burnout, they have no energy reserve for robust behavioural regulation or motivation to act when prompted. This can be perceived as rudeness. Incivility can then become an emotional demand on others, and trigger their development of burnout.

Incivility

Low-intensity deviance behaviour with ambiguous intent to cause harm, characterised by rude or disrespectful verbal or non-verbal behaviours.

Antecedents of incivility. The antecedents of incivility have both situational and individual factors. Situational factors can be unresolved conflicts with other people, decisions made, processes, or policies. When issues are left unaddressed or resolutions are perceived to be unsatisfactory, it is likely that individuals will express frustration or disappointment through uncivil behaviours. As discussed in Chapter 2, healthcare organisations have to constantly adapt to new demands, including advances in technology, to stay relevant. Fast-paced ongoing changes in the name of optimisation are becoming the norm. Unlike the more overt and intense forms of conflict, such as aggression or abuse, incivility is difficult to legislate or prosecute, and becoming increasingly common and pervasive in the workplace (Leiter, 2019). Constant change is often a precursor to staff being uncivil in the workplace. As the current legislation and organisational policies prohibit any forms of aggression in the workplace, a lower-intensity deviance behaviour becomes the easy alternative to overt aggression. The ambiguous intent provides a certain level of deniability or protection from formal disciplines for people who engage in uncivil behaviours.

Incivility can also be triggered by personality factors, such as low emotional stability, agreeableness or openness. These traits play a role in an individual's tendency to engage in incivility, and influence how individuals perceive and interpret behaviours from others. People can mistakenly interpret, as incivility, ambiguous comments or behaviours that were not intended to cause harm, therefore causing and stimulating uncivil behavioural responses (Sliter et al., 2015). Liu et al. (2009) found that individuals who have a stronger focus on goal achievements are more likely to experience frustration with behaviours that are perceived to be non-productive towards goal attainment, which leads to uncivil behaviours. How confident a person feels about engaging in direct conflict also influences the likelihood of engaging in incivility.

Consequences of incivility. The reciprocity of social relationships drives the spiralling effect of incivility at work. People are more likely to engage in uncivil behaviours in response to incivility, seeking revenge. This effect is amplified when those involved value justice or when the workplace culture values fairness. Without appropriate intervention, it may escalate into more severe forms of conflict over time, such as aggression (Pearson et al., 2000). Incivility damages the psychological safety of the workplace, and causes psychological distress and withdrawal behaviours such as absenteeism or turnover (Leiter et al., 2011).

Incivility has a negative impact on all three aspects of motivational core needs: belongingness, autonomy and competence.

As a new graduate nurse at work, trying to speculate on the intent of an ambiguous comment or behaviour from a co-worker or supervisor can be emotionally draining, and is unlikely to be helpful in building positive relationships. It would be more effective to seek support from a mentor or senior colleague, and openly communicate with a positive attitude. Not only will taking this approach curtail the negative spiral of incivility, it will also help you to develop confidence in navigating relationship challenges at work and self-efficacy in emotional regulation, ultimately building your resilience against burnout. This is where the availability of dedicated support people and regular debriefing can be invaluable.

Case Study 11.3: Navigating relationship challenges

Felipe is nearing the end of his final clinical placement in the medical unit. On the whole he has really enjoyed the last eight weeks, although there is one member of staff, Helen, who he has found it difficult to build a relationship with. Felipe often catches Helen rolling her eyes when he makes a comment. She also excludes him when inviting people to join her during breaks. Helen has worked on the medical unit for many years but isn't in a senior position.

- What might be driving Helen's behaviour?
- How should Felipe handle this situation?
- What resources can Felipe draw on for support?

Causes of burnout and incivility

While there are individual and situational factors that pre-empt incivility, there are key reasons why we experience burnout and incivility in healthcare contexts. These include the imbalance between job demands and resources, and job–person fit. Knowledge and understanding of these factors and imbalances can enable new graduates to mitigate and/or manage their responses and the outcomes.

Job demands and resources

As discussed in the first part of this chapter, the motivation to satisfy core needs drives people to participate in the workplace and invest energy into work demands. Underlying that investment is a finite amount of energy that individuals can generate from the resources available to them. The idea of balancing job demands and resources is that job resources may buffer the impact of job demands. This is the central notion of the **Job Demands-Resources (JD-R) model** (Demerouti et al., 2001). This model suggests that burnout is the result of an imbalance between job demands and resources. Job demands deplete energy, evoke a stress process and are closely associated with the exhaustion dimension of burnout. Job resources provide the energy for people to engage in the work. Insufficient resources will cause productive individuals to retreat and withdraw, closely associated with the cynicism dimension of burnout (Bakker et al., 2005).

The JD-R model offers organisations a unique perspective in managing job demands in certain professions that are difficult to reduce or redesign. For example, the high emotional demands for nurses cannot be easily modified. Instead of trying to reduce the innate job demand, it can be compensated by increasing job resources available to nurses to help them cope. The key elements of the right workplace environment – positive leadership, collegial teams and a psychologically safe workplace culture – are all sources of job resources that can help individuals cope with various job demands. When these elements are absent, individuals are more likely to experience burnout as they can only rely on their intrinsic motivation, which depletes over time.

Job–person fit

Not all jobs are created equal, not all individuals have the same preferences. Minimising the discrepancies between what the job requires and what an individual has to offer or prefers to do is the idea behind the job–person fit framework. Better alignment between the two means less friction between the ability and motivation to fulfil the job responsibilities, hence less resources are

Job Demands-Resources (JD-R) model

A model which suggests that balancing job demands and resources influences burnout, whereby job demands deplete energy and evoke stress and job resources provide energy to work productively.

required. Jobs are unlikely to change significantly in a short period of time. If an individual is experiencing friction, the cumulative effort or resources required to manage the friction increase exponentially over time. Therefore, individuals who are working in a job that is not a good fit, are more likely to experience burnout.

Six areas of work life influence job–person fit (Maslach & Leiter, 1997). These are discussed below. They provide a useful evaluation model for you to assess if a workplace environment is right for you and to identify areas that are not helpful. As new graduates, this may be useful to help you make sense of interactions in the workplace and know when to seek clarification and support about what might be happening for you and around you in the workplace.

1. *Values.* The alignment between the individual and the job is the most important aspect in eliciting a positive attitude and prosocial behaviour at work. Values implicitly fulfil core needs and fuel the energy level of individuals. Further, values drive individual behaviours and decision-making: people who share similar values tend to experience less friction and are more likely to provide support for each other. When values do not align, individuals have to constantly seek reasons and intrinsic motivations to stay in the job, particularly during stressful times. During the process, individual work resources deplete.

2. *Workload.* This is an area directly associated with the exhaustion dimension of burnout. When the job demands more energy than the individual is willing or prepared to exert, exhaustion is experienced. However, if the individual values their job and perceives it as meaningful and important, their willingness and preparedness to take on higher workload increase.

3. *Control.* This is the level of agency that individuals seek in their job. While some prefer to participate in work-related decision-making processes or be integrated into a workgroup, others may be more comfortable to work independently.

4. *Reward.* This is the area concerned with receiving confirmation and recognition from others, which promotes positive behaviours. Individuals have different preferences about the form of reward. Some prefer extrinsically motivated rewards such as financial compensation or status promotion, while others prefer intrinsically motivated rewards such as more challenging tasks, or gratitude from others.

5. *Community.* This pertains to relationships at work and is directly related to the belongingness element of core needs. The quality of relationships determines the level of support individuals have during their times of need. Individuals have different attachment styles, therefore the fit between the individual and relationship styles in the community is important.

6. *Fairness.* This is often upheld by people as a fundamental value. Without fairness, individuals will experience less control as rules are not being followed. Injustices negatively impact motivation, so individuals have less energy to manage workload, exercise agency or maintain positive community relationships.

Preventing and mitigating negative phenomena

Burnout and incivility are not sudden-onset phenomena. Many environmental and dispositional triggers can ignite any of the three dimensions of burnout, and the reciprocity cycle of incivility. Its developmental nature means that mitigation and prevention processes go hand-in-hand. Mitigation is fixing what is wrong, prevention is building what is right. The effective mitigation of early symptoms will contribute to lessening the severity or breadth of impact to other areas of life. The processes need to be implemented at both individual and workgroup levels.

At the individual level

In order to conduct effective interventions, individuals must first be educated about incivility and burnout, know what they are, be aware that they exist in the workplace, and understand the mechanisms of how they can occur (Maslach & Leiter, 2017). As a new graduate, you may find this information useful as you begin your first year transition process.

Undertake accurate evaluation

Earlier we provided you with introductory knowledge about some of the negative situations you might encounter in the workplace, including the dimensions of burnout, the reciprocal nature of incivility, and how individual difference and environmental stressors may influence the impact of burnout and incivility. Awareness of your own default thought patterns and communication styles in such situations is as important as being aware of the issues. Understanding how your own style or preferences interact with the characteristics of the workplace environment is critical for you to be able to formulate personal strategies to prevent and mitigate negative situations.

Awareness and understanding are necessary, but alone are insufficient for effective intervention. It is relatively easy to read and even memorise a theoretical perspective; it is much harder to make a connection between the knowledge and the situation you experience in everyday interactions and observations at work. Contrary to the common belief of 'knowing is half of the battle', research in judgment and decision-making tells us that knowledge is rarely the central factor controlling human behaviour. Cognitive processes – how we think – like situation selection, habit formation and emotion regulation are important (Santos & Gendler, 2014). These cognitive processes, however, are plagued with insidious biases, making it difficult to convert explicit knowledge of theories into tacit knowledge. Explicit knowledge is recorded and communicated through physical mediums, such as libraries and databases. **Tacit knowledge** is the opposite and is difficult to codify or communicate through any medium. Tacit knowledge can only be communicated through consistent and extensive relationships or contact (such as learning, from a palliative care nurse, how to converse with a dying patient). Recognising real-life situations where the theories and knowledge might be applicable, and understanding how to use the knowledge in the situation, are needed for effective intervention.

Tacit knowledge

Knowledge that is implicit and communicated through consistent and extensive relationships, contact or experiences with others.

For example, a colleague rushes past you, glares and complains, 'Why are you just standing there? Everyone else is really busy – don't you have anything to do?' and rushes off before you have a chance to say anything. As a graduate nurse, new to the team, it is very easy to jump to the cognitive conclusion that you did something wrong, or that the colleague is a mean-spirited person. These cognitive conclusions trigger emotional, then behavioural, responses. For example, you might feel intimidated, sad or shameful, therefore you might behaviourally withdraw, become tentative or even cry. On the other hand, if you attribute the issue to the colleague, you may feel anger, injustice or resentment and might act on those feelings by complaining, by non-directive micro-aggressive outbursts or by uncivil behaviours targeted at the colleague.

The prevalent tendency to 'blame the person' is a premature closure in the reasoning process or evaluation of the event. It can be the consequence of our different **cognitive biases**: anchoring bias (heavy reliance on the first thought that came to mind); availability bias (favouring retrievable information – things that can be recalled are more important than those that cannot); and unpacking effect (the likelihood of an event increases as its description becomes more specific) (Tversky & Kahneman, 1974; Tversky & Koehler, 1994). Individuals commonly experience a combination of these, and in the moment it is extremely difficult to look beyond the immediate situation to the wider issues that may be the cause of the situation.

As a new graduate nurse, it is important to consider these factors when you are trying to make sense of and manage a difficult situation. The ability to recognise what you experienced as a possible symptom of something other than a thoughtless remark, is critical to interventions at the individual level. While this can be difficult when your personal resources might have been depleted by the physical and psychological demands of being a new graduate nurse, or you feel you are not in a position of power or confident to suggest or implement any meaningful changes, it is important. An accurate situational evaluation is necessary to create an effective plan, one that can help discern attribution and ameliorate negative feelings and behaviours that might arise.

Develop self-efficacy and confidence

A healthy level of **self-efficacy** and **confidence** can also help you make a more objective assessment of the situation. When a person (someone else or yourself) jumps into your mind as the cause of a negative experience, you can either reject the thought or wait and unpack the situation until you achieve a more comprehensive and objective assessment. As a result, you are more likely to recognise the root cause of what is happening rather than making a quick judgment on yourself or others. Awareness, understanding, cognitive processes and situational recognition all play a part. They operate like the gears, clutch, steering wheel and mirrors in driving: some are easier than others to grasp, but they all have to work in synchrony to achieve desired outcomes. Like driving, however, as someone new to your role in the workplace, the only way to develop your confidence and self-efficacy is through daily practice and repetition over

Cognitive bias

A bias in thinking that causes an error when an individual processes and interprets information.

Self-efficacy

A person's belief in their abilities to succeed in the situation or accomplish a task, and to exert control over their own motivation, behaviour and social environment.

Confidence

An attitude or feeling of trust, belief and assurance in yourself, in others and/or in plans for the future.

time. Practice is important, not only from a 'what to do' perspective but also from a 'how to do it' perspective, and can be loosely divided into remedial (corrective) and strengthening (extend). In reality there are no clear demarcations between the two. Like developing physical well-being involves reducing fat and building muscles, the two are interconnected – actions in one will make the effort for the other easier as well. In order to flourish, graduate nurses not only have to work through the negative experiences that are inherent to the current healthcare system, but also work to build their capability and satisfy their core needs as a new graduate nurse. Engaging in effective practice might mean that new graduate nurses seek support to remediate, particularly if individual resources can no longer meet work demands.

For any type of intervention to be effective for yourself or others, new graduates need well-developed **personal readiness** capabilities. Chapter 6 explained that personal readiness capabilities are those that represent who we are as individuals and our ability to manage our thoughts, emotions and behaviours when we undertake our role and interact with others. These are fundamental to being able to manage negative workplace phenomena. In the next section we will examine how these capabilities support you to prevent, mitigate and manage difficult workplace situations.

Personal readiness

The capability to manage the roles and responsibilities of a registered nurse, oneself and one's environment.

Communicate the experience

If you recognise that you are experiencing incivility or the symptoms of burnout, the first step is to communicate the experience. This could be with a support person or directly with the person involved. Clearly articulating your experience is critical for others who are trying to help. Be mindful that for some people, particularly those with high workload demand, providing support can be experienced as a work demand, depending on how it is communicated. Therefore, use appropriate language that shows respect, withhold judgments and assumptions when making statements, and have a consultative approach rather than simply venting. Ensure you actively listen to what the other person is saying, keeping in mind that the other person, despite their intention to help, might also make assumptions or premature judgments, or use politically correct language that makes their message ambiguous. Actively clarify what is said or meant to ensure that you understand – this also reflects your respect for them. If you have a high level of personal readiness, you may choose to communicate directly with the person involved in the situation. Again, be mindful of how you communicate your message, keeping in mind the person may be experiencing an imbalance in job-resources demand or experiencing burnout. Communicate clearly with an intent to voice your concerns, not attribute blame or induce negative emotions in the other person. This way you are being a positive influencer, cultivating a psychologically safe culture and healthy workplace environment.

 ## Portfolio Activity 11.4: Stop, reflect and think

Consider who you could go to for support, and how you would communicate your concerns, if you were experiencing difficult interactions with someone or you were given unfair or unmanageable workloads.

Be responsive to feedback

Feedback is an essential component of transitioning to work and your development as a registered nurse. While positive feedback is easier to process, it is often the feedback that identifies areas for remediation that contains the most important development signals. In an ideal situation, leaders and senior nurses would have sufficient time to ensure feedback is well constructed and you would receive adequate education and support. However, as we discussed in Chapter 2, with current healthcare demands, leaders and senior nurses are often focused on working efficiently, are time-challenged and may not have formal training on how to work with new graduate nurses; they rely instead on their own hands-on experiences. Therefore, it is even more important for new graduate nurses to be competent in processing and responding to feedback with positivity, when the feedback is not perfectly packaged or communicated efficiently.

Be flexible and generous

The reasons that incivility is so insidious and ubiquitous, as previously discussed, are its reciprocal effect and ambiguous intent where noise – random errors, unintended decisions or actions – comprises the ambiguous intent part of incivility. The tit-for-tat strategy models the reciprocal effect of incivility, where one person cooperates with another in their very first interaction and then each copies the other's previous decisions. If one person chooses to compete instead of cooperating, the act will trigger the other person to compete in the following move. Deciding when a person should cooperate or be selfish in an ongoing interaction with another person is key to reducing the pervasiveness of incivility. Some generosity towards an ambiguous act by a colleague under stress will contribute to the overall health of the workplace. The most successful approach in terms of overall outcomes, is the generous version of tit-for-tat. This strategy allows some cooperation even if the other person chooses to compete. This allowance prevents one negative act from echoing indefinitely. In multicultural countries like Australia and New Zealand, being flexible and generous are particularly important, as people are likely to have diverse social norms and acceptable practices. One act might be perceived as rude by one culture and as completely reasonable by other cultures. In addition to cultural differences, personal styles play a part in the gap between intention and perception.

Case Study 11.4: Mitigating incivility

Returning to Case Study 11.3, how might Felipe use the generous tit-for-tat strategy to respond to Helen's behaviour? Did your original answers account for this strategy?

At a workgroup level

It is important to recognise that individuals are part of the solution in combating negative workplace phenomena; however, individuals operate within the workplace context, and their behaviours are often a reflection of the organisational system. In a complex healthcare system, the people within the system are both autonomous independent agents and interdependent agents. Complexity theory characterises **complex systems** as diverse, adaptive and interconnected. Complex systems emphasise the quality of relationships and exhibit distributed control and emergent behaviours and outcomes, which can be non-linear and highly

Complex system

A system of diverse, adaptive and interconnected components emphasised by the quality of relationships, distributed control and emergent behaviours and outcomes that are highly dependent on the context and initial conditions.

dependent on context and initial conditions. Consequently, there is often no one best way to conduct interventions at an organisational or a group level.

Participate in interventions

The diversity of people in the group, and their connectedness, individual agency and unique adaptiveness determine the effectiveness of any given intervention (Thompson et al., 2016). So it is not surprising that burnout interventions, such as workshops, support groups, stress management or coping training, yield mixed results. Employee participation in the design and implementation of an intervention is a key determinant to the effectiveness of an intervention program (Leiter & Maslach, 2014). Employee collaboration and ownership of the intervention ensures the relevance and applicability of the intervention program to the workplace context. The success of an intervention program depends on the full participation of people involved, and having an active role in the process motivates employees to exercise their agency and competence. Emergent behaviours at the group level are more effective than prescribed activities.

Be a leader

Every nurse is recognised as a leader in patient care: they coordinate, manage and motivate not only the healthcare teams and services, but also families and patients to achieve health outcomes for patients and their wider communities. It is important for new graduate nurses to recognise this. As we discussed in Chapter 5, if you are developing your readiness capabilities, you are simultaneously building your capacity for leadership. Graduate nurses may not be in positions of authority; however, they are in a position to take the lead and make decisions that affect patient care and the operations of the healthcare team. The agency to influence positive change is an indication of nursing leadership. This agency develops from day-to-day practice in modelling positive behaviours, providing emotional or clinical support to those in need and, by the same token, proactively seeking support in challenging situations rather than waiting for others to notice the stressor or until the situation has deteriorated to the point of causing harm.

OXFORD UNIVERSITY PRESS

Portfolio Activity: Making the transition

Have you experienced any negative experiences during your professional experience placements? If so, what have you learnt about how you would contribute to a healthy workplace environment during your graduate year? What strategies will you use to prevent and mitigate negative phenomena?

Conclusion

A new graduate nurse's transition is contingent on the conditions within the workplace environment. A positive healthy environment cultivates a place where individuals feel supported and safe to work to the best of their ability. In these environments, new graduates can safely put their learning into practice, demonstrate their level of practice readiness and seek support to grow and develop in their role. In this way, the workplace environment supports new graduate nurses to evolve as registered nurses. Both individuals and the organisation play a part in creating a healthy workplace environment. Equipped with the knowledge of what a healthy workplace environment involves and the understanding of what can be done to manage negative workplace phenomena, graduate nurses can make a difference by communicating their observations, modelling positive behaviours, and fully participating at the individual level or in workgroup-level interventions. By understanding the psychological motivations for work, both collectively and individually, graduate nurses can build their confidence in managing challenges in the workplace environment.

Key summary points

- The key elements to a healthy workplace environment are positive leadership, collegial teams and psychologically safe workplace culture.

- Healthy workplace environments cultivate psychologically safe workplace cultures. They are reliant on the leadership within the workplace and sustained by the collective shared values and collaboration within the team.

- Effective communication and listening, responsiveness to feedback, and being flexible and generous, underlined by confidence, are the fundamental competencies for nursing leadership at any level.

- The signs of burnout can be categorised into cognitive, affective, physical, behavioural and motivational. The six areas of work life – workload, control, reward, community, fairness and value – can be used to assess the potential causes of burnout.

- Recognising negative workplace interactions requires awareness, understanding, cognition and, most importantly, practice over time.

- Intervention strategies for negative workplace interactions must incorporate both individual and workgroup-level issues to be effective.

- Well-structured, evidence-based support strategies are an important contributor in cultivating the right environment to flourish and are essential for new graduate registered nurses to manage their transition to practice effectively.

Critical thinking questions

1. What are the key characteristics of a healthy workplace environment?

2. What are some of the behavioural signs of a person who is experiencing burnout?

3. How does an individual's style of leadership impact on the workplace environment?

4. What would you do if a colleague made cynical remarks about organisational civility workshops that you are required to attend? What are some of the potential reasons for them to make these comments?

5. Why is a structured program of support during a graduate nurse's first year of practice an important contributor in cultivating the right environment to flourish?

OXFORD UNIVERSITY PRESS

6. How can cognitive bias influence workplace interactions and consequently team effectiveness?

7. In what ways do confidence and self-efficacy help to mitigate negative phenomena in the workplace?

References

Adams, J. E., & Gillman, L. (2016). Developing an evidence-based transition program for graduate nurses. *Contemporary Nurse*, *52*(5), 511–521. https://doi.org/10.1080/10376178.2 016.1238287

Africa, L. M. (2017). Transition to practice programs: Effective solutions to achieving strategic staffing in today's healthcare systems. *Nursing Economics*, *35*(4), 178–183.

Aggar, C., Bloomfield, J., Thomas, T. H., & Gordon, C. J. (2017). Australia's first transition to professional practice in primary care program for graduate registered nurses: A pilot study. *BMC Nursing*, *16*(14), 1–11. https://doi.org/10.1186/s12912-017-0207-5

Ainsworth, M. S. (1979). Infant–mother attachment. *American Psychologist*, *34*(10), 932–937. https://doi.org/10.1037//0003-066X.34.10.932

Ankers, M. D., Barton, C. A., & Parry, Y. K. (2018). A phenomenological exploration of graduate nurse transition to professional practice within a transition to practice program. *Collegian*, *25*(3), 319–325. https://doi.org/10.1016/j.colegn.2017.09.002

Bakker, A. B., Demerouti, E., & Euwema, M. C. (2005). Job resources buffer the impact of job demands on burnout. *Journal of Occupational Health Psychology*, *10*(2), 170–180. https://doi.org/10.1037/1076-8998.10.2.170

Bakon, S., Craft, J., Wirihana, L., Christensen, M., Barr, J., & Tsai, L. (2018). An integrative review of graduate transition programmes: Developmental considerations for nursing management. *Nurse Education Practice*, *28*, 80–85. https://doi.org/10.1016/j.nepr.2017.10.009

Baumeister, R. F., & Leary, M. R. (1995). The need to belong: Desire for interpersonal attachments as a fundamental human motivation. *Psychological Bulletin*, *117*(3), 497–529. https://doi.org/10.1037/0033-2909.117.3.497

Benner, P. (1984). *From novice to expert: Excellence and power in clinical nursing practice*. Addison-Wesley.

Boamah, S. A., Read, E. A., & Laschinger, H. K. S. (2016). Factors influencing new graduate nurse burnout development, job satisfaction and patient care quality: A time-lagged study. *Journal of Advanced Nursing*, *73*(5), 1182–1195. https://doi.org/10.1111/jan.13215

Bortolotto, S. J. (2015). Developing a comprehensive critical care orientation program for graduate nurses. *Journal for Nurses in Professional Development*, *31*(4), 203–210. https://doi.org/10.1097/NND.0000000000000139

Bowlby, J. (1969). *Attachment and loss: Vol. 1. Attachment*. Random House.

Bowlby, J. (1979). *The making and breaking of affectional bonds*. Routledge.

Bull, R., Shearer, T., Phillips, M., & Fallon, A. (2015). Supporting graduate nurse transition: Collaboration between practice and university. *Journal of Continuing Education in Nursing*, *46*(9), 409. https://doi.org/10.3928/00220124-20150821-03

Burton, J. (2010, February). *WHO healthy workplace framework and model: background and supporting literature and practices*. World Health Organization. https://www.who.int/occupational_health/healthy_workplace_framework.pdf

Cochran, C. (2017). Effectiveness and best practice of nurse residency programs: A literature review. *MedSurg Nursing, 26*(1), 53–63.

Collins, N. L., & Read, S. J. (1990). Adult attachment, working models, and relationship quality in dating couples. *Journal of Personality and Social Psychology, 58*(4), 644–663. https://doi.org/10.1037//0022-3514.58.4.644

D'Ambra, A. M., & Andrews, D. R. (2014). Incivility, retention and new graduate nurses: An integrated review of the literature. *Journal of Nursing Management, 22*(6), 735–742. https://doi.org/10.1111/jonm.12060

Dawson, A. J., Stasa, H., Roche, M. A., Homer, C. S. E., & Duffield, C. (2014). Nursing churn and turnover in Australian hospitals: Nurses' perceptions and suggestions for supportive strategies. *BMC Nursing, 13*, Article 11. https://doi.org/10.1186/1472-6955-13-11

Deci, E. L., & Ryan, R. M. (1985). The general causality orientations scale: Self-determination in personality. *Journal of Research in Personality, 19*(2), 109–134. https://doi.org/10.1016/0092-6566(85)90023-6

Demerouti, E., Bakker, A. B., Nachreiner, F., & Schaufeli, W. B. (2001). The job demands-resources model of burnout. *Journal of Applied Psychology, 86*(3), 499–512.

Duchscher, J. B. (2008). A process of becoming: The stages of new nursing graduate professional role transition. *Journal of Continuing Education in Nursing, 39*(10), 441–450. https://doi.org/10.3928/00220124-20081001-03

Duchscher, J. E. B. (2009). Transition shock: The initial stage of role adaptation for newly graduated registered nurses. *Journal of Advanced Nursing, 65*(5), 1103–1113. https://doi.org/10.1111/j.1365-2648.2008.04898.x

Duchscher, J. E. B. (2012). *From surviving to thriving: Navigating the first year of professional nursing practice* (2nd ed.). Nursing the Future.

Dulebohn, J. H., Bommer, W. H., Liden, R. C., Brouer, R. L., & Ferris, G. R. (2012). A meta-analysis of antecedents and consequences of leader–member exchange: Integrating the past with an eye toward the future. *Journal of Management, 38*(6), 1715–1759. https://doi.org/10.1177/0149206311415280

Edmondson, A. (1999). Psychological safety and learning behavior in work teams. *Administrative Science Quarterly, 44*(2), 350–383. https://doi.org/10.2307/2666999

Edmondson, A., & Lei, Z. (2014). Psychological safety: The history, renaissance, and future of an interpersonal construct. *Annual Review of Organizational Psychology and Organizational Behaviour, 1*(1), 22–43. https://doi.org/10.1146/annurev-orgpsych-031413-091305

Edward, K.-L., Ousey, K., Playle, J., & Giandinoto, J.-A. (2017). Are new nurses work ready? The impact of preceptorship: An integrative systematic review. *Journal of Professional Nursing, 33*(5), 326–333. https://doi.org/10.1016/j.profnurs.2017.03.003

Fletcher, D., & Sarkar, M. (2013). Psychological resilience: A review and critique of definitions, concepts, and theory. *European Psychologist, 18*(1), 12–23. https://doi.org/10.1027/1016-9040/a000124

Fowler, A. C., Twigg, D., Jacob, E., & Nattabi, B. (2018). An integrative review of rural and remote nursing graduate programmes and experiences of nursing graduates. *Journal of Clinical Nursing, 27*(5–6), e753–e766. https://doi.org/10.1111/jocn.14211

Furman, W., & Buhrmester, D. (2009). Methods and measures: The network of relationships inventory: Behavioral systems version. *International Journal of Behavioral Development, 33*, 470–478. https://doi.org/10.1177/0165025409342634

Furnham, A., & Boo, H. C. (2011). A literature review of the anchoring effect. *Journal of Socio-Economics, 40*(1), 35–42. https://doi.org/10.1016/j.socec.2010.10.008

Harrison, H., Birks, M., Franklin, R. C., & Mills, J. (2020). Fostering graduate nurse practice readiness in context. *Collegian, 27*(1), 115–124. https://doi.org/10.1016/j.colegn.2019.07.006

OXFORD UNIVERSITY PRESS

Hazan, C., & Shaver, P. R. (1990). Love and work: An attachment-theoretical perspective. *Journal of Personality and Social Psychology, 59*(2), 270–280. https://doi.org/10.1037/0022-3514.59.2.270

Henderson, A., Ossenberg, C., & Tyler, S. (2015). 'What matters to graduates': An evaluation of a structured clinical support program for newly graduated nurses. *Nurse Education in Practice, 15*(3), 225–231. https://doi.org/10.1016/j.nepr.2015.01.009

Hoare, K. J. (2016). Retaining new graduate nurses in practice: Underpinning the theory of reciprocal role modelling with 'routinisation' theory and transition shock. *Social Theory & Health, 14*(2), 224–238. https://doi.org/10.1057/sth.2015.30

Kahn, W. A. (1990). Psychological conditions of personal engagement and disengagement at work. *Academy of Management Journal, 33*(4), 692–724. https://doi.org/10.2307/256287

Kaiser, J. A. (2017). The relationship between leadership style and nurse-to-nurse incivility: Turning the lens inward. *Journal of Nursing Management, 25*(2), 110–118. https://doi.org/10.1111/jonm.12447

Kramer, M., Halfer, D., Maguire, P., & Schmalenberg, C. (2012). Impact of healthy work environments and multistage nurse residency programs on retention of newly licensed RNs. *Journal of Nursing Administration, 42*(3), 148–159. https://doi.org/10.1097/NNA.0b013e31824808e3

Kramer, M., Brewer, B. B., & Maguire, P. (2013a). Impact of healthy work environments on new graduate nurses' environmental reality shock. *Western Journal of Nursing Research, 35*(3), 348–383. https://doi.org/10.1177/0193945911403939

Kramer, M., Maguire, P., Schmalenberg, C., Halfer, D., Budin, W. C., Hall, D. S., Goodloe, L., Klaristenfeld, J., Teasley, S., Forsey, S., & Lemke, J. (2013b). Components and strategies of nurse residency programs effective in new graduate socialization. *Western Journal of Nursing Research, 35*(5), 566–589. https://doi.org/10.1177/0193945912459809

Laschinger, H. K. S., Cummings, G., Leiter, M., Wong, C., MacPhee, M., Ritchie, J., Wolff, A., Regan, S., Rhéaume-Brüning, A., Jeffs, L., Young-Ritchie, C., Grinspun, D., Gurnham, M. E., Foster, B., Huckstep, S., Ruffolo, M., Shamian, J., Burkoski, V., Wood, K., & Read, E. 2016). Starting out: A time-lagged study of new graduate nurses; transition to practice. *International Journal of Nursing Studies, 57*, 82–95. https://doi.org/10.1016/j.ijnurstu.2016.01.005

Laschinger, H. K. S., Wong, C. A., & Grau, A. L. (2012). The influence of authentic leadership on newly graduated nurses' experiences of workplace bullying, burnout and retention outcomes: A cross-sectional study. *International Journal of Nursing Studies, 49*(10), 1266–1276. https://doi.org/10.1016/j.ijnurstu.2012.05.012

Lee, R. T., & Ashforth, B. E. (1996). A meta-analytic examination of the correlates of the three dimensions of job burnout. *Journal of Applied Psychology, 81*(2), 123–133. https://doi.org/10.1037/0021-9010.81.2.123

Leiter, M. P. (2017). Burnout as a developmental process: Consideration of models. In W. B. Schaufeli, C. Maslach & T. Marek (Eds.), *Professional burnout: Recent developments in theory and research* (pp. 237–250). Routledge.

Leiter, M. P. (2019). Costs of incivility in workplaces and potential remedies. In R. Burke & A. Richardsen (Eds.), *Creating psychologically healthy workplaces* (pp. 235–250). Edward Elgar. https://doi.org/10.4337/9781788113427

Leiter, M. P., & Maslach, C. (2014). Interventions to prevent and alleviate burnout. In M. Leiter, A. B. Bakker & C. Maslach (Eds.), *Burnout at work: A psychological perspective* (pp. 153–175). Psychology Press.

Leiter, M. P., & Maslach, C. (2017). Motivation, competence, and job burnout. In A. J. Elliot, C. S. Dweck & D. S. Yeager (Eds.), *Handbook of competence and motivation: Theory and application* (2nd ed., pp. 370–384). Guilford Press.

Leiter, M. P., Day, A., & Price, L. (2015). Attachment styles at work: Measurement, collegial relationships, and burnout. *Burnout Research, 2*(1), 25–35. https://doi.org/10.1016/j.burn.2015.02.003

Leiter, M. P., Laschinger, H. K. S., Day, A., & Oore, D. G. (2011). The impact of civility interventions on employee social behavior, distress, and attitudes. *Journal of Applied Psychology, 96*(6), 1258–1274. https://doi.org/10.1037/a0024442

Lindberg, P., & Vingård, E. (2012). Indicators of healthy work environments: A systematic review. *Work, 41*(Supplement 1), 3032–3038. https://doi.org/10.3233/WOR-2012-0560-3032

Liu, W., Chi, S. C. S., Friedman, R., & Tsai, M. H. (2009). Explaining incivility in the workplace: The effects of personality and culture. *Negotiation and Conflict Management Research, 2*(2), 164–184. https://doi.org/10.1111/j.1750-4716.2009.00035.x

Maslach, C. (2003). *Burnout: The cost of caring*. Malor Books.

Maslach, C., & Leiter, M. P. (1997). *The truth about burnout: How organizations cause personal stress and what to do about it*. Jossey-Bass.

Maslach, C., & Leiter, M. P. (2008). Early predictors of job burnout and engagement. *Journal of Applied Psychology, 93*(3), 498–512. https://doi.org/10.1037/0021-9010.93.3.498

Maslach, C., & Leiter, M. P. (2017). New insights into burnout and health care: Strategies for improving civility and alleviating burnout. *Medical Teacher, 39*(2), 160–163.

Maslach, C., Schaufeli, W. B., & Leiter, M. P. (2001). Job burnout. *Annual Review of Psychology, 52*(1), 397–422.

Mikulincer, M., & Florian, V. (1995). Appraisal of and coping with a real-life stressful situation: The contribution of attachment styles. *Personality and Social Psychology Bulletin, 21*(4), 406–414.

Missen, K., McKenna, L., & Beauchamp, A. (2014). Satisfaction of newly graduated nurses enrolled in transition-to-practice programmes in their first year of employment: A systematic review. *Journal of Advanced Nursing, 70*(11), 2419–2433. https://doi.org/10.1111/jan.12464

Murray, M., Sundin, D., & Cope, V. (2020). Supporting new graduate registered nurse transition for safety: A literature review update. *Collegian, 27*(1), 125–134. https://doi.org/10.1016/j.colegn.2019.04.007

Paterson, K., Henderson, A., & Burmeister, E. (2015). The impact of a leadership development programme on nurses' self-perceived leadership capability. *Journal of Nursing Management, 23*(8), 1086–1093. https://doi.org/10.1111/jonm.12257

Pearson, C. M., Andersson, L. M., & Porath, C. L. (2000). Assessing and attacking workplace incivility. *Organizational Dynamics, 29*(2), 123–137. https://doi.org/ 10.1016/s0090-2616(00)00019-x

Phillips, C., Esterman, A., & Kenny, A. (2015). The theory of organisational socialisation and its potential for improving transition experiences for new graduate nurses. *Nurse Education Today, 35*(1), 118–124. https://doi.org/10.1016/j.nedt.2014.07.011

Phillips, C., Kenny, A., Esterman, A., & Smith, C. (2014). A secondary data analysis examining the needs of graduate nurses in their transition to a new role. *Nurse Education Practice, 14*(2), 106–111. https://doi.org/10.1016/j.nepr.2013.07.007

Rush, K. L., Janke, R., Duchscher, J., Phillips, R., & Kaur, S. (2019). Best practices of formal new graduate transition programs: An integrative review. *International Journal of Nursing Studies, 94*, 139–159. https://doi.org/10.1016/j.ijnurstu.2019.02.010

Ryan, R. M., & Deci, E. L. (2000). Self-determination theory and the facilitation of intrinsic motivation, social development, and well-being. *American Psychologist, 55*(1), 68–78. https://doi.org/10.1037//0003-066x.55.1.68

Sainfort, F., Karsh, B.-T., Booske, B. C., & Smith, M. J. (2001). Applying quality improvement principles to achieve healthy work organizations. *Joint Commission Journal on Quality Improvement, 27*(9), 469–483. https://doi.org/10.1016/s1070-3241(01)27041-2

Sansone, C., Morf, C. C., & Panter, A. T. (2003). *The Sage handbook of methods in social psychology.* Sage Publications.

Santos, L. R., & Gendler, T. (2014). *What scientific idea is ready for retirement? Knowing is half the battle.* https://stage.edge.org/response-detail/25436

Sliter, M., Withrow, S., & Jex, S. M. (2015). It happened, or you thought it happened? Examining the perception of workplace incivility based on personality characteristics. *International Journal of Stress Management, 22*(1), 24–45. https://doi.org/10.1037/a0038329

Smith, P., Farmer, M., & Yellowley, W. (2013). Leadership. In P. Smith, M. Farmer & W. Yellowley (Eds.), *Organizational behavior* (pp. 93–111). Routledge. https://doi.org/10.4324/9780203765326

Snarr, R. L., Elias, C. M., Eckert, R. M., Williams, T., & Casey, J. C. (2017). Strength and conditioning professional burnout: Warning signs, prevention, and recovery. *Journal of Australian Strength and Conditioning, 25*(5), 27.

Spector, N., Blegen, M. A., Silvestre, J., Barnsteiner, J., Lynn, M. R., Ulrich, B., Fogg, L., & Alexander, M. (2015). Transition to practice study in hospital settings. *Journal of Nursing Regulation, 5*(4), 24–38. https://doi.org/10.1016/S2155-8256(15)30031-4

Stanley, D., & Stanley, K. (2018). Clinical leadership and nursing explored: A literature search. *Journal of Clinical Nursing, 27*(9–10), 1730–1743. https://doi.org/10.1111/jocn.14145

Sweet, L., & Broadbent, J. (2017). Nursing students' perceptions of the qualities of a clinical facilitator that enhance learning. *Nurse Education Practice, 22*, 30–36. https://doi.org/10.1016/j.nepr.2016.11.007

Thompson, D. S., Fazio, X., Kustra, E., Patrick, L., & Stanley, D. (2016). Scoping review of complexity theory in health services research. *BMC Health Services Research, 16*(1), 87. https://doi.org/10.1186/s12913-016-1343-4

Tversky, A., & Kahneman, D. (1974). Judgment under uncertainty: Heuristics and biases. *Science, 185*(4157), 1124–1131. https://doi.org/10.1126/science.185.4157.1124

Tversky, A., & Koehler, D. J. (1994). Support theory: A nonextensional representation of subjective probability. *Psychological Review, 101*(4), 547–567. https://doi.org/10.1037/0033-295X.101.4.547

Tyndall, D. E., Firnhaber, G. C., & Scott, E. S. (2018). The impact of new graduate nurse transition programs on competency development and patient safety: An integrative review. *Advances in Nursing Science, 41*(4), E26–E52. https://doi.org/10.1097/ANS.0000000000000217

Vaughn, V. Saint, S., Krein, S. L., Forman, J. H., Meddings, J., Ameling, J., Winter, S., Townsend, W., & Chopra, V. (2018). Characteristics of healthcare organisations struggling to improve quality: Results from a systematic review of qualitative studies. *BMJ Quality & Safety, 28*(1), 74–84. http//doi.org/10.1136/bmjqs-2017-007573

Walker, A., Costa, B. M., Foster, A. M., & de Bruin, R. L. (2017). Transition and integration experiences of Australian graduate nurses: A qualitative systematic review. *Collegian, 24*(5), 505–512. https://doi.org/10.1016/j.colegn.2016.10.004

World Health Organization. (2019, May 28). *Mental health: Burn-out an 'occupational phenomenon': International classification of diseases.* https://www.who.int/mental_health/evidence/burn-out

Wu, C.-H., & Parker, S. K. (2012). The role of attachment styles in shaping proactive behaviour: An intra-individual analysis. *Journal of Occupational and Organizational Psychology, 85*(3), 523–530. https://doi.org/10.1111/j.2044-8325.2011.02048.x

Wu, C.-H., & Parker, S. K. (2017). The role of leader support in facilitating proactive work behavior: A perspective from attachment theory. *Journal of Management, 43*(4), 1025–1049. https://doi.org/10.1177/0149206314544745

Chapter 12

Executing a Career Plan

Kylie Ward, Kylie Hasse, Tania Dufty and Helena Harrison

Learning Outcomes

Upon completion of this chapter, you will be able to:

1. Discuss the different career opportunities available for registered nurses.
2. Examine ways to advance your nursing career.
3. Evaluate the factors influencing new graduate employment.
4. Explain the preparation required for a successful job application.
5. Identify resources to support career development.

Key terms

Assessment continuum	Curriculum Vitae	Organisational fit
Career plan	Leadership	Practice readiness
Coaching	Lifelong learning	Professional portfolio
Consortium	Management	Resume
Cover letter	Mentor	Selection criteria

Introduction

In this chapter we will explore how to plan for a purposeful and fulfilling career as a registered nurse who is recognised as a leader in the profession. We begin the chapter by discussing career planning and the different career pathways open to registered nurses. We will then look at how you can best prepare an application for a new position, and factors influencing your success in securing a new graduate position. We close the chapter with some strategies to develop, sustain and advance your career beyond your graduate year. As we move through the chapter, keep in mind that planning your future and starting a new career are significant milestones. Many new graduates begin their career with a linear path in mind; however, highly experienced registered nurses will tell you that their careers have followed anything but a linear path, and that the direction they took was not what they had initially imagined or expected. Consider this when planning your career as a registered nurse. Leave your options open, seek opportunities in areas that interest you, but also accept challenges that move you out of your comfort zone and, as we have suggested throughout this text, cultivate a supportive network of professionals to guide you.

Case Study 12.1: Introducing Ellie

Ellie went straight to university after leaving school and has enjoyed her nursing degree. At 21, Ellie is excited about her future career and ambitious to do well. She is feeling a bit confused about what to do when she finishes her graduate year program and is looking for some advice.

Career planning – positioning yourself for success

Now that you have chosen your profession, it is important you take some time to consider the direction you would like to take after graduation. This is an exciting time in your career, one that is full of different options. It is likely that when you started your nursing program, your goal or plan was 'to be a nurse'. However, being a nurse does not just happen once you have completed your nursing program and registered. Being a nurse is an ongoing path of transition, growth and development that continues as you move from one role and context of practice to the next.

Planning your career path will enable you to focus and structure your professional growth and development in an area of nursing that interests and inspires you. A **career plan** allows you to set your goals, determine your skills and interests, and implement actions to reach your goals. Careful consideration and planning about where, with whom and what work you would like to do, will help you prepare effectively and optimise the experience for positive outcomes. As a result, a career plan can help ensure you enjoy your experiences and find them fulfilling and rewarding. In summary, a career plan will:

Career plan

A continuous practical strategy that outlines a person's short- and long-term career goals and the actions to take to achieve those goals.

- *Help you identify and attain your goals.* Planning steers us in a direction of our choice. When we work where we want to work, doing what we want to do, we are more inspired and committed to be the best we can be. This gives our work meaning and purpose.

- *Support you to grow and develop.* Continuing professional development is essential to your registration as a nurse. It keeps us motivated, confident, safe and satisfied.

- *Identify areas for development and improvement.* When considering a career path, we need to think about our capabilities and how they align (or not) with where we want to work. We can then determine areas of strength to build on, areas to develop and actions to take to improve and progress.

- *Secure the right position.* When you plan where you are headed and what you need to do, you address your learning needs and leverage your strengths. As a result, you will be prepared, confident and more likely to succeed in securing the position you are seeking.

Exploring career options

The first step in planning and developing your career is to consider where you want to work as a registered nurse. Although this might change over time, you have to start somewhere. As a nurse, you have joined a profession that offers multiple options for a career that will extend over decades. Nursing has such diversity that there are no clear boundaries for your future career. Wherever people live or congregate, care will be required across their lifespan. Nurses can specialise in a limitless choice of areas from disease or diagnosis, to contexts such as rural and remote care, retrieval and disaster nursing. An aged care nurse can work in acute and community care and an acute care surgical nurse can work in a hospital in the home program. It's exciting when you think about the career possibilities that await you, but it can also be a little overwhelming!

While it is important to think about this early in your nursing program, your final year is a good time to crystallise your ideas and set plans in motion to get you started. By your final year you have accumulated a range of experiences to draw upon and help you make some decisions about where you would like to work, and why. While some of your choices may be limited by your current level of experience, you still have many options available. On graduating, your priority is to secure a position to consolidate what you have learnt during your nursing program. With your first year completed and your fundamental nursing practice established, many more opportunities will open up for you to advance your career.

Career pathways for registered nurses

You will be aware by now that nursing is a career that offers almost limitless opportunities to work in different specialties and settings. In Chapter 1, we outlined the five broad areas in which nurses in Australia and New Zealand generally focus their practice, in addition to some of the specialty areas in which nurses work. In this next section we will review these in more detail so that you have a good understanding of the choices and terrific opportunities ahead of you.

Nurses tend to follow different career pathways which cover five broad areas of practice – clinical, management, education, research, and policy. Leadership capabilities are required in all five areas of practice. The pathways span different contexts: rural and remote healthcare, community, acute and primary care such as schools and general practice clinics, and different services and sectors such as aged care and the Australian Defence Force (ADF). The World Health Organization (WHO), the International Council of Nurses (ICN) and the Australian College of Nursing (ACN) employ a range of registered nurses to support the professional development of nurses, and in policy development areas to lobby for and promote the nursing profession (ACN, 2020a). Some examples of different areas of practice are highlighted in Appendix 14.

Each career pathway offers many different avenues to specialise and advance your career and each can overlap the others. For example, you can be a leader and manager in nurse education working in a health service or higher education institution. Similarly, you may be a registered nurse who works in research, within a policy division of a health department.

 Portfolio Activity 12.1: Stop, reflect and think

As you read about the different pathways in the following section, consider the multifaceted clinical roles and levels of practice available to you as a registered nurse. For those that interest you, think about the knowledge, skills, attributes and experience required to work in that area. What would you need to do in the next few years to secure a position in one of these pathways?

Clinical pathway

A clinical pathway offers the opportunity to work in varied nursing roles in different settings. Registered nurses in clinical roles provide direct clinical care, have oversight and coordinate clinical care, research clinical care and/or educate others in a clinical area. There are three forms of clinical practice: generalist, specialty and advanced practice. Like most nurses, the clinical nurse's career pathway commences in the graduate year, consolidating foundational knowledge as a generalist and building on this to a more advanced level of practice, in a generalist or specialist context of practice. In any area that you begin practice you will consolidate and advance your foundational nursing practice while developing capabilities specific to the area of practice in which you are working.

Generalist practice encompasses the provision of a comprehensive scope of clinical care for people with different health needs. It takes place in diverse healthcare settings and requires a broad depth and breadth of capabilities. Generalist practice encompasses a continuum level of practice from beginning to advanced (Australian Nursing and Midwifery Federation [ANMF], 2016). A foundational, beginner level of generalist practice is the basis for all types and levels of clinical practice. Due to the nature of their work, nurses working in rural and remote locations develop an advanced level of generalist practice. As noted in Chapter 2, healthcare services in rural and remote locations can be limited, with reduced access to allied health, medical and specialist services. Registered nurses need to be able to provide care across the lifespan continuum for varied clinical scenarios. Therefore they require a broad depth and breadth of capability to meet the healthcare needs of the people in their communities.

Specialty practice focuses on a specific area of nursing, directed towards a defined population or a defined area of activity. Specialty practice builds on generalist preparation and occurs at any point on a continuum from beginning to advanced practice, where the registered nurse develops capabilities related to the specialty area and becomes more advanced in this type of nursing practice (ANMF, 2016). Nurses who become nurse specialists complete postgraduate education and practice in a specialty field (ACN, 2019b). As we identified in Chapter 1, healthcare is becoming more specialised, thus demand for more specialty nurses is growing. This presents new, unique avenues for nurses to grow their career.

Advanced practice builds on generalist and specialist preparation. Advanced practice nursing is the culmination of sufficient experience, education and knowledge to practise at the full capacity of the registered nurse scope of practice (ACN, 2019b; Nursing and Midwifery Board of Australia [NMBA], 2016a). Advanced practice nursing is characterised by a deeper depth and breadth of knowledge and level of clinical practice that involves cognitive and practical integration of knowledge and skills from the clinical, health systems, education and research domains of nursing (NMBA, 2016a). Nurses who perform at this level of clinical practice are clinical leaders in nursing and healthcare (ACN, 2019b). Nurse practitioners (NPs) are an example of registered nurses who are advanced practice nurses (APNs). NPs are highly skilled, autonomous registered nurses who have the legal authority, under national laws, to practise beyond the level of a registered nurse (NMBA, 2016b). In both Australia and New Zealand, NPs are endorsed by their regulatory board, after completing an approved program of study at a master level in a specific area and having direct clinical contact that demonstrates advanced competency in practice within their scope (NMBA, 2016b; Ministry of Health, 2016). Many nurses develop advanced practice and may not be in a specific advanced practice role. These are often senior nurses working in a specialist or generalist capacity, within a department, clinic, unit or ward, who have significant clinical experience and education that enables them to function at an advanced practice level.

Case Study 12.2: Exploring options

Ellie has been researching her options. Ellie really enjoyed helping her peers in their study groups and explaining things to patients during her professional experience placements. She also has a keen interest in Indigenous health, and knows that working in a specialist service away from where she now lives would be the best way to gain experience in this area. This worries her as she has never been away from home and would miss her family. She is not sure what to do.

- What is Ellie's greatest risk at this point in time?

- What would you advise Ellie to do to help make an informed decision?

- How common do you think it is for new graduates to feel confused about what comes next in their career?

Management pathway

A management pathway in nursing offers a wide variety of options. The terms 'leadership' and 'management' are often used indiscriminately or interchangeably. In actual fact they are two very distinct concepts that share a synergistic relationship where elements of each combine to play an important role in

Leadership

The ability to influence and guide others toward achieving a common goal in a way that leaves them feeling motivated and accomplished.

Management

The process of planning, coordinating, leading and controlling resources to achieve specific goals.

achieving different outcomes in different situations. More broadly, **leadership** is described as a way of inspiring, motivating and mobilising people to achieve and bring about constructive change, whereas management is often associated with creating structure, order, consistency and efficiency in mobilising and controlling resources toward a goal. Being a successful manager in health requires leadership capabilities, and being a successful leader requires the capacity to manage yourself and available resources effectively. Each amplifies the other. A **management** position is commonly a formally recognised position of seniority within an organisation's hierarchy (ACN, 2016). It can be within a clinical, education, research or policy area in any setting. Registered nurses often begin their management career in the clinical area, taking on leadership roles including being a preceptor or clinical nurse guiding others, as a nurse in charge or as the nursing unit manager (NUM).

Effective managers are acutely aware of the internal and external pressures that shape healthcare. They have the capability to simultaneously manage people, resources, situations and environments. Thus, managers require knowledge and skills in financial, quality and human resource management and a sound knowledge of the system, organisational structure and culture in which they work (ACN, 2016; Day & Leggat, 2015). Managers need to have an understanding of their influence and use it to facilitate change and promote positive workplace environments. Therefore, an accomplished manager will have leadership capabilities. How individuals lead and manage can influence the culture of a workplace environment and the outcomes for staff and patients. Managers with strong leadership capabilities mobilise people to accomplish goals, promote greater job satisfaction, reduce staff turnover and motivate teams to reach their potential. In healthcare environments, this leads to safe, effective and high-quality care that improves patient outcomes (ACN, 2016; Health Workforce Australia [HWA], 2013).

Education pathway

An education pathway also offers a range of different roles for nurses. Education is a responsibility of all registered nurses and is explicit in our standards for practice, hence, like management, we begin our nursing careers with some capacity to educate. Registered nurses who are in formal education roles teach undergraduate and postgraduate nurses, and other staff. The roles, responsibilities and scope of nurse education and hence nurse educator practice is wide-ranging: the roles vary according to context, organisational structures and responsibilities. Nurse educators teach in tertiary, vocational education and training (VET) and all clinical contexts. Education is delivered online, face-to-face or using blended approaches. Hence, most registered nurses would not consider a job in education without substantial clinical experience and gaining further qualifications, specifically in education, teaching and learning. Nurse education can be formal and informal and has a significant cascading impact on healthcare and patient outcomes. Many educators begin their career through roles in their clinical area such as preceptoring or supervising nursing students, before progressing to a clinical educator or clinical coaching role. Within a healthcare setting, educators provide education to the healthcare team on all aspects related to the provision of care. Their expertise contributes to how the area functions, the professional development of others, and patient outcomes. From these initial roles, they might progress to nurse educator and then a management role in nurse education with a portfolio and responsibility for education across a service, facility, healthcare organisation or community. Alternatively, they may expand to different contexts such as teaching in the university setting, in a college or within the government sector, contributing to health and policy development at a more strategic level.

Research pathway

The research pathway offers a broad scope of unique opportunities. Registered nurse researchers are at the forefront of the development of knowledge and evidence. Primarily investigating, developing, promoting and translating knowledge and evidence to practice, nursing researchers can explore a range of topics and work in a variety of national and international contexts – universities, government departments, colleges, hospitals, community clinics, research laboratories and more. Those in a formal research position will have a PhD and/or a master's degree, and experience in research. Having a comprehensive and thorough understanding of the research process, being organised and able to manage projects and work collaboratively within teams are some of the key capabilities of nurse researchers. As research involves a number of different activities, from synthesising evidence for practice, collecting, analysing and interpreting data and translating evidence to practice, many registered nurses participate in research without being in a formal role. This is a good way to gain insight and experience in research. Working as a research assistant is also a good starting point if you are interested in research, as this allows you to experience different research activities and methods, and to develop research skills (Lee, 2017).

Policy pathway

The policy pathway offers several different career opportunities. Given the size of the healthcare industry and the scale and complexity of health needs, there is increasing need for health professionals to develop, consult on and contribute to healthcare policy. Nurses can make a significant contribution to improving healthcare systems and patient outcomes, through health service planning and developing policies to guide preparation of healthcare professionals, care delivery systems, healthcare financing and ethics, and addressing the determinants of health (Smith, 2014). A good example is the response to the COVID-19 pandemic where nurses across all contexts of practice and positions contributed to the development of polices, protocols, education and similar. This involved policy and advocacy related to staff, patients, community, clinical practice, systems and processes.

All nurses can contribute to policy-making at many levels, from working on policies and protocols in their workplaces, nursing or health organisations, through to influencing policy-making at local, national or international levels (Smith, 2014). Often the first way to get started and gain experience is in your area of practice, your organisation or an affiliated professional body or organisation. Professional bodies ensure that nurses' expertise and experience are both heard and recognised through professional representation on national boards or committees. Your professional organisation also offers opportunities to participate in expert groups such as policy chapters or working groups focusing on specific issues. The ICN and the ACN are examples of professional bodies that shape health policy through collaborative action, engagement of members and stakeholders, and advocating for consumers, patients and members of the profession (ACN, 2020a).

Portfolio Activity: Making the transition

With the options available, choosing a career pathway in nursing can be equally exciting and perplexing. Use the reflective activity (Appendix 15) to assist you in selecting an area of practice in which you might like to work. While you may have already made a decision, working through this activity will confirm and refine your choice or highlight some other options. Take some time to work through the activity. Consider the questions carefully, make notes as you go and refer back to what you have read in this chapter to help you clarify your thoughts and ideas.

New graduate employment opportunities

Higher education providers and healthcare services are responsible for ensuring you receive a quality education that meets regulatory requirements for registered nurses, and that you are eligible to register as a nurse and are ready for practice. Universities and healthcare services are not, however, responsible for securing your employment as a new graduate nurse – this is up to you. As we stated in Chapter 4, your first year of practice as a nurse is an exciting time in your career but is also a significant period of transition and learning that can be challenging and, at times, overwhelming. As this is the final phase of your learning to become a registered nurse, it is important that you take time to assess the options available and secure the right position.

As you explore your options, it is important to have realistic expectations. You are competing with other graduates who are also seeking their first position, thus not every graduating registered nurse will acquire the position they want. Therefore, keep an open mind when seeking a new position. Your first year of practice sets the foundation for your future career, therefore it is important to get a job; however, it is equally important to have a rewarding and enjoyable experience. Consider all options and be aware that while some opportunities offered to you may not be exactly what you are seeking, they may give you just the experience you need.

New graduate nurse consortiums

Consortium

An association of individuals and organisations whose objective is to pool their resources and activities toward a common purpose.

In Australia and New Zealand, most new graduate nurses are employed into registered nurse positions through an online **consortium** application process. A consortium application process offers a coordinated recruitment strategy where new graduate nurses are able to submit one application for a graduate nurse position to a group of healthcare services, which employ new nurses as part of a structured transition program that, as discussed in Chapter 11, is designed to support their transition and consolidate their pre-registration education.

In Australia, state and territory governments have consortiums for new graduates to apply for registered nurse positions in structured transition to practice (TTP) or graduate nurse transition programs (GNTP). These positions commonly last for 12 months to accommodate the transitional period, can be part- or full-time, and are offered at a range of different hospital and health services in various locations. Most graduate programs offer rotational experiences through different specialty areas, differing in length and number. The allocation of the rotations varies and it may be set or flexible. Larger tertiary and secondary teaching hospitals employ greater numbers of new nurses and may offer more rotations and/or selection of areas to work; however, smaller rural, remote and regional facilities can often provide unique experiences not available in larger metropolitan areas, such as generalist positions with Indigenous communities or community clinics.

New Zealand has a national system known as the Nursing Advanced Choice of Employment (ACE) system, whereby new graduate nurses can apply to multiple district health boards (DHBs) using one application (Ministry of Health, 2019). DHBs employ new graduates into first year practice programs known as nurse entry to practice (NETP) and nurse entry to specialty practice (mental health) (NESP). The programs are delivered collaboratively by DHBs and local primary and aged care providers, and usually provide credit toward a postgraduate university degree (Ministry of Health, 2019).

While each consortium has specific criteria that a new graduate nurse must meet to be eligible to apply, most applications require you to submit a resume or curriculum vitae (CV), university transcripts and a graduate summary that details your clinical placements and work preferences. For most applications, nursing students can identify two or three preferred healthcare facilities and clinical practice settings. In New Zealand, these include primary and aged residential care. Once submitted, consortium members review the applications of graduates who identified them as a preferred employer. The applications are shortlisted. In Australia, new graduates are invited for interview; in New Zealand, the DHBs notify the ACE system of their preferred candidates and the system matches graduate preferences with DHB preferences.

Alternatives to the consortium

While completing a structured transition program is strongly encouraged, it is not mandatory. If you miss out or decide not to apply for a transition program because the area you have in mind is not part of the consortium, or personal commitments mean you need to delay your start time, you can still seek employment as a nurse once you are registered. As most healthcare services are part of graduate consortiums, you may need to consider working in clinical areas and geographic locations that are not your first choice. When looking for positions in these situations, keep in mind the key elements you need to complete your transition continuum: adequate support and good learning opportunities to consolidate what you have learnt in your nursing program. Also consider employers outside the public health system including private hospitals, private primary and community health providers, and aged care facilities. Where possible, try to avoid working in positions where you may not have new graduate specific support mechanisms (such as those discussed in Chapter 11) or you are the sole provider of care for a shift; for example, being the only nurse in a remote area clinic or general practice. As a new nurse, your education and experience are not quite enough to work in a fully autonomous role just yet, even if the service would like to employ you. As you are aware, your first year is a steep learning curve: an adequate support structure will guide you to safely and independently manage the full scope of registered nurse responsibilities.

International nursing graduates

If you are a non-resident nursing student who has studied in Australia or New Zealand and are seeking employment, check your eligibility for available positions. Along with your registration, you must hold a current working visa to be employed, and meet the English language requirement as specified by the health service and professional body. Ensure you review these details during your final year before you put forward an application for a position.

Preparation for employment

Securing a position in a competitive environment requires planning and effort. Your entire nursing program is your preparation for practice as a registered nurse, therefore everything you do throughout your degree is vital to securing the position you are seeking to advance your career. Keeping a record of this is essential. There are, however, key activities you can do, particularly in your final year, to prepare and secure the job you are seeking.

- Know the critical points of assessment as a potential employee.
- Demonstrate a commitment to nursing.
- Network and seek a mentor.
- Research and know your preferences.

The assessment continuum

Assessment continuum

The processes, sources and types of assessments healthcare services undertake to assess new graduate nurses for evidence of practice readiness.

While it is important to make a good impression and demonstrate your level of capability at all times during your nursing program, your final year is a decisive timepoint. This is the critical time when employers are continually assessing you as a potential candidate for new graduate positions. In this **assessment continuum**, there are key points of assessment and processes which healthcare services use to gather information about performance (Harrison et al., 2020a). These are illustrated in Figure 12.1.

Future employers seek new graduate nurses who are practice ready. This means that you are able to register and work at the level of a novice–beginner registered nurse in a healthcare environment. Employers will look for the capabilities associated with the four domains of readiness discussed in Chapter 5 that indicate you are able to work independently, providing a basic level of safe, competent and efficient healthcare with support and minimal to no supervision (Harrison et al., 2020a).

Assessments of **practice readiness** are informal processes rather than formal processes such as assessments of your clinical care in the university or workplace. While these are very important, your overall experience, performance and interactions with the healthcare service, patients and staff are equally important. As Figure 12.1 indicates, these assessments begin well before your entry to the workplace. Usually they occur in third year during your professional experience placements and when you first contact a healthcare service to seek information about employment in their GNTP (Harrison et al., 2020a). Your interactions with the healthcare service when you investigate their graduate programs are critical, along with your employment application and the interview process. These formal and informal assessments tell the healthcare service about your personal, professional and industry readiness capabilities, how enthusiastic and keen you are and your desire and commitment to do well. Most importantly, do not underestimate the value of your final year professional experience placements. These provide the opportunity for you to interact with potential employers and showcase your capability in all the domains of readiness, and your ability to practise independently and know when to seek support and escalate concerns. They allow your facilitators to report on your level of competence and readiness for practice, and a potential employer to assess your performance as a future employee (Harrison et al., 2020b).

The written application you submit for a new graduate program is another significant assessment opportunity of your practice readiness. Applications are forwarded via the consortium to the healthcare services or DHB identified in your preference list. Healthcare professionals assess each application, focusing on how it is presented and on key areas of content – specifically your background, education, and work or clinical placement experiences (Harrison et al., 2020a). They are seeking new graduate nurses who have experiences that align with their needs and demonstrate good outcomes. Along with the other assessments, the healthcare service is determining your **organisational fit**; that is, your compatibility with the organisation – how well your beliefs, values and experience align with and complement the organisation's vision, mission, values and organisational culture (Herkes et al., 2019a). As discussed in Chapter 11, sound person–job fit yields productivity and effective teamwork, and contributes to job satisfaction, retention, and improved patient outcomes. Collectively, this cultivates a positive workplace culture (Herkes et al., 2019a, 2019b).

Practice readiness

The necessary capabilities to work as a novice–beginner registered nurse in a healthcare environment and provide a basic level of safe, competent and efficient healthcare in a complex and dynamic environment.

Organisational fit

A person's compatibility with an organisation based on the alignment between the person's beliefs, values, needs and goals and the organisation's vision, mission, values and needs.

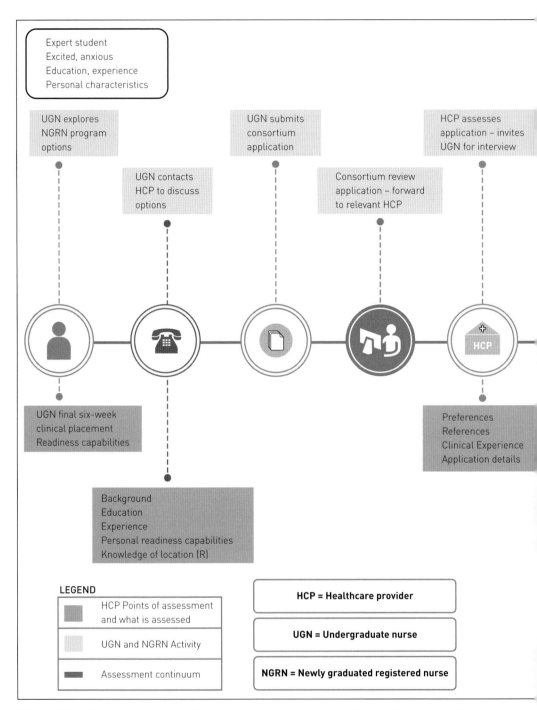

Figure 12.1 The assessment continuum: processes, sources and types of assessments of newly graduated registered nurses for evidence of practice readiness (Harrison et al., 2020a, p. 6)

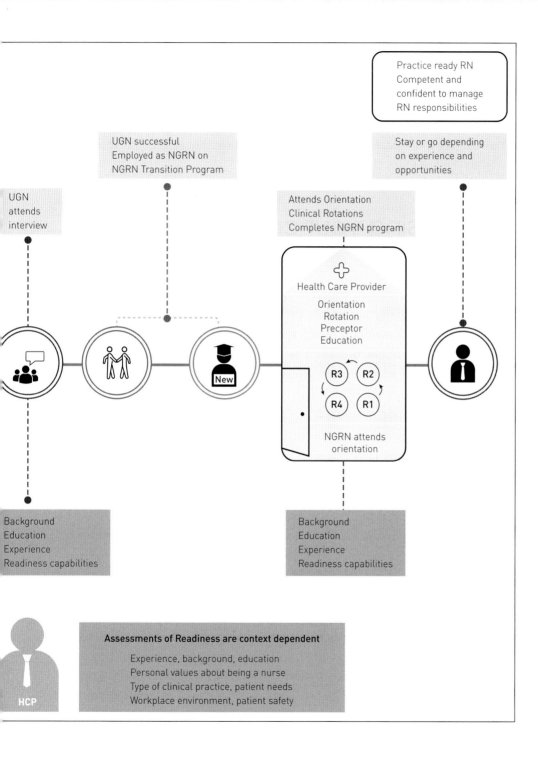

Practice ready RN
Competent and
confident to manage
RN responsibilities

UGN successful
Employed as NGRN on
NGRN Transition Program

Stay or go depending
on experience and
opportunities

UGN
attends
interview

Attends Orientation
Clinical Rotations
Completes NGRN program

Health Care Provider

Orientation
Rotation
Preceptor
Education

R3   R2

R4   R1

NGRN attends
orientation

New

Background
Education
Experience
Readiness capabilities

Background
Education
Experience
Readiness capabilities

HCP

Assessments of Readiness are context dependent

Experience, background, education
Personal values about being a nurse
Type of clinical practice, patient needs
Workplace environment, patient safety

 ## Portfolio Activity 12.2: Stop, reflect and think

Consider an organisation where you hope to work on completion of your studies. Based on what you know about that organisation, do you feel you will be a good fit? If necessary, research the organisation to confirm that your personal values and goals align with those of the organisation.

Showcasing your capability and commitment

Healthcare services seek new graduates who are keen and enthusiastic, open to learning and developing, and safe in their practice. There are certain ways you can demonstrate and maintain these capabilities during your nursing program and in your first year of practice. These actions will support your application for a nursing position and are informally assessed by potential employers during your final year (Harrison et al., 2020a). They will also help you to cope better with your first-year transition experiences.

Professional portfolio

An organised collection of evidence that maps and validates an individual's personal and professional learning and development, capabilities and achievements over time.

1. *Maintain a professional portfolio.* In Chapter 3 we discussed **professional portfolios** and their importance to you and your professional development as a registered nurse. A professional portfolio showcases your learning and development over time and demonstrates how you meet the standards of practice of your profession (Cusack & Smith, 2020). The beginning of your nursing program is the starting point of your learning and development, therefore keeping a record of what you do in your degree is essential. When considering your career and securing your first position as a nurse, an up-to-date portfolio serves as a means to convey your engagement and hence commitment to nursing and, importantly, it presents evidence to validate this. During your nursing program you would have been encouraged to keep a portfolio with records of your clinical experiences, feedback, learning and development and achievements. Now is the time to evaluate your portfolio and make sure it is updated and well presented. If you don't have a portfolio, we encourage you to develop one and collate your evidence, as you will need aspects of it for your application process. Organisations such as the ACN

have a professional portfolio process that can assist you to bring together your professional development activities and showcase your achievements and goals (ACN, 2020b).

2. *Engage in **lifelong learning**.* Completing a pre-registration program is only the first step in your development. Ongoing learning and professional growth are vital, and require lifelong commitment. As lifelong learners, nurses commit to continually improving professional practice and actively seek opportunities to learn. This is expected in the nursing profession as it directly impacts on your performance in the workplace, your patients and consumers and your professional growth. As noted in Chapter 2, healthcare environments are dynamic, and change is a constant part of our professional life as registered nurses. Maintaining patient safety and optimising healthcare outcomes rely on registered nurses engaging with change, and continually learning and developing to ensure competence and currency in practice. Demonstrating your commitment to lifelong learning by openly seeking learning opportunities, being enthusiastic and positive, and completing the required continuing professional development (CPD) indicates your personal and professional readiness.

   > **Lifelong learning**
   >
   > Self-directed deliberate pursuit of education that promotes ongoing personal and/or professional learning and development.

   By investing in education, you are investing in yourself, your career, your profession and those who you care for. You are committing to providing better outcomes for healthcare systems. During your first year of practice as a registered nurse, moderate your choices as the year is already characterised by significant learning and development and you do not want to overwhelm yourself with too much more. Consider shorter courses, workshops and inservices that are relevant to your area of work – this will help consolidate and progress your current practice. Try to avoid taking on anything new until your second year. By the time you enter your second year of nursing, consider some postgraduate education – explore opportunities to progress your career in the direction you are seeking, which aligns with your career goals.

3. *Acquire professional memberships.* Joining a professional organisation related to nursing, or a particular area of nursing, is an important aspect of your career. These memberships can help keep you current in professional standards and clinical practice, keep you connected professionally and provide opportunities for professional development, mentoring and involvement in policy and research. A good starting point is to choose a national organisation that

represents and promotes the professional aspects of nursing and provides membership for nursing students, such as the ACN (ACN, 2020a). The ACN embraces nursing students as part of the profession and future leaders in nursing, and provides access to courses and career coaching. There are over 50 specialty organisations in clinical, education, management and research areas of the profession. Early in your final year, explore and join those organisations that might be relevant to your potential areas of career interest, and record this in your portfolio and CV.

4. *Develop leadership capability.* In Chapter 11 we discussed leadership: its impact in the workplace environment and the importance of developing your leadership capabilities to enhance your readiness for practice and fulfil your registered nurse responsibilities. Leadership is fundamental to effective nursing, and nurses are recognised as leaders in patient care and at the forefront of initiatives to improve healthcare safety and quality. Nurses are an integral part of leadership teams within organisations at every level (ACN, 2019a). As a nurse you are constantly leading, as you will implement goal-driven interventions to improve patients' health status and comfort.

As you progress in your development as a registered nurse you will be coordinating and motivating care teams, families and patients to support patients' well-being (ACN, 2016). Developing your leadership alongside your personal and professional capabilities will not only help you advance your career, it will help you manage workload pressures and challenges in the workplace (Kaiser, 2017; Laschinger & Grau, 2012). These particular capabilities enable you to manage multiple priorities, cope with change and, if needed, address conflict. Therefore, it is important to continue to develop your leadership capabilities. Seek supported opportunities to participate in roles where you take the lead. While it is prudent to wait until later in or after your first year, there may be smaller leadership roles you can take on to enhance your skills. You can also undertake leadership education through short workshops in skill development or similar. Again, the ACN has specific programs aimed at developing leadership that you might like to join in the second year of practice as a registered nurse (ACN, 2020c). Let your manager, preceptor or mentor know you are interested in developing your leadership capability and they can help support you.

 Portfolio Activity 12.3: Stop, reflect and think

Throughout this text we have made the point that nurses are leaders, regardless of area of practice. Do you consider yourself a leader? How have your leadership capabilities improved since commencing your nursing studies? If you feel a little unconfident in your leadership abilities, what resources can you access to develop your skills in this area?

Promote a professional profile

Having a professional profile encompasses how you 'brand' yourself – in other words, how you portray and present yourself to others. Promoting your brand depends on how you communicate and raise your profile in larger networks. When done professionally, this can offer support and opportunities that help extend and advance your career.

1. *Branding.* Throughout every stage of your career, establishing credibility is important. In an increasingly connected and accessible world, you must think about the personal and professional image you portray to others in person and online, and particularly in relation to your patients, colleagues and future employers. People will make assumptions, judgments and decisions about you based on messages conveyed through several aspects of your presentation.

    • Personal appearance and behaviours

    • Verbal and non-verbal communication

    • Social media platforms

    • Professional portfolio

    • Job application

    Collectively these factors establish your 'brand': how you choose to portray yourself and what you represent – you are choosing what people see and how you want to be known. As a professional you need to ensure this is done astutely, professionally and authentically. There are three ways to correctly brand yourself as a nurse: be authentic, be known for something and watch your online presence (Sherman, 2015). Being authentic means being true to yourself. Avoid trying to imitate someone else. The essence of being authentic is consistency, which is easy when you are being true to what and who you are. Being known for something is about what you represent and how people around perceive and describe you.

> As CEO of the Australian College of Nursing I get hundreds of LinkedIn requests per month. I never accept anyone without a valid photo or someone who has a photo that is glamour, casual or non-professional. I do not want to see someone with a beer or wine glass in their hand, party clothes or with friends. It shows me they are not professional and do not understand the importance of the image of professionalism, especially if they are representing the nursing profession (Adjunct Professor Kylie Ward, CEO, ACN).

Monitor your online presence for what you endorse and present as your personal and professional brand. In Chapter 7 we discussed the use of social media as part of professional readiness. Social media profiles including Facebook, LinkedIn and Instagram can be very revealing. Potential employers will check these platforms for information about you, so it is essential that they reveal what you would like a potential employer to see. At all times, be aware of adhering to your professional standards in regard to social media use. When using social media profiles, you might want to consider some of the following.

- Use a professional photo.

- Maintain a polite presence and be authentic.

- Consider connections carefully: be discerning.

- Engage regularly.

- Respond to requests and information promptly.

- Check spelling, grammar and privacy settings.

2. *Networking.* Networking with other professionals and building productive relationships and connections can present unique opportunities to shape and grow your career. Professional relationships can link you to employment opportunities, and help you develop your career, complete job applications and prepare for interview. Many employers use their networks and seek referrals from others, such as employees or organisations in their community. Networking occurs through many avenues: your university, professional

Portfolio Activity: Making the transition

Think about your social media profiles and the pictures and comments you share. What do your social media profiles say about you? Are they authentic and represent what you want to portray and be known for? Do you need to change some of them, or are they a true reflection of you? If you have a LinkedIn page, see what your friends, peers and colleagues have endorsed about you. If you haven't looked at your social media platforms in a while, perhaps now is the time for a refresh. If they are not an accurate reflection of you, or reveal too much that might put a potential healthcare employer off, maybe they need to be adjusted and refined to align more with your brand.

memberships, peers and colleagues you have met through work and during professional experience placements. Formal networking events are also very useful for meeting people at different levels of an organisation, and other nurses who share your interests. These opportunities help you explore other people's experiences and inform your decisions. Before a networking event, do your research to understand the host organisation and who is likely to attend. Prepare a few questions to start a conversation and gather information. Have a brief pitch ready to summarise your skills, experience and interests. Dress professionally and have your contact details on hand to share.

3. *University and clinical placement experiences.* As discussed in Chapter 10, one of the best opportunities to create a good impression, demonstrate your capability and build relationships is throughout your nursing program. Every clinical placement experience puts you front and centre to a prospective employer. This is particularly important if the area you are placed is where you are interested in working as a registered nurse and/or pursuing as your career. Liaising with your facilitator, preceptor or clinical coach and the healthcare team offers critical moments to showcase your capability and build relationships that will support your career. Make every moment count. Individuals such as a clinical coach or facilitator, preceptor or nurse unit manager, could be an excellent referee for you.

Preparing and submitting your application

The next significant step is to prepare and submit your application for a position. Again, impressions are important and how you present your application is part of your branding – it says something about who you are, what you represent and, in this instance, tells your story and the quality of your work. This impression can lead to an interview.

Research your preferences

Recruitment for new graduate positions generally occurs in July–August for the subsequent year, so it is important that you begin preparing at the start of the final year of your nursing program. Prior to submitting your application, research your preferences to ensure the healthcare service meets your needs and provides some of the choices you are seeking for your career. Do some fact-finding about the healthcare service's transition program to see if it provides the elements you are looking for to support you in your first year of practice.

As part of your fact-finding, contact the healthcare service and speak with the individuals who coordinate the GNTP and/or manage the recruitment processes. Similarly, if you choose an alternative to the consortium approach, phone to ask about a position. Keep in mind that this is often the first point of assessment of you as a potential employee and your readiness for practice, even if you have had professional experience placements, so it is important you make a professional impression and are prepared for the conversation. This interaction can generate specific evidence about your confidence, personality, communication and knowledge of the healthcare service (Harrison et al., 2020a). It can convey how well you know the organisation and your commitment to it and to the profession of nursing. It also provides the opportunity for the healthcare staff to explain different aspects of the service and prepare you for the experience of being employed there. The information you discover will be useful for you during the application and interview process.

Application

Applying for a new position requires time and organised, detailed preparation. While the prospect of a new position is exciting, the application process and thought of an interview can be daunting and, for some, anxiety-provoking. Key elements of your application include writing a cover letter and CV or resume and addressing selection criteria. Take time to analyse the job description – don't just assume you know what a position is about. Write a rough draft of how you meet the requirements, work out what information you need. If you have an up-to-date portfolio, use it, as it will make the process more efficient and save you some time.

Cover letter

A **cover letter** accompanies your CV or resume and is a potential employer's first introduction to who you are. It is an opportunity to make an impression – make it count. Potential employers use cover letters and selection criteria responses to screen applications for their suitability for the position, and consequently for an interview. An employer might request a stand-alone cover letter or one that includes your responses to the selection criteria. In either case, your cover letter needs to be succinct, focusing on key information that conveys a clear message about your suitability for the position. Ensure your letter is well presented and has no spelling or grammatical errors. Organise the information logically, and use some formality in how you address the person in the letter and how you sign off. Include your contact details, the position title and the position number for which you are applying. Keep in mind that your CV and selection criteria responses already include a lot of information. Avoid repeating what is in your supporting documents – reframe your information in a way that complements rather than repeats it. Where appropriate, you can refer to the information in those documents rather than rewriting it.

In a consortium application, there may be specific documents or an electronic interface where you input your information. Follow these instructions carefully. If you have the option, upload a document you have created as that gives you more control over how the information is presented. We suggest that even if a cover letter is not required, include a brief one with your selection criteria.

Cover letter

A document that accompanies a person's resume or CV. It provides additional detail about their background, experiences and suitability for a position.

Selection criteria

Selection criteria

Essential qualifications, experience and capabilities (knowledge, abilities and attributes) an individual must demonstrate to be considered eligible for a job.

The second document you need to prepare for your application is a statement addressing the **selection criteria**. The employer will use it to screen and determine a candidate's eligibility for interview. It is an opportunity for you to impress and assert your suitability for a position. Keep your responses succinct and organised. Candidates can easily be disregarded if their responses to selection criteria are not on-topic or are poorly written. Responding to selection criteria provides an opportunity to articulate your strengths, attributes, experience and knowledge to promote yourself as the perfect candidate. The selection criteria relate directly to the capabilities and experience required for a position, and are often broken into 'essential' and 'desirable' requirements. Essential criteria are compulsory to perform the role being advertised, such as being a registered nurse in order to apply for that role. Desirable criteria are attractive but not mandatory for the role; for example, previous experience working as an assistant in nursing. Your responses to the selection criteria tell readers that you have the necessary capability to fulfil the responsibilities of the position. Therefore, your responses need to be convincing. You should not only provide information about your capability, but also include examples that validate what you state and exemplify how you meet the criteria.

Curriculum Vitae

A detailed, comprehensive summary of an individual's experiences, capabilities and achievements over time.

Portfolio Activity: Making the transition

Consider positions you have applied for in the past. How will your applications for positions as a registered nurse differ from these? What have you learnt from the process that you can apply to future applications?

Resume

A document that presents a succinct summary of an individual's personal details, and their professional qualifications, capabilities, experiences and achievements over time.

CV or resume

In launching your new nursing career, your **CV** or a **resume** (a summarised version of your CV) allows you to present yourself and communicate your professional qualifications, employment and experience, achievements and capabilities. This is your opportunity to clearly articulate what you can bring to an employer.

There is no single winning design for a CV or resume and there are many templates available. Whatever style you choose – keep it simple. Create a clean, organised and logical document with essential information: this will be a mix of standard content and content that is tailored to the position for which you are applying, and that you want the employer to know. Use headings, continuity of style and layout throughout – these make it easy for those reading your document to find information. If the employer requires a set style and template, use that: this is not the best time to stand out for not following directions. Describe yourself accurately. Do not include information about yourself that is not true or implies that you are something you are not. Those reading your document will understand you are starting your career and won't expect you to have an abundance of qualifications and experience. A standard CV or resume structure should include the elements listed in Table 12.1. These are explained in more detail in Figure 12.2. We have included some tips to help you put together an effective CV or resume that is fit for your purpose.

 ## Portfolio Activity 12.4: Stop, reflect and think

If you already have a CV or resume, review its structure and content in light of the tips provided in this chapter. In what ways can it be improved? If you don't already have a resume, construct one using the information provided. If you are stuck on how to start, there are numerous templates available on the internet.

The interview

Presenting yourself to future employers always requires care and commitment, particularly when securing your first nursing position. Preparation will give you the confidence to answer any on-the-spot questions, and confirms that you are resourceful and serious about your application.

Preparation

Interviews can be intimidating and anxiety-provoking experiences, but with good preparation and practice that familiarises you with the feelings, thoughts and behaviours of the interview experience, you can manage the process to

Table 12.1   Structured outline for a standard CV or resume

Header	• Name • Professional registrations (letters)
Content	• Contact details • Professional summary or career statement • Professional qualifications • Continuing education • Professional employment and experience • Early career history • Professional affiliations • Referees
Other potential inclusions	These are items to consider including for different positions, particularly after you gain experience and acquire more qualifications. They should be placed prior to your list of referees. Additional inclusions could be: • Professional accreditation or expertise • Awards • Research experience • Publication list • Teaching and learning experience

Tips for an effective CV or resume
◊   Describe yourself accurately. Avoid using words unless you can demonstrate the descriptions. Commonly overused words include 'leader', 'problem solver', 'innovator', 'motivated team player'.
◊   Articulate your capabilities to match the position requirements.
◊   Use professional language – do not use colloquial words or expressions.
◊   When using abbreviations, write them out in full, then abbreviate.
◊   There is no requirement to include a photo or your date of birth, age, marital status, nationality, sexual orientation and so forth.
◊   Ensure your personal and employer details are correct.
◊   Make your document clear and easy to read: keep it simple and uncluttered.
◊   Proofread! There is nothing more unprofessional, and for some readers irritating, than grammatical errors and spelling mistakes.
◊   Ask someone you trust to read your document together with the job description and selection criteria to check for errors and ensure you have adequately addressed the requirements.
◊   Discuss salary only if it relates to a negotiation outside an industrial award.
◊   Check if the process uses applicant tracking system software. Ensure your resume is compatible with this system to read and process your application.
◊   Check your voicemail. A potential employee may be disappointed or put off if they are unable to leave a message or reach a voicemail that is inappropriate, childish or incoherent.

OXFORD UNIVERSITY PRESS

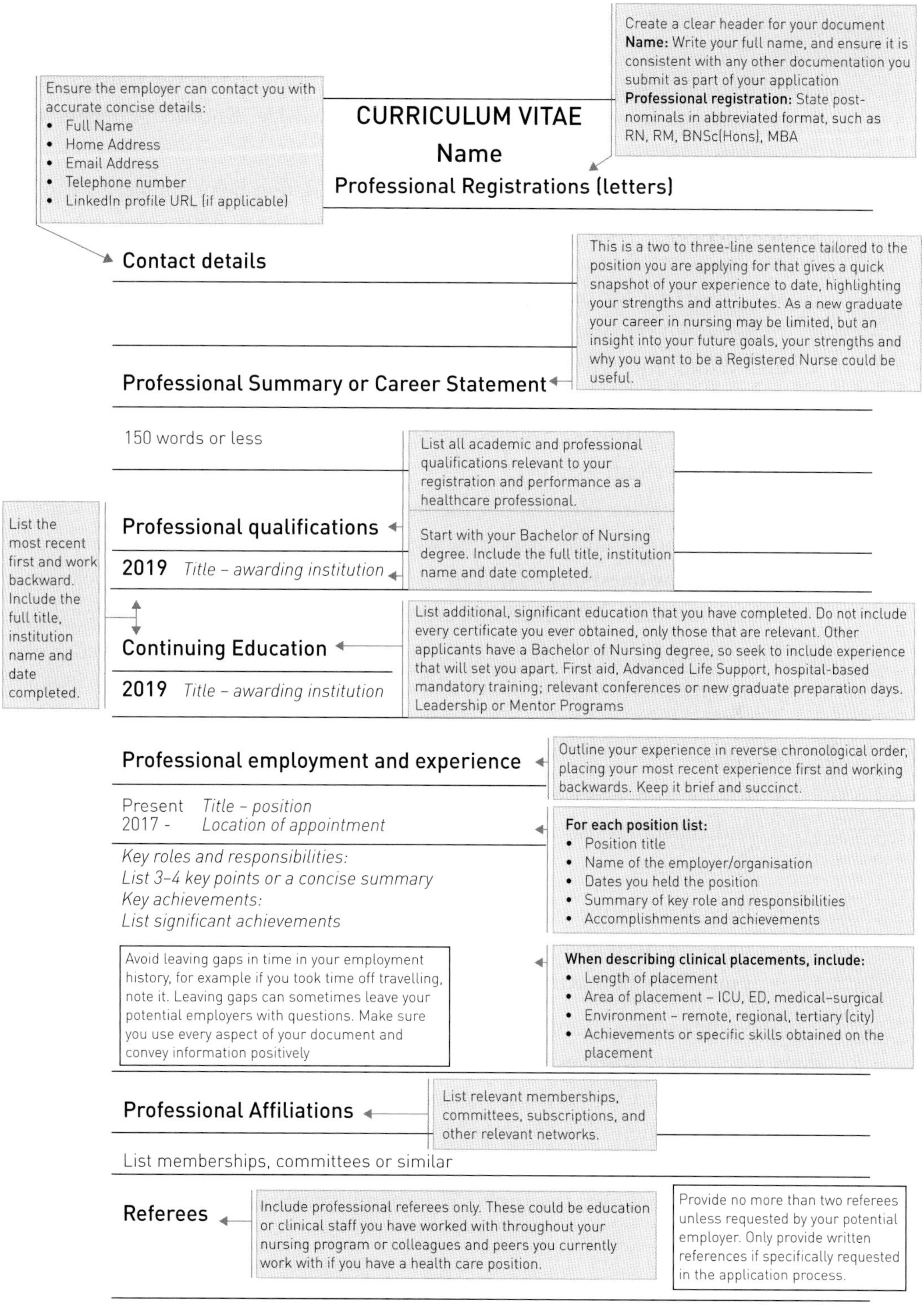

Create a clear header for your document
Name: Write your full name, and ensure it is consistent with any other documentation you submit as part of your application
Professional registration: State post-nominals in abbreviated format, such as RN, RM, BNSc(Hons), MBA

Ensure the employer can contact you with accurate concise details:
- Full Name
- Home Address
- Email Address
- Telephone number
- LinkedIn profile URL (if applicable)

CURRICULUM VITAE
Name
Professional Registrations (letters)

Contact details

This is a two to three-line sentence tailored to the position you are applying for that gives a quick snapshot of your experience to date, highlighting your strengths and attributes. As a new graduate your career in nursing may be limited, but an insight into your future goals, your strengths and why you want to be a Registered Nurse could be useful.

Professional Summary or Career Statement

150 words or less

List all academic and professional qualifications relevant to your registration and performance as a healthcare professional.

List the most recent first and work backward. Include the full title, institution name and date completed.

Professional qualifications

2019   *Title – awarding institution*

Start with your Bachelor of Nursing degree. Include the full title, institution name and date completed.

Continuing Education

2019   *Title – awarding institution*

List additional, significant education that you have completed. Do not include every certificate you ever obtained, only those that are relevant. Other applicants have a Bachelor of Nursing degree, so seek to include experience that will set you apart. First aid, Advanced Life Support, hospital-based mandatory training; relevant conferences or new graduate preparation days. Leadership or Mentor Programs

Professional employment and experience

Outline your experience in reverse chronological order, placing your most recent experience first and working backwards. Keep it brief and succinct.

Present   *Title – position*
2017 -   *Location of appointment*

For each position list:
- Position title
- Name of the employer/organisation
- Dates you held the position
- Summary of key role and responsibilities
- Accomplishments and achievements

Key roles and responsibilities:
List 3–4 key points or a concise summary
Key achievements:
List significant achievements

Avoid leaving gaps in time in your employment history, for example if you took time off travelling, note it. Leaving gaps can sometimes leave your potential employers with questions. Make sure you use every aspect of your document and convey information positively

When describing clinical placements, include:
- Length of placement
- Area of placement – ICU, ED, medical–surgical
- Environment – remote, regional, tertiary (city)
- Achievements or specific skills obtained on the placement

Professional Affiliations

List relevant memberships, committees, subscriptions, and other relevant networks.

List memberships, committees or similar

Referees

Include professional referees only. These could be education or clinical staff you have worked with throughout your nursing program or colleagues and peers you currently work with if you have a health care position.

Provide no more than two referees unless requested by your potential employer. Only provide written references if specifically requested in the application process.

Figure 12.2   A standard CV structure and inclusions (©Harrison, Birks & Mills, 2020)

showcase your true potential. The best preparation relies on two key things: your knowledge and how you communicate that knowledge. Knowledge relates to three areas.

1. *Know the employer.* Prior research on the organisation helps you get to know the employer and anticipate likely interview questions. What you discover can be incorporated into your responses to demonstrate that you are serious about working for the organisation. At a minimum you should know some things about the organisation you are applying to, such as its vision, mission and values, the type of organisation and what it is known for (Gibson, 2020). If possible, visit and familiarise yourself with the organisation: walk the corridors, visualise yourself being in uniform and walking those same corridors as a staff member.

2. *Know the position.* Read about the position you are applying for and know the key accountabilities associated with it. This can guide you on the focus of the interview questions related to the role and responsibilities. The position description and selection criteria are the best sources of information for this.

3. *Know yourself.* This is a vital element in an interview. It involves knowledge of your capabilities and experience and your ability to speak confidently about yourself. Documents that provide a good foundation for your interview include:

   - CV or resume: reviewing these can help you summarise your experiences and capabilities so that you are succinct when responding to questions about them.

   - Responses to the selection criteria: these provide examples of how you fulfil the responsibilities of the role, and explain your experience and capabilities in practice.

The other source of information in an interview is communicated through how we present ourselves – our verbal and non-verbal behaviours. During an interview we need to respond to questions in an unfamiliar context and under pressure – conditions that commonly trigger a stress response. So, while we have the relevant knowledge, how do we move to sharing this in a calm, logical and conversational manner? The answer is authentic practice.

Authentic practice involves anticipating and practising answering questions as though you were in the interview, similar to the simulation experiences in your nursing program. In anticipating the questions, review the position description and selection criteria for possible areas of focus. Make up a few questions that might align with the position. Generally, interviews will be structured around five areas of questioning.

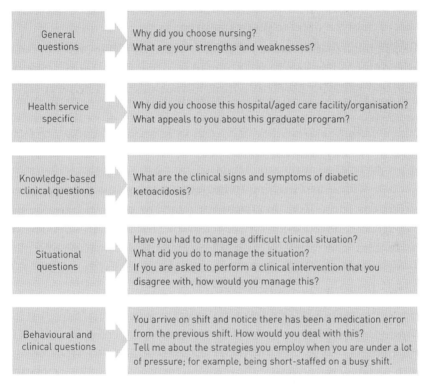

| General questions | Why did you choose nursing?
What are your strengths and weaknesses? |

| Health service specific | Why did you choose this hospital/aged care facility/organisation?
What appeals to you about this graduate program? |

| Knowledge-based clinical questions | What are the clinical signs and symptoms of diabetic ketoacidosis? |

| Situational questions | Have you had to manage a difficult clinical situation?
What did you do to manage the situation?
If you are asked to perform a clinical intervention that you disagree with, how would you manage this? |

| Behavioural and clinical questions | You arrive on shift and notice there has been a medication error from the previous shift. How would you deal with this?
Tell me about the strategies you employ when you are under a lot of pressure; for example, being short-staffed on a busy shift. |

Figure 12.3 Five areas of interview questioning

Once you have worked out some questions, practise answering them on your own or with a trusted colleague, mentor, supervisor or senior nurse. Try to make the experience as authentic as possible and monitor your language, speech, pace and tone and your body language. Interviews are very revealing situations and many organisations use behavioural interview techniques to gauge an individual's performance. According to the University of Sydney (2019), behavioural interviewing is common among internship and graduate recruiters. In asking about your experience and achievements, the potential employer is testing your specific skills and competencies required for the role. The idea behind this type of interview questioning is that past behaviour is an indicator of future performance, and how you respond in content and behaviour indicates something about you (University of Sydney, 2019). Questions often start with phrases like 'Tell me about a time when …', 'Describe a situation where …' and 'Give an example of …', prompting you to talk about a specific situation in your answer. Think about some situations that could be applied to these types of answers to assist the panel to get to know you.

Keep in mind that the art of an effective interview is how well you can have a conversation. While knowledge is important, your ability to stay calm under pressure and talk with people is critical to your success. When you are calm, you will think and recall information more effortlessly. Practising the interview as authentically as possible immerses you in the experience so that you can familiarise yourself with your emotional responses. Even in a practice situation, many people will feel anxious or nervous. Getting to know this response, being comfortable with it and devising strategies to manage it will help you master such reactions during your interview. An interview coach can also be useful. Several agencies offer fee-for-service interview coaching. An interview coach can assist with your responses, overall image and body language, offer tips on using voice control and pitch to convey confidence, and assist with relaxation techniques to manage interview nerves.

The final step of preparation, after researching the position and the organisation and preparing your responses to potential questions, is to confirm the logistics of the interview process. Your interview may be face-to-face or via a virtual medium. Regardless of the medium, there are key factors applicable to all approaches, as shown.

- Confirm the interview timing and location and, if possible, discover the names of the interviewers.

- Dress appropriately and professionally: neat and tidy, including shoes that cover your toes.

- Avoid wearing long jewellery, earrings or necklaces that you might subconsciously fiddle with during the interview.

- Arrive at the interview at least 15 minutes early.

- If the interview is conducted virtually via videoconference, ensure the background is professional.
- Acknowledge and/or shake hands firmly, with good posture and eye contact.
- Remain courteous throughout the interview.
- Thank the interviewer/s for their time at completion.

At the end of the interview, it is reasonable to ask questions. Most interview panels will offer you this opportunity. If you do have questions, prepare these ahead of time. You could ask what support is offered for you as a new graduate or early career nurse, or about something specific such as study support, leadership opportunities, or a particular clinical practice you would like to learn. Asking a prepared question shows you are interested in your professional growth and development, are aware you will need some support and are comfortable asking questions. You can also ask when you would be likely to hear about the interview outcome and if they are open to you seeking feedback on your interview. Alternatively, if you do not have questions – state this and be sure to indicate that everything has been covered in the pre-information provided, your research and during the interview.

Post interview

After the interview, take some time to reward yourself and debrief positively. Try to avoid thinking about all the things you could have said or could have said better, would have said, or forgot to say. Coach yourself to think about what went well! When you recognise things that may have improved your responses or demonstrated your knowledge or abilities better, consider them positively, without chastising yourself. Remember – a successful interview is not just about securing a position. There will be times when you may not be the preferred candidate. In that instance, being successful may mean that you acquitted yourself well – you presented yourself professionally, communicated clearly and answered the questions with relevant responses. Success can also mean that you learnt from the experience and have improved in managing your anxiety to respond effectively. These are great achievements to reflect upon and learn from.

Case Study 12.3: The interview experience

Ellie has been invited to interview for the graduate nurse program at the hospital of her choice. She is really hoping that she will be offered a rotation in the renal dialysis unit as she enjoyed her final placement there and would like to work in Indigenous health in the future. During the interview Ellie is asked a question about how she would respond if a patient demonstrated symptoms of shock during dialysis. Ellie was very nervous and 'went blank'. She stumbled through her answer and forgot to include some of the important clinical signs and symptoms of a deteriorating patient that would trigger escalation. After the interview, Ellie broke down in tears and had a sleepless night worrying that she might not be offered a position.

- What would you advise Ellie to do in this situation?

- Who could Ellie seek advice from?

- What are the key lessons that Ellie can take away from this interview experience?

Registering as a nurse

Before you commence working as a nurse you must register with the Nursing and Midwifery Board of Australia or the New Zealand Nursing Council, as appropriate. This is a straightforward process; however, your application for registration cannot be finalised until your undergraduate degree is conferred and the registering authorities have assessed your documents. TTPs or GNTPs commence in January and February and will require your registration details prior to employment, therefore it is important not to delay the process. Registration can be completed online. It requires payment of a registration fee, submission of specified documents and evidence that you meet English language registration standards if required. If you are organised, you will be able to avoid any errors that might delay the process by having the relevant documents prepared.

Continue building your career – find a mentor or coach

In both Australia and New Zealand, many organisations encourage the use of mentors and coaches to support the professional development of their nursing staff. These individuals, particularly those with experience and professional development in education, coaching or supervision, can provide guidance, knowledge and experience to help increase your confidence and capability as you consolidate your skills (Aspex Consulting, 2017).

An important way to build your career is to be coached by an experienced, knowledgeable leader. **Mentors** are experienced and trusted individuals, chosen by less experienced individuals to support their career development. Mentors motivate and encourage their mentees to achieve goals, and provide advice, information and feedback on their performance. Mentoring has long been an important part of career development. In nursing, the use of mentors has become an important method to facilitate professional development and effectively lead and manage health.

Coaching is a structured, focused process that uses strategies and techniques to promote sustained change. Coaching is about helping others find the answers within themselves, gain a better understanding of their circumstances and take action to move through their challenges (Cox et al., 2018). When promoting growth and development, the coach gives praise, instruction and advice. Coaching is recognised as a powerful vehicle for optimising personal effectiveness and enhancing increasing performance to achieve results (Cox et al., 2018). As discussed in Chapter 11, clinical coaches have been introduced as a way to support new graduates during their first year of practice as a nurse (Kelton, 2014; Martyn et al., 2019). They will be an important source of guidance in helping you to navigate the healthcare environment and your new responsibilities, or when seeking opportunities to develop your clinical practice or during times where you might feel challenged or overwhelmed (Martyn et al., 2019). A trusted peer can also be a helpful support. They can help you to organise workloads, find relevant learning opportunities and offer a chance to debrief, voice concerns and identify stressors (Ankers et al., 2018; Ketelaar et al., 2015).

Mentor

An experienced and trusted individual, chosen by a less experienced individual to provide guidance, advice and support.

Coaching

A structured, focused process that uses strategies and techniques to promote sustained change.

Finding a mentor, coach or a trusted peer within or outside your workplace is useful, particularly if you are not in a structured transition program. Reaching out to your professional organisations can be useful. Many, such as the ACN, provide avenues to network and source mentors. They also offer access to education and continuing professional development in a range of different areas such as developing your clinical practice, or building resilience and conflict resolution.

Conclusion

This chapter has explored the essential things to consider in developing your career as a registered nurse. Given the choices open to new nurses, a good career plan will help guide your professional development. Scope the organisations you want to work for, seek relevant learning and development opportunities, accept challenges and commit to lifelong learning: all this will help ensure you establish a solid foundation to achieve your career goals. Prepare yourself well for your new job – think about what's available to you as a student to support you to be practice ready, prepare for interview and develop the capabilities that will support your entry to practice as a new registered nurse. Make a good impression while on clinical placement, seek the mentors you want to guide you in crafting your career pathway, plan your development and find innovative ways to achieve your goals. We wish you all the very best as you are embarking on your career in the world's most trusted and ethical profession.

Key summary points

- Career planning begins as a nursing student and continues throughout a registered nurse's career.
- Establishing a career plan early and seeking opportunities to progress goals as a student is an important step to being well prepared for transition to practice as a registered nurse.
- New nurses need to seek opportunities to integrate and consolidate their education into practice in the work environment, and to develop the necessary

personal, professional, clinical and industry readiness capabilities for practice.

- Interview preparation is essential to being authentic and communicating your readiness and suitability for a job.

- Spending time creating a succinct, organised and well-structured CV or resume is a vital part of the application process as it indicates your suitability for a position.

- Investing in self-directed lifelong learning will advance your career and ensure your practice remains contemporary, safe and relevant.

Critical thinking questions

1. Can you explain the difference between a mentor, preceptor and clinical supervisor, and the advantages each one might have at different stages of your career?

2. As a nursing student, what do you consider to be important steps in preparing for your role as a registered nurse and planning your development?

3. As a new nurse applying for a position on a graduate nurse program, what are the essential factors that will enable you to be the successful applicant who secures a job?

4. What is the difference between a resume and CV, and in what situation is each one most suitable?

5. Why do you think healthcare organisations are seeking new nurses with leadership capabilities? How might you demonstrate these to a potential employer in your cover letter and responses to selection criteria?

6. Write a list of potential employers who will help you achieve your career goals, as identified in your career plan. What information do you have about these organisations that will assist you to present yourself well during the application process?

7. What support strategies do you require to develop your personal readiness, clinical readiness, professional readiness and industry readiness during your final year as a nursing student and first year of employment?

References

Ankers, M. D., Barton, C. A., & Parry, Y. K. (2018). A phenomenological exploration of graduate nurse transition to professional practice within a transition to practice program. *Collegian*, *25*(3), 319–325. https://doi.org/10.1016/j.colegn.2017.09.002

Aspex Consulting. (2017). *Review of nursing and midwifery graduate transition to practice programs in Victoria: Final report*. https://www2.health.vic.gov.au/health-workforce/nursing-and-midwifery/whats-new

Australian College of Nursing. (2016). *Nurse leadership: A white paper by ACN 2015*. https://www.acn.edu.au/wp-content/uploads/2017/10/acn_nurse_leadership_white_paper_reprint_2017_web.pdf

Australian College of Nursing. (2019a). *Nurse executive capability framework: White paper*. https://www.acn.edu.au/wp-content/uploads/Nurse-Executive-Capability-Framework.pdf

Australian College of Nursing. (2019b). *A new horizon for health service: Optimising advanced practice nursing: White paper*. https://www.acn.edu.au/wp-content/uploads/white-paper-optimising-advanced-practice-nursing.pdf

Australian College of Nursing. (2020a). *About us*. https://www.acn.edu.au/about-us

Australian College of Nursing. (2020b). *ACN professional portfolio*. https://www.acn.edu.au/membership/acn-professional-portfolio

Australian College of Nursing. (2020c). *Emerging nurse leader program*. https://www.acn.edu.au/leadership/emerging-nurse-leader-program

Australian Nursing and Midwifery Federation. (2016). *Nursing specialty*. http://anmf.org.au/documents/policies/P_Nursing_specialty.pdf

Benner, P. E., Sutphen, M., Leonard, V., & Day, L. (2010). *Educating nurses: A call for radical transformation*. Jossey-Bass.

Cox, E., Bachkirova, T., & Clutterbuck, D. (2018). *The complete handbook of coaching* (3rd ed.). Sage Publications.

Cusack, L., & Smith, M. (2020). *Portfolios for nursing, midwifery and other health professions*. Elsevier Health Sciences.

Day, G. E., & Leggat, S. G. (Eds.) (2015). *Leading and managing health services: An Australasian perspective*. Cambridge University Press.

Gibson, A. (2020). *The complete guide to job interviews*. https://nurse.org/resources/job-interviews/

Harrison, H., Birks, M., Franklin, R., & Mills, J. (2020a). An assessment continuum: How healthcare professionals define and determine practice readiness of newly graduated registered nurses. *Collegian*, *27*(2), 198–206. https://doi.org/10.1016/j.colegn.2019.07.003

Harrison, H., Birks, M., Franklin, R., & Mills, J. (2020b). Fostering graduate nurse practice readiness in context. *Collegian*, *27*(1), 115–124. https://doi.org/10.1016/j.colegn.2019.07.006

Health Workforce Australia. (2013). *Health LEADS Australia: The Australian health leadership framework*. https://www.aims.org.au/documents/item/352

Herkes, J., Churruca, K., Ellis, L. A., Pomare, C., & Braithwaite, J. (2019a). How people fit in at work: Systematic review of the association between person–organisation and person–group fit with staff outcomes in healthcare. *BMJ Open*, *9*, Article e026266. https://doi.org/10.1136/bmjopen-2018-026266

Herkes, J., Ellis, L. A., Churruca, K., & Braithwaite, J. (2019b). A cross-sectional study investigating the associations of person–organisation and person–group fit with staff outcomes in mental healthcare. *BMJ Open*, *9*(e030696), 1–7. https://doi.org/10.1136/bmjopen-2019-030669

Kaiser, J. A. (2017). The relationship between leadership style and nurse-to-nurse incivility: Turning the lens inward. *Journal of Nursing Management, 25*(2), 110–118. https://doi. org/10.1111/jonm.12447

Kaiser, L., Bartz, S., Neugebauer, E., Pietsch, B., & Pieper, D. (2018). Interprofessional collaboration and patient-reported outcomes in inpatient care: Protocol for a systematic review. *Systematic Reviews, 7*(1), 126. https://doi.org/10.1186/s13643-018-0797-3

Kelton, M. F. (2014). Clinical coaching: An innovative role to improve marginal nursing students' clinical practice. *Nurse Education in Practice, 14*(6), 709–713. https://doi. org/10.1016/j.nepr.2014.06.010

Ketelaar, S. M., Nieuwenhuijsen, K., Frings-Dresen, M. H. W., & Sluiter, J. K. (2015). Exploring novice nurses' needs regarding their work-related health: A qualitative study. *International Archives of Occupational and Environmental Health, 88*(7), 953–962. https://doi.org/10.1007/s00420-015-1022-5

Laschinger, H. K. S., & Grau, A. L. (2012). The influence of personal dispositional factors and organizational resources on workplace violence, burnout, and health outcomes in new graduate nurses: A cross-sectional study. *International Journal of Nursing Studies, 49*(3), 282–291. https://doi.org/10.1016/j.ijnurstu.2011.09.004

Lee, G. (2017, 19 October). *Nursing in practice: How to become … a nurse researcher*. https://www.nursinginpractice.com/how-become%E2%80%A6-nurse-researcher

Martyn, J., Scott, J., van der Westhuyzen, J. H., Spanhake, D., Zanella, S., Martin, A., & Newby, R. (2019). Combining participatory action research and appreciative inquiry to design, deliver and evaluate an interdisciplinary continuing education program for a regional health workforce. *Australian Health Review, 43*(3), 345–351. https://doi.org/10.1071/AH17124

Ministry of Health. (2016). *New Zealand health strategy 2016*. https://www.health.govt.nz/about-ministry/what-we-do/new-zealand-health-strategy-update

Ministry of Health. (2019). *Recruitment of new graduate registered nurses: Summary*. https://www.health.govt.nz/our-work/nursing/developments-nursing/recruitment-new-graduate-registered-nurses

Minority Nurse. (2018). *Pursuing a career in public policy: No longer the road less travelled in nursing*. https://minoritynurse.com/pursuing-a-career-in-public-policy-no-longer-the-road-less-traveled-in-nursing/

Nursing and Midwifery Board of Australia. (2016a). *Fact sheet: Advanced nursing practice and specialty areas within nursing*. https://www.nursingmidwiferyboard.gov.au/Codes-Guidelines-Statements/FAQ/fact-sheet-advanced-nursing-practice-and-specialty-areas.aspx

Nursing and Midwifery Board of Australia. (2016b). *Nurse practitioner standards for practice*. https://www.nursingmidwiferyboard.gov.au/Codes-Guidelines-Statements/Professional-standards/nurse-practitioner-standards-of-practice.aspx

Nursing and Midwifery Board of Australia. (2016c). *Registration standard: Continuing professional development*. http://www.nursingmidwiferyboard.gov.au/Codes-Guidelines-Statements/Professional-standards.aspx

Sherman, R. (2015). *Building your own personal brand: Emerging nurse leader*. https://www.emergingrnleader.com/building-personal-brand/

Smith, S. (2014). Participation of nurses in health services decision-making and policy development. *International Journal of Evidence-Based Healthcare, 12*(3), 193. https://doi.org/10.1097/01.XEB.0000455187.34972.68

University of Sydney. (2019). *Behavioural interviews: Answering skills-based interview questions from your experience*. https://sydney.edu.au/careers/students/applyingfor-jobs/interview-tips/behavioural-interviews.html

Appendices

Appendix 1: Learning Plan

Commenced	Identified learning need	Strategies to address learning	Review dates	Reflection on progress	Relevance to professional practice	Completed
Date	What do you need to learn?	What activities will you do to help you learn and develop the capabilities you identified?	Timeframe to meet your learning goals	How am I going with my learning? What indicates I am achieving my goals?	What standard, competency, code or capability does this learning need align with?	Date
State the date you commenced your learning goal.	Describe your learning need – area of practice or capability that you need to develop or improve.	Describe the activity/ies you will engage in to address your learning need. This will also help your facilitator, lecturer or preceptor to find opportunities for you to develop.	Identify dates to review your progress with your learning and development.	Write a brief reflection that considers how this activity adds value to you, your client, your clinical practice, your profession and/or your organisation.	List the relevant guideline and include the weblink to the relevant document. You may need to explain why it is important for you to address this learning goal (this helps you link learning with practice).	State the date you achieved your goal.
Add additional rows as needed						

OXFORD UNIVERSITY PRESS

Appendix 2: Worksheet – Making the Transition

As you review Figure 1.1 and Table 1.1, consider the following ideas and make some notes in the sections below.

1. Are there similarities and/or differences between the two professional guidelines?

Registered nurse standards for practice – Australia	Competencies for registered nurses – New Zealand

2. Both of these guidelines were updated in 2016. Think about the practice of registered nurses you have witnessed during your clinical placement. Do you think the guidelines are still applicable to the practice of registered nurses? If so, why? If not, why not?

3. Now think about your education as a nurse in both the university and clinical contexts. Do you think you have the capabilities to meet the professional standards outlined in the guidelines that are relevant to your practice as a new registered nurse? In the space provided below, list the standard or area of competence that you think you might need to develop or improve to ensure you meet the professional standards of practice expected of you on graduation.

4. Next, visit the professional organisation that regulates your practice as a registered nurse in your country and find the standards or competencies for practice. Bookmark the page for later reference.
    a. Nursing and Midwifery Board of Australia (NMBA): https://www.nursingmidwiferyboard.gov.au/
    b. Nursing Council of New Zealand (NCNZ): https://www.nursingcouncil.org.nz/

5. Review the standard/s or domain/s of competency where you think you need to improve and develop to support your transition and subsequent practice as a registered nurse.

6. Using the learning plan provided, list each area and outline two goals with strategies to help you enhance your performance. If necessary, seek help from your university or clinical leaders to crystallise your ideas.

Appendix 3: The CPD Summary Template

Guidelines for completing the template

Item	What to include
Date	Insert the date the activity was undertaken. If it was over several dates, insert the date range.
Practice standard or competency	Check the standards or competencies for practice relevant to your country and identify the areas of practice you want to develop. Insert the practice standard number you plan to develop in the box. If it is for career advancement, you may choose to use the specialisations national practice standards or certification requirements.
Identified learning need	Insert a statement indicating the area of learning you need to develop.
Activity	State what you did to address your learning need.
Reflective evaluation	State what you learnt, how you plan to change your practice as a result of your learning, and what else you may need to learn.
Evidence	State the form of evidence that supports your claim of learning. Include the title or name of the evidence for easy reference.
Appendix number	Attach the evidence to the CPD summary as an appendix. State the appendix number and title for easy reference.
CPD hours	Number of hours spent on the CPD activity should be provided in this column.

CPD Summary Template

Name:

Date: *Insert year range: e.g. June 20-- to May 20--*

Date	Practice standard	Identified learning need	Activity	Reflective evaluation	Evidence	Appendix number	CPD hours

Source: Nursing and Midwifery Board of Australia. (2016). Continuing professional development. https://www.nursingmidwiferyboard.gov.au/Registration-Standards/Continuing-professional-development.aspx Accessed 23 October 2019

Appendix 4: Professional Portfolio Questionnaire

1.	I know what a professional portfolio is and what to include.			
	Select a response	Agree	Unsure	Disagree
2.	I have developed a professional portfolio and I feel confident with the content in my portfolio.			
	Select a response	Agree	Unsure	Disagree
3.	I have developed a professional portfolio, but I am not confident that the content in my portfolio is what I need.			
	Select a response	Agree	Unsure	Disagree
4.	As a registered nurse, I understand why a professional portfolio is important.			
	Select a response	Agree	Unsure	Disagree
5.	I know the different types of portfolios and which one is needed to demonstrate I meet my registration standards or competencies.			
	Select a response	Agree	Unsure	Disagree
6.	I am able to describe what is needed in a professional portfolio.			
	Select a response	Agree	Unsure	Disagree
7.	I have a lot of evidence for my portfolio, but I am not sure where it belongs.			
	Select a response	Agree	Unsure	Disagree
8.	I have a CV and a portfolio but I am not sure how they fit together.			
	Select a response	Agree	Unsure	Disagree
9.	I know what 'quality' evidence means in a professional portfolio.			
	Select a response	Agree	Unsure	Disagree
10.	I could use my current portfolio to apply for a graduate position.			
	Select a response	Agree	Unsure	Disagree

Appendix 5: Capability – Domains of Practice Readiness

Personal	Clinical	Professional	Industry	
1.	1.	1.	1.	
2.	2.	2.	2.	
3.	3.	3.	3.	
4.	4.	4.	4.	
5.	5.	5.	5.	
Reflection	**Reflection**	**Reflection**	**Reflection**	
Reflection – how will these capabilities benefit me as a new nurse working in contemporary healthcare systems?	Reflection – how will these capabilities benefit me as a new nurse working in contemporary healthcare systems?	Reflection – how will these capabilities benefit me as a new nurse working in contemporary healthcare systems?	Reflection – how will these capabilities benefit me as a new nurse working in contemporary healthcare systems?	

OXFORD UNIVERSITY PRESS

Appendix 6: Domain 1 – Personal Readiness

Rate your confidence and competence – plan learning goals – identify support

In the following table, reflect on and rate your current level of competence and confidence in the domain of personal readiness. If needed, make any notes about your capability and confidence in the comments section. Once you have finished, save the document to discuss with your clinical facilitator or university lecturer. This will help you plan your self-directed learning to improve your practice readiness and preparation for your first year of practice.

Confidence and competence level From 5 (very confident) to 1 (not confident and need help)	5 Very confident and competent	4 Confident and competent	3 Somewhat confident and competent	2 Not very confident or competent	1 Not confident or competent: need help	Score 3, 4, 5 Practise independently	Score 1 or 2 Seek help Plan learning	Comments
Personal readiness attitudes								
Commitment								
Resilience								
Compassion								
Tolerance								
Confidence								
Personal readiness skills								
Respectful communication								
Effective interaction								
Relationship management								
Emotional intelligence								
Self-management								

Appendix 7: Domain 2 – Professional Readiness

Rate your confidence and competence – plan learning goals – identify support

In the following table, reflect on and rate your current level of competence and confidence in the domain of professional readiness. If needed, make any notes about your capability and confidence in the comments section. Once you have finished, save the document to discuss with your clinical facilitator or university lecturer. This will help you plan your self-directed learning to improve your practice readiness and preparation for your first year of practice.

Confidence and competence level From 5 (very confident) to 1 (not confident and need help)	5 Very confident and competent	4 Confident and competent	3 Somewhat confident and competent	2 Not very confident or competent	1 Not confident or competent: need help	Score 3, 4, 5 Practise independently	Score 1 or 2 Seek help Plan learning	Comments
Adhere to professional standards								
Functioning within scope of practice								
Critical thinking								
Reflective practice								
Continuing professional development								
Professional integrity								
Professional accountability								
Honesty and trust								
Professional presence								
e-professionalism								
Effective resource management								
Time management								
Prioritisation								
Delegation								

Appendix 8: Domain 3 – Clinical Readiness

Rate your confidence and competence – plan learning goals – identify support

In the following table, reflect on and rate your current level of competence and confidence in the domain of clinical readiness. If needed, make any notes about your capability and confidence in the comments section. Once you have finished, save the document to discuss with your clinical facilitator or university lecturer. This will help you plan your self-directed learning to improve your practice readiness and preparation for your first year of practice.

Confidence and competence level From 5 (very confident) to 1 (not confident and need help)	5 Very confident and competent	4 Confident and competent	3 Somewhat confident and competent	2 Not very confident or competent	1 Not confident or competent: need help	Score 3, 4, 5 Practise independently	Score 1 or 2 Seek help Plan learning	Comments
Appreciate the 'why' of clinical nursing								
Fundamental clinical knowledge								
Evidence base for practice								
Other – add here								
Knowing 'how' to nurse clinically								
Basic clinical skills								
Safe, quality care								
Other – add here								
Understanding 'what' needs to be done								
Translating knowledge and skills into practice								
Pulling it all together								
Other – add here								

Appendix 9: Domain 4 – Industry Readiness

Rate your confidence and competence – plan learning goals – identify support

In the following table, reflect on and rate your current level of competence and confidence in the domain of industry readiness. If needed, make any notes about your capability and confidence in the comments section. Once you have finished, save the document to discuss with your clinical facilitator or university lecturer. This will help you plan your self-directed learning to improve your practice readiness and preparation for your first year of practice.

Confidence and competence level From 5 (very confident) to 1 (not confident and need help)	5 Very confident and competent	4 Confident and competent	3 Somewhat confident and competent	2 Not very confident or competent	1 Not confident or competent: need help	Score 3, 4, 5 Practise independently	Score 1 or 2 Seek help Plan learning	Comments
Industry readiness knowledge								
Healthcare systems and organisations								
Industry and organisational regulations								
Industry readiness attributes								
Adaptation to reality								
Appropriate workplace behaviour								
Industry readiness abilities								
Critical self-assessment								
Self-development planning								

Appendix 10: Industry Readiness Self-Assessment Checklist 1

Rate your current level of competence using the following scale:

1 = Not competent, 2= Developing Competence, 3 = Competent, 4 = Highly Competent

Knowledge of healthcare system and organisations		1	2	3	4
I know and understand the regulations that govern healthcare in Australia or New Zealand.	Current Competence:	☐	☐	☐	☐
I know and understand the relevant award of registered nurses working within healthcare.	Current Competence:	☐	☐	☐	☐
I know and understand the responsibilities and expectations of registered nurses working within healthcare.	Current Competence:	☐	☐	☐	☐
I am aware of the realities of healthcare environments including the pace and shift work.	Current Competence:	☐	☐	☐	☐
I am aware of the complexities in managing clients, colleagues and other healthcare professionals.	Current Competence:	☐	☐	☐	☐
I am familiar with my organisational work environment and how it functions and operates its services.	Current Competence:	☐	☐	☐	☐
I have a good understanding of my organisation's values and its culture.	Current Competence:	☐	☐	☐	☐
I have a good understanding of how to work effectively as a team member in my organisation.	Current Competence:	☐	☐	☐	☐
I have a good understanding of my ward's routines.	Current Competence:	☐	☐	☐	☐
I understand the risks in my workplace.	Current Competence:	☐	☐	☐	☐
I understand the KPIs of my area and my role in meeting these.	Current Competence:	☐	☐	☐	☐
I feel competent and able to work within highly specialised ward environments.	Current Competence:	☐	☐	☐	☐

Source: Caballero & Walker, 2020.

Appendix 11: Industry Readiness Self-Assessment Checklist 2

Rate your current level of competence using the following scale:

1 = Not competent, 2= Developing Competence, 3 = Competent, 4 = Highly Competent

Knowledge of industry and organisational regulations	1	2	3	4
I have a solid understanding of the organisational regulations, policies, practices, protocols and frameworks that are critical to my nursing work within my organisation. Current Competence:	☐	☐	☐	☐
I understand the importance of adhering to/working in alignment with the organisational regulations, policies, practices, protocols and frameworks relevant to nursing in my organisation. Current Competence:	☐	☐	☐	☐
I understand and can confidently explain how the hospital ward where I work as a nurse functions. Current Competence:	☐	☐	☐	☐
I understand how my role contributes to the effective functioning of the ward in which I work. Current Competence:	☐	☐	☐	☐
I am well acquainted with the physical layout of my organisation and understand where the major functions/units of the organisation are located. Current Competence:	☐	☐	☐	☐
I am familiar with where and how to access resources and information that are important in my work as a nurse in my organisation. Current Competence:	☐	☐	☐	☐
I have a solid understanding of the size of my organisation and the resourcing capacity it has to service the local community. Current Competence:	☐	☐	☐	☐
I have a solid understanding of the community my healthcare organisation services. Current Competence:	☐	☐	☐	☐
I have identified formal mentors who I can go to for assistance and support to help me perform my role effectively. Current Competence:	☐	☐	☐	☐
I have identified informal mentors who I can go to for assistance and support to help me perform my role effectively. Current Competence:	☐	☐	☐	☐

Source: Caballero & Walker, 2020.

OXFORD UNIVERSITY PRESS

Appendix 12: Industry Readiness Self-Assessment Checklist 3

Rate your current level of competence using the following scale:

1 = Not competent, 2= Developing Competence, 3 = Competent, 4 = Highly Competent

Attributes for adaptation to reality		1	2	3	4
I understand the expectations and requirements of a registered nurse in the healthcare system/my organisation.	Current Competence:	☐	☐	☐	☐
I understand and can confidently explain the realities and complexities of nursing work in the healthcare system/my organisation.	Current Competence:	☐	☐	☐	☐
I have identified the personal impacts and challenges that shift work may have on my life.	Current Competence:	☐	☐	☐	☐
I feel prepared to effectively manage the personal impacts and challenges associated with nursing shift work.	Current Competence:	☐	☐	☐	☐
I feel confident about working in a fast-paced nursing work environment.	Current Competence:	☐	☐	☐	☐
I understand how to demonstrate agility in my nursing work.	Current Competence:	☐	☐	☐	☐
I understand the stress that stems from working as a nurse in the healthcare system/my organisation.	Current Competence:	☐	☐	☐	☐
I feel prepared to effectively manage the stress of working as a nurse in the healthcare system/my organisation.	Current Competence:	☐	☐	☐	☐
I understand the importance of demonstrating flexibility and being able to adapt quickly in my work as a nurse.	Current Competence:	☐	☐	☐	☐
I feel prepared to adapt my skills and knowledge in order to manage different situations and contexts within the healthcare system/my organisation.	Current Competence:	☐	☐	☐	☐

Source: Caballero & Walker, 2020.

Appendix 13: Industry Readiness Self-Assessment Checklist 4

Rate your current level of competence using the following scale:

1 = Not competent, 2= Developing Competence, 3 = Competent, 4 = Highly Competent

Attributes for appropriate workplace behaviour		1	2	3	4
I understand the behaviours I need to demonstrate in order to align to my organisation's values.	Current Competence:	☐	☐	☐	☐
I understand how a professional work ethic is defined in my organisation.	Current Competence:	☐	☐	☐	☐
I feel confident that I am able to demonstrate a professional work ethic in my approach to work as a nurse in my organisation.	Current Competence:	☐	☐	☐	☐
I understand the behaviours I am required demonstrate professional workplace behaviour.	Current Competence:	☐	☐	☐	☐
I feel confident in being able to identify when an individual is not demonstrating professional workplace behaviour.	Current Competence:	☐	☐	☐	☐
I feel confident in managing the unprofessional workplace behaviour of others.	Current Competence:	☐	☐	☐	☐
I understand the importance of taking a self-directed approach to my learning and development as a graduate nurse, rather than relying on others to direct me.	Current Competence:	☐	☐	☐	☐
I am aware of the behaviours my manager and co-workers would describe as being proactive and taking initiative.	Current Competence:	☐	☐	☐	☐
I feel confident to demonstrate initiative in my work and in my learning and development.	Current Competence:	☐	☐	☐	☐
I understand how to engage in self-assessment to help me continuously improve my professional practice	Current Competence:	☐	☐	☐	☐
I have identified a professional development process to assist me to continuously improve my professional practice.	Current Competence:	☐	☐	☐	☐
I am comfortable receiving all types of feedback (i.e. positive, constructive).	Current Competence:	☐	☐	☐	☐
I understand how to ask for feedback on my performance from my managers, peers, formal and informal mentors in order to further my learning.	Current Competence:	☐	☐	☐	☐
I regularly ask for feedback and ways I can improve my performance from my managers, peers, formal and informal mentors.	Current Competence:	☐	☐	☐	☐
I am clear on what I need to do in order to implement feedback to improve my performance.	Current Competence:	☐	☐	☐	☐

Source: Caballero & Walker, 2020.

OXFORD UNIVERSITY PRESS

Appendix 14: Different Areas of Practice

Australian Defence Force nursing

The Australian Defence Force (ADF) offers unique positions for nurses in the Royal Australian Navy, Australian Army and Royal Australian Air Force (RAAF). ADF nurses work all over the world in challenging roles that require leadership, a strong work ethic and a desire to serve the nation. They can work full- or part-time as reservists on short-term contracts (20 days minimum per year) fitting in with current work commitments. You can enter the Army or RAAF as a sponsored undergraduate from the second year of your Bachelor of Nursing. You are paid while you study and carry out a two-year graduate program prior to entering the ADF as an Army or RAAF Nurse. Alternatively, the graduate scheme requires a minimum of two years as a registered nurse, to gain direct entry as an officer. Most services require postgraduate experience and qualification in a military-related area such as emergency, intensive care or perioperative nursing, with a strong interest in mental health, primary health or aeromedical retrieval.

Aged care

Nurses in this specialty area advocate and care for the health and well-being of older persons. Aged care is provided in a range of contexts – aged care facilities, acute care hospitals, community settings or nursing homes. In aged care, a registered nurse can fulfil a number of roles: a provider of direct specialist care, teacher of aged care nursing, or nurse manager of a specific area, service or facility. As advocates, nurses support older adults to maintain dignity, independence and autonomy as an individual. At any one time a nurse in this specialty will often undertake parts or all of these roles. With longer life expectancy, the number of older adults with comorbidities that require more specialist complex care is growing, therefore this specialty is growing and expanding with new knowledge and practice, models of care and healthcare services focused on wellness. It is an exciting area of healthcare to choose as a future career. Further, older persons are present in all healthcare settings, therefore core skills in aged care are extremely vital in any area of nursing practice.

Community health

Nurses in community health work in a variety of roles within specific organisations, communities and locations – at home, in general practice clinical, in schools or with a public health organisation that services a population area. These nurses are primary healthcare providers, offering preventive and community-based intervention services to individuals and groups. An understanding of primary healthcare is important for these nurses to be effective in the role. A community health nurse is knowledgeable and skilled in health promotion and disease prevention, multidisciplinary teamwork, case management, planning, policy development, and working with culturally diverse populations. Practice areas include school health, community nursing, sexual health, general practice and Indigenous health.

Mental health

Working in partnership with the patients, their families, partners and the community, mental health nursing is a specialised field that aims to provide care for individuals with mental illness or mental health problems. As a mental health nurse, you can specialise in a range of areas and settings: children and adolescents, adults, those in the justice system, community and more. Your undergraduate degree prepares you with foundational knowledge in mental health, which enables you to work in this area; however, to advance your level of practice in mental health, gaining experience and postgraduate qualifications is required. Interprofessional practice is a significant element in mental health issues, as mental health nurses work with a range of diverse healthcare professionals in a variety of settings.

Appendix 15: Reflective Activity – Determining Your Specialty

There are many exciting areas in which you can choose to work as a registered nurse. This reflective activity will assist you to select an area of practice and location where you might like to work. You may already have decided on your area of choice; if so, working through this exercise will confirm and refine your choice.

Take some time to work through the steps and consider the questions carefully. Make notes as you go, to refer back to at a later time. If you need to, refer back to Chapter 12 and Chapter 1 to help clarify your choices and your career path.

Reflect on the following questions and make some notes on your responses.

1. **Consider what you have learnt in the different subjects in your nursing program.**
   - What aspects did you enjoy the most, what came to you naturally and made you want to know more?
   - Which clinical skills did you most enjoy and achieve your best practice in?
   - Did you find it easy to teach others, research information and write or perhaps solve problems?
   - Was there something about Indigenous health (for example) that led you to want to understand and research more?
   - What about the things that challenged you or that you dislike and find hard to understand? List them.

2. **Consider your professional experience placements.**
   - What aspects of the healthcare environment and nursing practice were most and least appealing?
   - Was there a particular unit, ward or department that you seem to have a natural aptitude for?
   - Do you like a drama, moving at a quick pace? Or do you prefer a quieter environment or more one-on-one activities?
   - Would you like to be in charge or lead the clinical care?

3. **Consider the individuals you have worked with on your placements (clients and staff).**
   - Which clients did you most enjoy caring for? For example, adults or children, old or young, those with chronic or acute illnesses.
   - What about the staff? Was there one nurse or other health professional who you admired or disliked? What was it about their practice and manner that caught your attention?

After you have made some notes in response to these questions, see if you can identify any consistent themes – positive and negative. These could be related to knowledge, skills, practices and behaviours or attitudes. They could be things about the environment, and client descriptions. Perhaps there is a challenge you enjoy or an area that you consistently identify that you dislike. **Highlight this.** It will give you a sense of what you might enjoy or may not enjoy.

Refer back to Chapter 1 and some of the specialty areas we highlighted. Review the different areas of practice described in Appendix 14. Think about some of the areas you have worked or know about in the healthcare system. Consider the five broad areas of practice – are there any areas that seem to align with your points/ideas and thoughts? Make a note of these **and move to the next part of the exercise.**

4. **Now think about the physical environments you would enjoy and/or have enjoyed working in.**
   - Describe this environment – conduct an imaginary environmental scan. Is it warm or cool? Is it wet or dry? Rainforest, tropical beach or big open spaces?
   - Do you enjoy quiet times or busy urban areas with lots of people to look at and talk to?
   - Do you like to drive or fly? Do you like telecommunication, IT and computers?
   - Think about what you enjoy around you when you are working.

   Are there any locations that could potentially align with your description? These could be capital cities, remote, regional or rural locations or international locations or perhaps an office. It could be your current location. Wherever it might be – use the internet, investigate the health services in the area and see if any match your preferences and might be able to provide you with more information.

5. **During your investigation, see if you can find a position description for your chosen area of practice.** This can give you a good idea about the knowledge, skills and roles of the nurse. It can also lead you to more information about the practice area from professional organisations linked to the area.
   - See what it says about the role, accountabilities and responsibilities.
   - What skills and knowledge are required for the nurse in this role? Do these interest you?
   - Do you need to be a member of any specific professional groups or organisations?
   - Are there any specific competencies that you need to demonstrate?

6. **During your investigation, look for the models of care the service uses in its approach.**
   Does IT play a significant role? Are there clinical pathways to guide nursing care? Do these align with your ideas about the goals of nursing care – does their way of working resonate with your ideals and goals?

7. **Finally, consider what courses are available that might provide you with the specific knowledge and skills relevant to the area you are interested in.**
   Start with your university and the Australian College of Nursing, look at the postgraduate courses and short courses for continuing professional development. While you may not be thinking of studying just yet, this part of the activity will give you information about the capabilities (knowledge, abilities and attributes) specific to a broad area of practice such as leadership and management or education, or a specialty area such as mental health or aged care. This can motivate you and help you plan experiences that support your development in the direction you want to take your nursing career. Some guiding questions you might like to consider:
   - Are any short courses available? Check the universities in the locations you think you might like to work in. Are online courses available?
   - If you're thinking of a specialty area, what subjects and clinical placements are you completing this year that might link to your area of interest?
   - If your clinical portfolio is up-to-date with highlights of your practice, review it to see what skills you have developed that might suit this area.

Hopefully, in completing these steps you have determined an area of nursing that interests you. The following steps will be useful in planning the pathway to working in your area of practice. Take note that if you begin working in an area and find it is not working out for you, you can always change to a different area. One of the benefits of nursing is the range of areas in which you can practise. Your capabilities are transferable across a wide context of practice and offer the opportunity to move between locations and settings.

a. Consider talking to senior clinical nurses, specialists and managers in various fields to get some ideas about working in that particular area and the type of nursing practices, models of care or similar that are involved in it. It is best to have a prepared list of questions and to ask what they like about that specialty.

b. Set a goal of working in the area you are interested in, to be achieved by a certain date. Your goal could be 'I will work in a remote location as a specialist nurse in paediatrics by ...'

c. Consider your final professional experience placement. Could you complete this in an area where you are interested in working? This will help determine if it is an area you enjoy and want to pursue as part of your career pathway. Remember to take an active role while on placement. Be interested and enthusiastic about your work, ask questions, seek answers and know what you want to achieve in regard to the subject and your goals. Talk with the staff, reflect on what you're doing and learning – find out as much as you can about the area of practice and how what you have learnt applies to that area of practice.

d. Investigate the specialty areas further. Start with the internet and your local facility. Consider the notes you have already made in this reflective activity. Find and research the areas that spark your interest or make you curious.

e. Attend conferences and seminars that relate to your area of practice. While you're studying or during your first year of practice this might be difficult but it is doable. At times, scholarships or opportunities are provided – look out for them. When you have completed your degree and are working, development activities become a great source of inspiration, updating and development. If you are linked to a professional organisation relevant to your specialty area, you will get advance notice of many additional activities – and at cheaper prices. You can join professional associations now. Often they will send interesting pieces of information or new directions for your specialty area.

f. When you have graduated, aim to do one personal development course each year. This is so that you are achieving your life AND career goals, and therefore are maintaining a healthy balance.

OXFORD UNIVERSITY PRESS

Glossary

Advocacy

Publicly speaking up and supporting an individual, cause or course of action.

Assessment continuum

The processes, sources and types of assessments healthcare services undertake to assess new graduate nurses for evidence of practice readiness.

Attachment style

The pattern of behaviour an infant develops in response to stress, which is determined by the emotional bond and the consistency of supportive care provided by the caregiver.

Attitude

A person's disposition or state of mind, how they carry themselves and respond to an object, issue, situation or other people.

Attribute

Inherent characteristics or qualities of a person.

Burnout

A state of physical, mental and emotional exhaustion that stems from chronic workplace stress that is not successfully managed.

Career plan

A continuous practical strategy that outlines a person's short- and long-term career goals and the actions to take to achieve those goals.

Clinical readiness

The capability to provide a safe, basic level of clinical care within one's scope of practice.

Coaching

A structured, focused process that uses strategies and techniques to promote sustained change.

Cognitive bias

A bias in thinking that causes an error when an individual processes and interprets information.

Commitment

Acceptance of the obligations inherent in the professional role.

Complex system

A system of diverse, adaptive and interconnected components emphasised by the quality of relationships, distributed control and emergent behaviours and outcomes that are highly dependent on the context and initial conditions.

Confidence

An attitude or feeling of trust, belief and assurance in yourself, in others and/or in plans for the future.

Consortium

An association of individuals and organisations whose objective is to pool their resources and activities toward a common purpose.

Continuing professional development

Engagement in learning activities that ensure currency of practice and promote professional growth.

Cover letter

A document that accompanies a person's resume or CV. It provides additional detail about their background, experiences and suitability for a position.

Critical thinking

The structured approach to analysis and interpretation of information as a basis for understanding and responding to a range of simple to complex situations.

Culture

Shared attitudes, social conventions, values, goals and practices that characterise a group or situation.

Curriculum Vitae

A detailed, comprehensive summary of an individual's experiences, capabilities and achievements over time.

Delegation

Allocation of prioritised activities to another person to ensure timely completion.

Digital health

The collective use of digital technologies to deliver, manage, and improve healthcare and promote wellness.

Emotional intelligence

A high level of self-awareness of your own and others' emotions and the ability to manage these emotions to enhance interpersonal relationships.

Employment awards

Agreements between industry bodies and unions that determine employment levels and remuneration.

E-portfolio

A digital approach to the structure, storage and presentation of materials that demonstrate an individual's knowledge, skills and experiences.

Evidence
Artefact used to substantiate a claim of knowledge, skill or experience.

Evidence-based practice
The use of available, reliable and current evidence to support the delivery of nursing care.

Healthcare system
An organised, interconnected arrangement of individuals, institutions, organisations and resources that provide healthcare services to meet the health needs of a population.

Healthy workplace environment
The outcome of a collaborative, interrelated system of people, structure and practices that enables others to engage effectively in work processes and relationships to meet the core and subjective needs of all employees.

Incivility
Low-intensity deviance behaviour with ambiguous intent to cause harm, characterised by rude or disrespectful verbal or non-verbal behaviours.

Industry readiness
The capability to navigate the healthcare system, organisations, healthcare parameters and resources in the provision of care.

Interprofessional practice
Two or more health professionals collaborating as a team toward a common purpose with a mutual respect for each other's expertise and a commitment toward achieving this purpose.

Job Demands-Resources (JD-R) model
A model which suggests that balancing job demands and resources influences burnout, whereby job demands deplete energy and evoke stress and job resources provide energy to work productively.

Leadership
The ability to influence and guide others toward achieving a common goal in a way that leaves them feeling motivated and accomplished.

Level of practice readiness
The extent to which a graduate nurse is prepared for the professional role in personal, professional, clinical and industry domains.

Lifelong learning
Self-directed deliberate pursuit of education that promotes ongoing personal and/or professional learning and development.

Management

The process of planning, coordinating, leading and controlling resources to achieve specific goals.

Mentor

An experienced and trusted individual, chosen by a less experienced individual to provide guidance, advice and support.

Organisational fit

A person's compatibility with an organisation based on the alignment between the person's beliefs, values, needs and goals and the organisation's vision, mission, values and needs.

Personal readiness

The capability to manage the roles and responsibilities of a registered nurse, oneself and one's environment.

Person-centred care

An approach to practice whereby the individual is the focus of healthcare and an active partner in their healthcare decisions.

Policies and procedures

A set of instructions used to determine what action is required, or to provide a framework on which to base your clinical reasoning.

Practice readiness

The necessary capabilities to work as a novice–beginner registered nurse in a healthcare environment and provide a basic level of safe, competent and efficient healthcare in a complex and dynamic environment.

Prioritisation

Process of ordering work tasks according to their level of importance.

Profession

An occupation, practice or vocation that requires mastery of a complex set of knowledge and skills developed through formal accredited education and/or practical experience, and is governed by its own professional body.

Professional accountability

Taking responsibility for your decisions and actions.

Professional portfolio

An organised collection of evidence that maps and validates an individual's personal and professional learning and development, capabilities and achievements over time.

Professional readiness

The capability to work efficiently and provide care in accordance with registered nurse standards and codes of practice.

Professional workplace behaviour

The ability to consistently engage in professional workplace behaviour and manage the unprofessional behaviour of others.

Psychological safety

The experience of feeling safe to express yourself without fear of being negatively judged or ridiculed.

Quality evidence

Evidence for a portfolio that is tangible, suitable, relevant to purpose and from a range of sources.

Reflection

An organised, deliberate process of thinking that examines past experiences to understand what happened, gain insight and develop a range of new or different actions for a specific situation.

Reflective practice

The formal or informal process of reviewing and evaluating events for the purpose of improving future outcomes.

Resilience

The ability to respond and adapt to changing and challenging situations.

Resume

A document that presents a succinct summary of an individual's personal details, and their professional qualifications, capabilities, experiences and achievements over time.

Role transition

The process of moving from one role and responsibilities to another.

Scope of practice

The range of responsibilities and activities that nurses are educated, competent and permitted by law to undertake.

Selection criteria

Essential qualifications, experience and capabilities (knowledge, abilities and attributes) an individual must demonstrate to be considered eligible for a job.

Self-determination

The concept that people are motivated to participate and engage in activities because of their inherent human needs and intrinsic motives.

Self-efficacy

A person's belief in their abilities to succeed in a situation or accomplish a task, and to exert control over their own motivation, behaviour and social environment.

Self-management

The ability to manage aspects of ourselves and our lives that promote our own well-being and that of our relationships.

SMART goals

Goals that are written in terms that are specific, measurable, achievable, relevant and time-bound.

Supernumerary

When a person is not included in the rostered numbers to cover the clinical area but makes an active contribution to care delivery.

Supervision

Oversight of the activities of another person or group of people to ensure they function safely and effectively.

Tacit knowledge

Knowledge that is implicit and communicated through consistent and extensive relationships, contact or experiences with others.

Tolerance

The ability to accept the values, beliefs and practices of others without judgment.

Transferable skills

Skills and abilities that are relevant and able to be applied across different areas. They are sometimes referred to as portable skills.

Transition

A non-linear evolutionary and transformative journey that features a complex exchange between emotion and intellect, relational dynamics, and context along a continuum.

Transition continuum

Practice readiness develops over a period of time, commencing on the first day of nursing studies and continuing through to the end of the first year of practice.

Transition shock

A new nurse's response to the acute and turbulent relationship between the roles, responsibilities, relationships and knowledge required of a new nurse.

OXFORD UNIVERSITY PRESS

Index

OXFORD UNIVERSITY PRESS